THIRD EDITION

MEDICAL LANGUAGE

FOCUS ON TERMINOLOGY

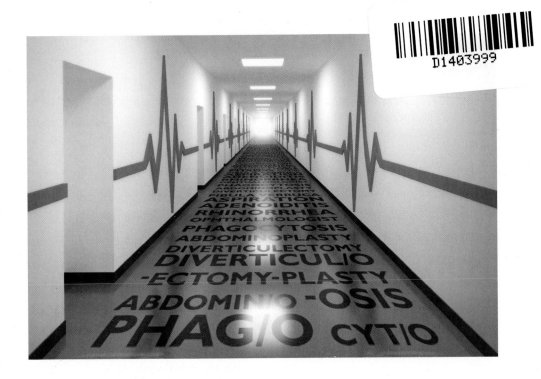

Marie A. Moisio, MA, RHIA
formerly of Northern Michigan University, Marquette, Michigan

Elmer W. Moisio, PhD, RN
formerly of Northern Michigan University, Marquette, Michigan

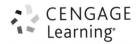

CENGAGE
Learning®

Australia • Brazil • Mexico • Singapore • United Kingdom • United States

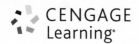
CENGAGE
Learning·

Medical Language: Focus on Terminology, Third Edition

Marie A. Moisio and Elmer W. Moisio

SVP, GM Skills & Global Product Management: Dawn Gerrain

Product Director: Matthew Seeley

Associate Product Manager: Laura Stewart

Senior Director, Development: Marah Bellegarde

Product Development Manager: Juliet Steiner

Senior Content Developer: Debra M. Myette-Flis

Product Assistant: Deborah Handy

Vice President, Marketing Services: Jennifer Ann Baker

Marketing Manager: Jonathan Sheehan

Senior Production Director: Wendy Troeger

Production Director: Andrew Crouth

Content Production Management and Art Direction: Lumina Datamatics, Inc.

Cover image(s): ©Eugene Sergeev/Shutterstock.com

For product information and technology assistance, contact us at
Cengage Learning Customer & Sales Support, 1-800-354-9706

For permission to use material from this text or product,
submit all requests online at **www.cengage.com/permissions.**
Further permissions questions can be e-mailed to
permissionrequest@cengage.com

Library of Congress Control Number: 2014952391

ISBN: 978-1-285-85421-2

Cengage Learning
20 Channel Center Street
Boston, MA 02210
USA

Cengage Learning is a leading provider of customized learning solutions with office locations around the globe, including Singapore, the United Kingdom, Australia, Mexico, Brazil, and Japan. Locate your local office at: **www.cengage.com/global**

Cengage Learning products are represented in Canada by Nelson Education, Ltd.

To learn more about Cengage Learning, visit **www.cengage.com**

Purchase any of our products at your local college store or at our preferred online store **www.cengagebrain.com**

Notice to the Reader

Printed in the United States of America
Print Number: 01   Print Year: 2015

CONTENTS

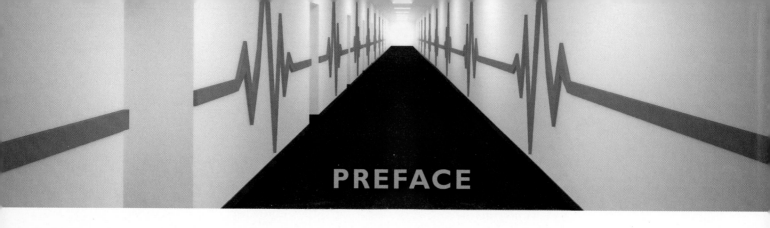

PREFACE

Introduction

Medical terminology is the language of the health care industry. Successful functioning of health care workers in any position related to the industry requires a working knowledge of this language. *Medical Language: Focus on Terminology, Third Edition,* provides basic information about the structures and functions of each body system and numerous reinforcement exercises designed to assist the student in mastering the meaning and spelling of literally thousands of medical terms.

The text is designed for use by educational programs in the areas of medical assisting, medical transcription, medical coding, health insurance billing, nursing, surgical technician, health unit coordinating, and other health-related professions. It can also be used for in-service training and professional development.

Objectives

The primary objective of this text is to provide students with a clear, concise understanding of commonly used medical terms by:

- Introducing students to the foundations of medical terminology
- Presenting techniques for breaking complex medical terms into roots, prefixes, and suffixes
- Providing a variety of reinforcement exercises to enable students to learn to spell, define, and use medical terms

Features of the Text

This text has many features designed to encourage student success in learning medical terminology.

- Learning objectives identify expectations for each chapter.
- Numerous reinforcement exercises following each major chapter topic were field-tested by medical terminology students.
- Medical reports provide an opportunity to learn medical terms in context.
- End-of-chapter reviews include objective and subjective measures of student comprehension.
- Challenge exercises encourage students to use the Internet for further study.
- Appendices include word elements and abbreviations.

Changes to the Third Edition

Medical Language: Focus on Terminology is the new title of the former Moisio/Moisio *Medical Terminology: A Student Centered Approach* textbook. This title reflects the authors' pedagogy that learning medical terminology is like learning a new language. Developing the ability to use and understand medical language goes beyond rote memorization of lists of terms. Every exercise associated with this new edition is structured to reinforce the learner's understanding of the foundations of medical terms; the body system associated with each term; and how the terms are used as medical language in various medical documents.

- New illustrations and photos in each chapter to visually reinforce all aspects of medical language—from body system structure and function to medical diseases, procedures, and treatments.
- Updated definitions and descriptions as recommended by nearly a dozen external reviewers from a variety of health care disciplines.

Instructor Resources

Learning Lab

The Medical Terminology Learning Lab is an online homework solution that allows your students to practice the most difficult concepts associated with their Cengage Learning textbooks in a simulated real-world environment.

Developed to help you improve program quality and retention, the Learning Lab prepares your students for their career by *increasing comprehension and critical thinking skills*.

Instructor Companion Site

The powerful resources for instructors are available to assist you with teaching medical terminology and assessing your students' mastery of the material. The Instructor Companion Site contains:

- **The Instructor's Manual** is designed to help you with lesson preparation and performance assessment. It includes:

  - Fifteen- and Ten-Week Course Schedules
  - Generic Lecture Plans
  - Suggested Classroom Activities
  - Chapter Quizzes with Answer Keys
  - Final Exam with Answer Keys
  - Case Reports
  - Answers to review exercises in the text

- **Cognero Online Testbank** contains questions you can use as is, and you can add your own questions to create review materials or tests.
- **PowerPoint® Presentations** designed to aid you in planning your class presentations. If a learner misses a class, a printout of the slides for a lecture makes a helpful review page.

MindTap

MindTap is a fully online, interactive learning experience built upon authoritative Cengage Learning content. By combining readings, multimedia, activities, and assessments into a singular learning path, MindTap elevates learning by providing real-world application to better engage students. Instructors customize the learning path by selecting Cengage Learning resources and adding their own content via apps that integrate into the MindTap framework seamlessly with many learning management systems.

The guided learning path demonstrates the relevance of medical terminology to health care professions through engagement activities and interactive exercises. Learners apply an understanding of medical terminology through scenarios. These simulations elevate the study of medical terminology by challenging students to apply concepts to practice.

To learn more, visit www.cengage.com/mindtap.

Building Blocks of Medical Terminology

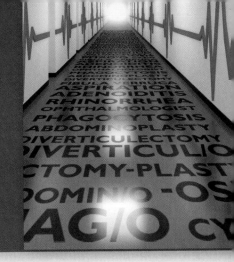

OBJECTIVES

At the completion of this chapter, the student should be able to:

1. Briefly define roots, prefixes, suffixes, combining forms, and combining vowels.
2. Analyze medical terms by identifying the root, prefix, and suffix.
3. Combine roots and suffixes accurately.
4. Build medical terms using roots, prefixes, suffixes, and combining vowels.

OVERVIEW

Learning medical terminology is very much like learning a foreign language. You begin by studying the rules of the language, progress to learning words, move on to putting the words together to form sentences, and finally, develop the ability to communicate using the language.

It is virtually impossible to "memorize" a language, but you can, and must, memorize the rules and word parts associated with the language. For example, in Spanish the word parts -*a* (pronounced "ah") and -*ita* (pronounced "eetah") represent the female gender. Seño*ra* is an adult or married woman and seño*rita* is a young or unmarried woman. One rule of the Spanish language states that *el* precedes a singular male noun and *la* precedes a singular female noun (*los* and *las* are used for plural male and female nouns, respectively). Therefore, the correct way to write *the young girl* in Spanish is *la señorita*.

Most medical terms are derived from Greek and Latin. Fortunately, you do not need to learn those languages to understand medical terminology. The Greek and Latin bases for medical terms are included in all medical dictionaries. As you look up the definitions for medical terms, you will notice that the Greek and Latin foundations are included in the definitions.

An **eponym** (**EP**-oh-nim) or **acronym** (**ACK**-roh-nim) may also be used as medical terms. An eponym is a disease, structure, operation, or procedure named for the person who discovered or described it first. For example, *Alzheimer's disease* is named for German neurologist Alois Alzheimer.

An acronym is a word formed from the first letter of each part of a compound word or phrase. For example, the word **laser** is an acronym for the phrase **l**ight **a**mplification by **s**timulated **e**mission of **r**adiation.

Medical terminology is the language of the health care industry. To use this language, you must memorize the word parts and rules. Many medical words, like English words, are made up of three basic parts: roots, prefixes, and suffixes. Various combinations of these components determine the meaning of the words.

In the English language, the root word *cycle* takes on a new meaning when combined with the prefixes *bi-*, *tri-*, and *uni-*. Bicycles, tricycles, or unicycles are vehicles with wheels and pedals that require "person-power" to move. Combining the root word *cycle* with another root, *motor,* results in the term *motorcycle.* A motorcycle is a vehicle with wheels and pedals that is powered by a motor or engine. If you know the meaning of the roots, prefixes, and suffixes, you are able to understand the word.

This chapter introduces roots, prefixes, and suffixes as they apply to medical terminology (Figure 1-1). Rules for combining the word parts, also called **word elements**, are presented as well.

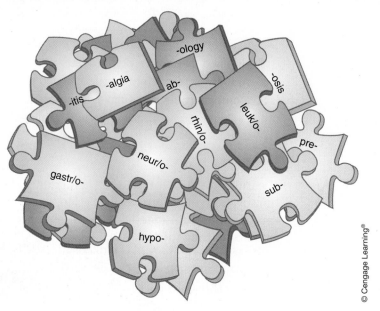

© Cengage Learning®

Figure 1-1 Roots, prefixes, suffixes, and combining forms are used to create many medical terms.

Roots

A **root** is the foundation of a medical term. Medical terms usually have at least one root. Roots usually identify a part of the body or a color and always keep the same meaning. Prefixes and suffixes change the meaning of words that have the same root. Some of the more common body part roots are as follows:

- arthr = joint
- cardi = heart
- derm or dermat = skin
- gastr = stomach

All medical term roots have a **combining form** that is created when a root is combined with a vowel. The vowel, called the **combining vowel**, is usually an *o* and occasionally an *i* or *e*. The combining vowel is used to join word elements and helps ease the pronunciation of medical terms. The combining form of a root is written with a slash followed by the combining vowel. Review the following examples of combining forms:

- arthr**/o** = joint
- cardi**/o** = heart

- dermat/**o** = skin
- gastr/**o** = stomach

The combining form of a root is used when joining roots with roots or combining roots with suffixes that begin with a consonant. In this text, word roots are introduced with the appropriate body system. For example, *cardi/o* means "heart" and is included with other word roots in the cardiovascular system chapter; *gastr/o* means "stomach" and is included with other word roots in the digestive system chapter.

Roots that identify color are found throughout each body system chapter. The combining form of these roots are listed here:

- cyan/o = blue; bluish
- eosin/o = rosy red; rosy
- erythr/o = red
- leuk/o = white
- melan/o = black
- xanth/o = yellow

Prefixes

A **prefix** is a word element or part that is added to the beginning of the word root. Not all medical terms have a prefix. In a list of word parts, prefixes are easily identified because they are written with a hyphen after the prefix. Many prefixes associated with medical terms keep their English meaning. For example, pre- (before), post- (after), and anti- (against) are commonly used medical terminology prefixes that retain the English meaning. Review the following examples of prefixes:

- ante- = before; forward
- hemi- = half
- multi- = many
- neo- = new
- sub- = under; below

Prefixes are added to a word root without additional vowels or combining forms. Commonly used prefixes are presented later in this chapter. You must memorize these prefixes so that you can apply their meaning to the medical terms presented in the body system chapters.

Suffixes

A **suffix** is a word element or part that is added to the end of the word root. All medical terms must have a suffix to complete the term, except in those rare instances when the root can stand alone as a word. In a list of word parts, suffixes are easy to recognize because they are written with a hyphen preceding the suffix.

As with prefixes, suffixes change the meaning of the medical term. In addition, suffixes indicate whether a medical term is a noun or an adjective. Remember that a noun identifies a person, place, animal, or thing and an adjective is a word that describes a noun. Review the following examples of adjective suffixes:

- -ac; -al; -ar; -ary = pertaining to; like
- -ic; -iac = pertaining to
- -oid = like; resembling

Adjective suffixes have the same meaning both for English words and for medical terms. For example, circul**ar** driveway means that your driveway is like a circle; a theatric**al** event means that the event pertains to the theater; an andr**oid** is an object that resembles a human. A few noun suffixes and their meanings are presented here:

- -ectomy (ek-toh-mee) = surgical removal; excision
- -itis (igh-tis) = inflammation of
- -megaly (meg-ah-lee) = enlargement
- -pathy (path-ee) = disease

Commonly used suffixes are also presented later in this chapter. You must memorize these suffixes so that you can apply their meaning to the medical terms presented in the body system chapters.

EXERCISE 1

Fill in the blanks.

1. Word parts that make up medical terms are also called

   _____.

2. A/An _____ is the foundation of a medical term.

3. _____ are added to the end of word roots.

4. A/An _____ is added to the beginning of a word root.

5. Most medical terms have a/an _____ and a/an

   _____.

6. The _____ is used to join word elements and help the pronunciation of medical terms.

7. A/An _____ is created when a root is combined with a vowel, usually *o* or sometimes an *i* or *e*.

8. Suffixes indicate whether a medical term is a/an _____ or a/an _____.

EXERCISE 2

Write the meaning of the listed word elements.

1. arthr/o   _____

2. gastr/o   _____

3. ante-   _____

4. multi-   _____

5. -oid   _____

6. -ic   _____

7. -megaly   _____

8. -pathy   _____

Combining Roots, Prefixes, and Suffixes

Combining roots, prefixes, and suffixes is the basic way to create medical terms. A few rules apply to this process. Review the following rules and examples and complete the exercises.

1. *When combining more than one root in a medical term, the combining form of the root is usually used between the roots.*
   Example: **cardi**o**gastric** (**kar**-dee-oh-**GASS**-trik) = pertaining to the heart and stomach.
   Note that the combining form *cardi/o* is used to join the roots *cardi* and *gastr*.
2. *When combining a root with a suffix that begins with a consonant (any letter other than a, e, i, o, u, and y), the combining form of the root must be used to connect the suffix and root.*
   Example: **gastr**o**megaly** (gass-troh-**MEG**-ah-lee) = enlarged stomach or enlargement of the stomach.
   The root *gastr* means stomach, and the suffix -*megaly* means enlarged. Note how using the combining form gastr/o aids in the pronunciation of this term. Imagine how difficult it would be to say gastrmegaly!
3. *When combining a root with a suffix that begins with a vowel, the combining form is not used.*
   Example: **gastrectomy** (gass-**TREK**-toh-mee) = surgical removal of the stomach. Because the suffix -*ectomy*, which means surgical removal, begins with a vowel, the root *gastr* is used to create the medical term. Pronunciation is much smoother without the combining vowel.
4. *There will always be some exceptions to these rules. For example, when combining word roots and one of the roots begins with a vowel, the combining vowel is retained.*
   Example: **gastr**o**enterology** (**gass**-troh-en-ter-**ALL**-oh-jee) = the study of the stomach and intestines, which are the major organs of the digestive system. The root *gastr* means stomach and the root *enter* means intestine. To ease pronunciation of this term, the combining vowel *o* is retained with the root *gastr*.

Pronunciation Rules

Pronouncing medical terms seems difficult at times because medical terms are often very long. A comprehensive medical dictionary is a valuable tool for learning the pronunciation and meaning of medical terms. You should have this type of dictionary available at all times while you are learning this "language." In addition, there are several rules that provide guidance for term pronunciation. These rules are presented here. Note that in this text, pronunciations are written phonetically (by sound) with the primary accented syllable presented in bold, uppercase letters. Secondary accented syllables are presented in bold, lowercase letters.

1. *Medical terms with two syllables are usually accented on the first syllable.*
   Example: gastric = **GASS**-trik; pertaining to the stomach
2. *Medical terms with more than two syllables are usually accented on the third to last or next to last syllable.*
   Example A: gastritis = gass-**TRY**-tis = inflammation of the stomach
   Example B: gastromegaly = gass-troh-**MEG**-ah-lee = enlarged stomach
   Example A illustrates the next to last syllable accent rule. Example B illustrates the third to last syllable accent rule.

3. *The vowel in the accented syllable is pronounced with the long vowel sound when the syllable ends with the vowel.*
   Example: gastritis = gass-**TRY**-tis. The accented syllable *tri* is pronounced with the long *i* sound.
4. *The vowel in the accented syllable is pronounced with the short vowel sound when the syllable ends with a consonant.*
   Example: cardiomegaly = **kar**-dee-oh-**MEG**-ah-lee. The accented syllable *meg* is pronounced with the short *e* sound.
5. *There will always be exceptions to these rules.*

Singular and Plural Words

In the English language, singular words are often made plural by adding *s* or *es* to the word, for example, tree (singular), trees (plural); and box (singular), boxes (plural). Because medical terms are often derived from Latin, the plural forms of many medical terms follow Latin rules. You are already familiar with these rules and may not even be aware of it. For example, the word *data* is actually the plural form of the word *datum*; *alumnus* is the singular form of *alumni*. Table 1-1 lists several singular medical terms with examples of the plural forms. Note that the word ending changes to form the plural.

TABLE 1-1 SINGULAR AND PLURAL ENDINGS

Singular Ending	Plural Ending	Singular Example	Plural Example
-a	-ae	papilla (pah-**PILL**-ah) a small nipple-shaped projection	papillae (pah-**PILL**-ay)
-en	-ina	lum*en* (**LOO**-men) cavity or channel of an organ or structure	lum*ina* (**LOO**-min-ah)
-ex; -ix	-ices	ap*ex* (**AY**-pecks) top, end, or tip of a structure	ap*ices* (**AY**-pih-seez)
-ies	-ietes	par*ies* (**PAIR**-ee-ess) wall of an organ or cavity	par*ietes* (pah-**RIGH**-ih-teez)
-is	-es	diagnos*is* (digh-ag-**NOH**-sis) name of a disease or condition	diagnos*es* (digh-ag-**NOH**-seez)
-is	-ides	epididym*is* (**ep**-ih-**DID**-ih-miss) coiled duct of the testicle	epididym*ides* (**ep**-ih-did-ih-**MY**-deez)
-nx	-nges	lary*nx* (**LAIR**-inx) voice organ of the throat	lary*nges* (lah-**RIN**- jeez)

(continues)

TABLE 1-1   SINGULAR AND PLURAL ENDINGS (continued)

Singular Ending	Plural Ending	Singular Example	Plural Example
-on	-a	gangli*on* (**GANG**-lee-on) knot or knotlike mass	ganglia (**GANG**-lee-ah)
-um	-a	atri*um* (**AY**-tree-um) upper chamber of the heart	atria (**AY**-tree-ah)
-us	-i	bronch*us* (**BRONG**-kus) air passage of the respiratory system	bronch*i* (**BRONG**-kigh)
-us	-era	visc*us* (**VISS**-kuss) internal organ	visc*era* (**VISS**-eh-rah)
-us	-ora	corp*us* (**KOR**-pus) body	corp*ora* (**KOR**-por-ah; kor-**POR**-ah)

© 2016 Cengage Learning®

EXERCISE 3

Correctly combine each root with the suffix to form a medical term. You must decide whether or not to use the combining form.

EXAMPLE:	ROOT	SUFFIX	TERM
	arthr/o	-megaly	arthromegaly

	ROOT	SUFFIX	TERM
1.	arthr/o	-itis	_____
2.	arthr/o	-ectomy	_____
3.	arthr/o	-pathy	_____
4.	dermat/o	-itis	_____
5.	dermat/o	-pathy	_____
6.	gastr/o	-ic	_____
7.	gastr/o	-ectomy	_____
8.	gastr/o	-megaly	_____
9.	cardi/o	-megaly	_____
10.	cardi/o	-pathy	_____

EXERCISE 4

Based on the meaning of the roots and suffixes, write a definition for each term you created in Exercise 3.

1. _____
2. _____
3. _____
4. _____

5. _____

6. _____

7. _____

8. _____

9. _____

10. _____

EXERCISE 5

Write the plural form for the following singular terms.

1. ampulla   _____

2. fornix   _____

3. foramen   _____

4. ovum   _____

5. phalanx   _____

6. testis   _____

7. thrombus   _____

Analyzing Medical Terms

Once you have mastered the meanings of roots, prefixes, and suffixes, you are able to analyze a medical term and arrive at a basic definition of the term. For example, *arthr/o* means joint and *itis* means inflammation; *arthritis* is briefly defined as inflammation of a joint.

To analyze a medical term, identify the root(s), prefix, and suffix. Most medical terms have a root and a suffix, but might not have a prefix. Once you have identified the word elements, recall the meaning of each element. When you write the brief definition, begin with the meaning of the suffix first, the prefix second, and the root last. Some of the longest or most complicated-looking medical terms can be defined with this technique. See Figure 1-2 for a brief definition of **otorhinolaryngology** (**oh**-toh-**righ**-noh-**lair**-in-**GOL**-oh-jee). The best place to find the complete definition of any medical term is, of course, in a medical dictionary.

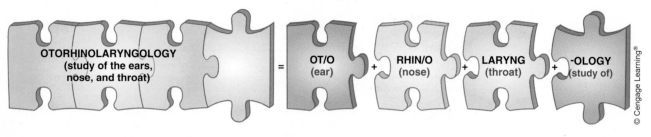

Figure 1-2 To find the basic meaning of a medical term, begin with the suffix first.

Practice analyzing medical terms by completing the following exercise. Table 1-2 lists the meanings of the roots, prefixes, and suffixes for the medical terms included in the exercise.

TABLE 1-2   ROOTS, PREFIXES, SUFFIXES, AND MEANINGS

Root	Meaning	Prefix	Meaning	Suffix	Meaning
arteri/o	artery	endo-	within	-algia	pain
arthr/o	joint	epi-	above, upon	-ic	pertaining to
cardi/o	heart	hemi-	half	-itis	inflammation
derm/o; dermat/o	skin	hypo-	below, deficient	-megaly	enlarged
gastr/o	stomach	peri-	around	-osis	abnormal condition
hepat/o	liver	poly-	many	-pathy	disease
myc/o	fungus			-plasty	repair
oste/o	bone			-sclerosis	abnormal hardening

© 2016 Cengage Learning®

EXERCISE 6

Analyze each medical term. Write a brief definition for the term based on the meaning of each word part. If a word part is not used in a given term, write none in the space.

EXAMPLE: hemigastrectomy
ROOT: gastr = stomach
PREFIX: hemi- = half
SUFFIX: -ectomy = surgical removal
DEFINITION: surgical removal of half the stomach

1. arthralgia
   ROOT: _arthr_____   PREFIX: _arthr_____   SUFFIX: _algia_____

   DEFINITION: _____

2. endocarditis
   ROOT: _____   PREFIX: _____   SUFFIX: _____

   DEFINITION: _____

3. hemigastroplasty
   ROOT: _____   PREFIX: _____   SUFFIX: _____

   DEFINITION: _____

4. hepatomegaly
   ROOT: _____   PREFIX: _____   SUFFIX: _____

   DEFINITION: _____

5. hypogastric

ROOT: _____ PREFIX: _____ SUFFIX: _____

DEFINITION: _____

6. osteoarthritis

ROOT: _____ PREFIX: _____ SUFFIX: _____

DEFINITION: _____

7. osteopathy

ROOT: _____ PREFIX: _____ SUFFIX: _____

DEFINITION: _____

8. pericarditis

ROOT: _____ PREFIX: _____ SUFFIX: _____

DEFINITION: _____

9. polyarthritis

ROOT: _____ PREFIX: _____ SUFFIX: _____

DEFINITION: _____

10. hepatitis

ROOT: _____ PREFIX: _____ SUFFIX: _____

DEFINITION: _____

11. arteriosclerosis

ROOT: _____ PREFIX: _____ SUFFIX: _____

DEFINITION: _____

12. mycosis

ROOT: _____ PREFIX: _____ SUFFIX: _____

DEFINITION: _____

Building Medical Terms

A working knowledge of roots, prefixes, and suffixes allows you to analyze and define many medical terms. That same knowledge can also help you build medical terms from a definition. It is important to remember that not all terms can be created from a definition. Many medical terms are not built from prefixes or suffixes, and there are many instances when the basic definition based on prefixes and suffixes does not provide a full or completely accurate definition. For example, in this chapter, the definition of gastrectomy, based solely on the meaning of the root and suffix, is surgical removal or excision of the stomach. In practice, the term *gastrectomy* commonly means surgical excision of *part* of the stomach. However, analyzing, defining, and building medical terms with roots, prefixes, and suffixes provides an excellent foundation for developing a working knowledge of medical terminology.

Practice building medical terms by completing the following exercise. Refer to Table 1-2 for a list of the roots, prefixes, and suffixes included in the exercise.

EXERCISE 7

Read each definition. Write the name of the body part, the combining form for the root, the suffix, and the prefix on the lines provided. Using the rules for word building, write a medical term for each definition.

EXAMPLE:

DEFINITION:	inflammation of joints
BODY PART:	joints
ROOT:	arthr/o
SUFFIX:	-itis
PREFIX:	none
MEDICAL TERM:	arthritis

1. DEFINITION: disease of the heart

   BODY PART: _____

   ROOT: _____

   SUFFIX: _____

   PREFIX: _____

   MEDICAL TERM: _____

2. DEFINITION: surgical repair of the liver

   BODY PART: _____

   ROOT: _____

   SUFFIX: _____

   PREFIX: _____

   MEDICAL TERM: _____

3. DEFINITION: stomach pain

   BODY PART: Sto   _____

   ROOT: _____

   SUFFIX: _____

   PREFIX: _____

   MEDICAL TERM: _____

4. DEFINITION: skinlike; resembling skin

   BODY PART: _____

   ROOT: _____

   SUFFIX: _____

   PREFIX: _____

   MEDICAL TERM: _____

5. DEFINITION: pertaining to the area around the heart

   BODY PART: _____

   ROOT: _____

   SUFFIX: _____

   PREFIX: _____

   MEDICAL TERM: _____

6. DEFINITION: inflammation of bone

   BODY PART: _____

   ROOT: _____

   SUFFIX: _____

   PREFIX: _____

   MEDICAL TERM: _____

7. DEFINITION: surgical repair of the skin

   BODY PART: _____

   ROOT: _____

   SUFFIX: _____

   PREFIX: _____

   MEDICAL TERM: _____

8. DEFINITION: pain in many joints

   BODY PART: _____

   ROOT: _____

   SUFFIX: _____

   PREFIX: _____

   MEDICAL TERM: _____

9. DEFINITION: under the liver

   BODY PART: _____

   ROOT: _____

   SUFFIX: _____

   PREFIX: _____

   MEDICAL TERM: _____

Prefixes

Prefixes and their meanings should be memorized early in your study of medical terminology. In this section, commonly used prefixes are presented and defined. Exercises focus on mastering the meaning of each prefix. Memorization is often boring. To make learning the prefixes less so, it is helpful to use gamelike formats. For example:

Create flashcards with the prefix or suffix on one side and its meaning on the other. Place the cards on a smooth surface, prefix/suffix side up, and with several other students see how many cards each of you can "capture" by giving the correct meaning for the prefix or suffix. Ask a friend or partner to help you complete various flashcard drills. Think of words you already know that include the prefixes given in this section.

Prefixes can be divided into four categories: general, negative, numeric, and problem or disease prefixes. Each category of prefixes is presented individually.

General Prefixes

General prefixes make up the largest number of prefixes presented in this text and often refer to size, shape, direction, and location. The first set of general prefixes is listed in Table 1-3. Note that the table includes the meaning of the prefix and an example of a medical term containing the prefix. Some examples include an everyday word with the prefix. Learn this group of prefixes and complete the exercises.

TABLE 1-3 GENERAL PREFIXES

Prefix	Meaning	Examples
ab-	away from	**ab**normal = away from being normal **ab**duct (ab-**DUCT**) = to move away from the body
ad-	to; toward	**ad**dendum = in addition to; added to **ad**duct (ad-**DUCT**) = to move to or toward the body
ante-	before	**ante**room =a room or area before a larger room or area **ante**febrile (an-tee-**FEE**-brill) = before a fever
astr-	star	**astr**ology = study of the stars **astr**ocyte (**ASS**-troh-sight) = star-shaped cell
auto-	self	**auto**biography = story written by yourself about your life **auto**graft (**AH**-toh-graft) = surgical transplant of one's own tissue
brady-	slow	**brady**cardia (bray-dih-**KAR**-dee-ah) = slow heart rate
ect-	outside; outer	**ect**oderm (**EKT**-oh-derm) = outermost layer of the skin
en-	within; in	**en**trails = organs within or inside a human or animal **en**tropia (en-**TROH**-pee-ah) = turning in of the eyes
endo-	within; inner	**endo**cardium (**en**-doh-**KAR**-dee-um) = within the heart; inner lining of the heart
epi-	above; upon	**epi**gastric (ep-ih-**GAS**-trik) = above the stomach
ex-	out; outer	**ex**it = to go out; passage/doorway used to go out **ex**icision (ek-**SIH**-zhun) = taking out; cutting away
hemi-	half	**hemi**sphere = half of a sphere **hemi**plegia (**heh**-mih-**PLEE**-jee-ah) = paralysis of one side (half) of the body
infra-	below; inferior	**infra**orbital (in-frah-**OR**-bih-tal) = below the eye socket

(continues)

TABLE 1-3   GENERAL PREFIXES (continued)

Prefix	Meaning	Examples
inter-	between; among	**inter**mission = time period between events or periods of activity
		interstitial (**in**-ter- **STISH**-al) = between parts of a tissue
intra-	within	**intra**state = existing or occurring within a state
		intracellular (**in**-trah-**SELL**-yoo-lar) = within the cells
iso-	same; equal	**iso**metric (eye-soh-**MET**-rik) = having the same length or dimension

© 2016 Cengage Learning®

EXERCISE 8

Read each sentence. Write the prefix and its definition for each italicized medical term. Using your medical dictionary, write a brief definition of the term.

EXAMPLE: *Macroglossia* is associated with a specific type of birth defect.
PREFIX: macro- = large   DEFINITION: hypertrophied or large tongue

1. *Autoimmune* diseases are difficult to treat.

    PREFIX: _____   DEFINITION: _____

2. The *endocardium* includes the heart valves.

    PREFIX: _____   DEFINITION: _____

3. *Abduction* is the opposite of adduction.

    PREFIX: _____   DEFINITION: _____

4. *Adduction* is the opposite of abduction.

    PREFIX: _____   DEFINITION: _____

5. An *intradermal* injection is often used to administer a TB test.

    PREFIX: _____   DEFINITION: _____

6. *Bradykinesia* might be a side effect of some medications.

    PREFIX: _____   DEFINITION: _____

7. An *ectopic* pregnancy often occurs in the fallopian tubes.

    PREFIX: _____   DEFINITION: _____

8. An *astrocyte* is a specific cell of the nervous system.

    PREFIX: _____   DEFINITION: _____

9. The brain is divided into a right and left *hemisphere*.

    PREFIX: _____   DEFINITION: _____

10. *Epigastric* pain caused a restless evening for the patient.

    PREFIX: _____   DEFINITION: _____

EXERCISE 9

Match the prefix in Column 1 with the meaning in Column 2.

COLUMN 1

_____ 1. ab-

_____ 2. ante-

_____ 3. astr-

_____ 4. auto-

_____ 5. brady-

_____ 6. ect-

_____ 7. epi-

_____ 8. infra-

_____ 9. inter-

_____ 10. intra-

_____ 11. iso-

COLUMN 2

a. above; upon

b. away from

c. before

d. below; inferior

e. between

f. within; in

g. same; equal

h. self

i. slow

j. star

k. outside; out

EXERCISE 10

Write the prefix for each meaning.

1. above; upon   _____

2. away from   _____

3. before   _____

4. below; inferior   _____

5. between   _____

6. half   _____

7. out; outer   _____

8. outside; outer   _____

9. same; equal   _____

10. self   _____

11. slow   _____

12. star   _____

The last set of general prefixes is listed in Table 1-4. Note that the table includes the meaning of the prefix and an example of a medical term containing the prefix. Some examples also include an everyday word with the prefix. Learn this group of prefixes and complete the exercises.

TABLE 1-4 GENERAL PREFIXES

Prefix	Meaning	Examples
macro-	large	**macro**cyte (**MAK**-roh-sight) = abnormally large red blood cell
meta-	change; after; beyond	**meta**plasia (met-ah-**PLAY**-zee-ah) = change from one type of growth to another
micro-	small	**micro**cyte (**MY**-kroh-sight) = abnormally small red blood cell
multi-	many	**multi**lobular (mull-tigh-**LOB**-yoo-lar)= having many lobes
neo-	new	**neo**plasm (**NEE**-oh-plazm) = new growth
pan-	all	**pan**carditis (**pan**-kar-**DIGH**-tiss) = inflammation of the entire heart
para-	near; beside	**para**nasal (**pair**-ah-**NAY**-sal) = near or beside the nose
peri-	around; surrounding	**peri**meter = boundary surrounding a specific location **peri**cardium (**pair**-ih-**KAR**-dee-um) = membrane around the heart
poly-	many	**poly**arthritis (**pall**-ee-ar-**THRIGH**-tiss) = inflammation of many joints
post-	after	**post**partum (post-**PAR**-tum) = after giving birth
pre-	before; in front of	**pre**natal (pre-**NAY**-tal) = before giving birth
retro-	behind; backward	**retro**spect = looking back at past events **retro**grade (**REH**-troh-grayd) = moving backward
semi-	half	**semi**lunar (sem-eye-**LOO**-nar) = half-moon shaped
sub-	below; under	**sub**hepatic (**sub**-heh-**PAT**-ik) = below or under the liver
super-	above; over; excess	**super**ior (soo-**PEER**-ee-or) = above or toward a higher place
supra-	above; on top of	**supra**spinal (**soo**-prah-**SPIGH**-nal) = above the spine
sym-	with; association	**sym**pathy = having an association with another's feelings **sym**biosis (sim-bee-**OH**-siss) = living with or in close association
syn-	together; with; union	**syn**chronize = to move or operate together or in unison **syn**ergistic (sin-er-**JISS**-tik) = related to working together
tachy-	fast	**tachy**cardia (**tak**-ih-**KAR**-dee-ah) = fast heart rate

© 2016 Cengage Learning®

EXERCISE 11

Read each sentence. Write the prefix and its definition for each italicized medical term. Using your medical dictionary, write a brief definition of the term.

1. A caterpillar experiences *metamorphosis* to become a butterfly.

   PREFIX: _____ DEFINITION: _____

2. The laboratory technician uses a *microscope* to examine tissue samples.

   PREFIX: _____ DEFINITION: _____

3. Some heart valves are *semilunar* in shape.

   PREFIX: _____ DEFINITION: _____

4. *Tachycardia* might cause the patient to feel dizzy.

   PREFIX: _____   DEFINITION: _____

5. *Substernal* chest pain is a sign of "heartburn."

   PREFIX: _____   DEFINITION: _____

6. A *neoplasm* can be cancerous or noncancerous.

   PREFIX: _____   DEFINITION: _____

7. The adrenal glands are also known as the *suprarenal* glands.

   PREFIX: _____   DEFINITION: _____

8. Humans are *multicelluar* organisms.

   PREFIX: _____   DEFINITION: _____

9. *Retroflexion* prevents an organ from functioning properly.

   PREFIX: _____   DEFINITION: _____

10. The patient's *postoperative* course was uneventful.

    PREFIX: _____   DEFINITION: _____

EXERCISE 12

Match the prefix in Column 1 with the meaning in Column 2.

COLUMN 1

_____ 1. pan-

_____ 2. para-

_____ 3. peri-

_____ 4. poly-

_____ 5. post-

_____ 6. pre-

_____ 7. meta-

_____ 8. super-

_____ 9. sym-

_____ 10. syn-

COLUMN 2

a. above; over; excess

b. after

c. all

d. around; surrounding

e. before; in front of

f. change

g. many

h. near; beside

i. together; with; union

j. with; association

EXERCISE 13

Write the prefix for each meaning.

1. above; on top of   _____

2. above; over; excess   _____

3. behind; backward   _____

4. change   _____

5. fast   _____

6. half   _____

7. large   _____

8. near; beside   _____

9. new   _____

10. together; with; union   _____

Negative, Numeric, and Disease Prefixes

Negative and numeric prefixes are self-explanatory. **Problem** or **disease prefixes** provide some information about an abnormal structure or function. Learn this group of prefixes, listed in Table 1-5, and complete the exercises.

TABLE 1-5 NEGATIVE, NUMERIC, AND DISEASE AND PROBLEM PREFIXES

NEGATIVE PREFIXES

Prefix	Meaning	Example
a; an; ana	no; not; without	**an**archy = without laws or government **an**algesia (an-al-**JEE**-zee-ah) = without pain; no sensation of pain
anti-	against	**anti**fungal (an-tigh-**FUNG**-al) = against fungus
contra-	against; opposite	**contra**ception (con-trah-**SEP**-shun) = against conception
non-	not	**non**functioning = does not function

NUMERIC PREFIXES

Prefix	Meaning	Example
bi-	two; double; both	**bi**lateral (bigh-**LAT**-er-al) = both sides; two sides
centi-	hundred; hundredth	**centi**meter (**SEN**-tih-**me**-ter) = one hundredth of a meter
dec-	ten	**dec**aliter (**DEK**-ah-**lee**-ter) = 10 liters
milli-	one thousandth	**milli**liter (**MILL**-ih-**lee**-ter) = one thousandth of a liter
quadr-	four	**quadr**iplegia (**kwod**-rih-**PLEE**-jee-ah) = paralysis of all four limbs
tri-	three	**tri**cuspid (trigh-**KUSS**-pid) = having three flaps
uni-	one	**uni**lateral (yoo-nih-**LAT**-er-al) = one side

DISEASE AND PROBLEM PREFIXES

Prefix	Meaning	Example
carcin-	cancerous	**carcin**oma (kar-sin-**OH**-mah) = cancerous tumor
dys-	difficult; painful	**dys**uria (dis-**YOO**-ree-ah) = painful urination
hyper-	above; excessive; increased	**hyper**thyroidism (**high**-per-**THIGH**-royd-izm) = excessive thyroid activity
hypo	deficient; below; decreased	**hypo**thyroidism (**high**-poh-**THIGH**-royd-izm) = deficient thyroid activity
mal-	bad; poor; abnormal	**mal**absorption (mal-ab—**SORP**-shun) = abnormal absorption

EXERCISE 14

Read each sentence. Write the prefix and its definition for each italicized medical term. Using your medical dictionary, write a brief definition of the term.

1. The *bicuspid* valve in the heart is also called the mitral valve.

   PREFIX: _____   DEFINITION: _____

2. *Antibiotic* medications are an effective treatment for some diseases.

   PREFIX: _____   DEFINITION: _____

3. *Hypertension* can be successfully treated and controlled.

   PREFIX: _____   DEFINITION: _____

4. Squamous cell *carcinoma* might involve the cervix.

   PREFIX: _____   DEFINITION: _____

5. *Hypothyroidism* often responds to medication therapy.

   PREFIX: _____   DEFINITION: _____

6. A stroke sometimes results in *dysphagia*.

   PREFIX: _____   DEFINITION: _____

7. Some procedures are done with local *anesthesia*.

   PREFIX: _____   DEFINITION: _____

8. Some birth defects are characterized by *malformation* of an organ or limb.

   PREFIX: _____   DEFINITION: _____

9. Most medications have at least one *contraindication*.

   PREFIX: _____   DEFINITION: _____

10. After taking fertility medications, Helen gave birth to *quadruplets*.

    PREFIX: _____   DEFINITION: _____

EXERCISE 15

Write the prefix for each definition.

1. above; excessive   _____

2. against   _____

3. against; opposite   _____

4. bad; poor; abnormal   _____

5. cancerous   _____

6. deficient; below   _____

7. difficult; painful   _____

8. hundred; hundredth   _____

9. no; not; without   _____

10. not   _____

11. one   _____

12. one thousandth   _____

13. ten   _____

14. three   _____

15. two; double; both   _____

Suffixes

Suffixes are added to the end of a word root and, as with prefixes, change the meaning of the medical term. When defining a medical term the meaning of the suffix is used first. Example: Cardiovascular means pertaining to (-ar) the heart (cardi/o) and vessels (vascul/o).

Suffixes identify a medical term as a noun or an adjective. Suffixes indicate if a term is related to a diagnosis, abnormal condition, procedure, or general medical processes and functions.

General Suffixes

General suffixes are used to describe general medical processes and functions and are the largest number of suffixes presented in this text. Review the suffixes and meanings in Table 1-6 and complete the exercises.

TABLE 1-6   GENERAL SUFFIXES

Suffix	Meaning	Example
-ac; -al; -ar; -ary	pertaining to	cardiovascular (kar-dee-oh-VASS-kyoo-lar) = pertaining to the heart and vessels
-crine	to secrete	endocrine (EN-doh-krin) = to secrete within, into
-crit	to separate	hematocrit (hee-MAT-oh-krit) = to separate blood
-cyte	cell	leukocyte (LOO-koh-sight) = white cell; white blood cell
-gen; -genesis; -genic	producing, forming	spermatogenesis (sper-mat-oh-JEN-eh-siss) = producing sperm
-globin; -globulin	protein	hemoglobin (HEE-mah-gloh-bin) = blood protein
-gram	record	venogram (VEE-noh-gram) = record of the veins
-graph	instrument for recording	cardiograph (KAR-dee-oh-graf) = instrument that records heart activity
-graphy	process of recording	cardiography (kar-dee-AH-grah-fee) = recording the activity of, or a picture of the heart
-iac; ic	pertaining to	cardiac (KAR-dee-ak) = pertaining to the heart
-oid	resembling; like	ovoid (OH-voyd) = resembling an oval or an egg
-(o)logist	specialist	dermatologist (der-mah-TALL-oh-jist) = physician specializing in the diagnosis and treatment of conditions related to the skin
-(o)logy	study of	dermatology (der-mah-TALL-oh-jee) = study of the skin
-ous	pertaining to	mucous (MEW-kuss) = pertaining to mucus
-pepsia	digestion	dyspepsia (diss-PEP-see-ah) = difficult or painful digestion

(continues)

TABLE 1-6   GENERAL SUFFIXES (continued)

Suffix	Meaning	Example
-phagia	eating; swallowing	**aphagia** (ah-**FAY**-jee-ah) = lack of the ability to swallow
-phonia	voice; sound	**aphonia** (ah-**FOH**-nee-ah) = lack of the ability to produce sound; lack of voice

EXERCISE 16

Read each sentence. Write the suffix and its definition for each italicized medical term. Using your medical dictionary, write a brief definition of the term.

1. *Endocrine* glands do not have ducts.

   SUFFIX: _____   DEFINITION: _____

2. Many bacteria are *pathogenic*.

   SUFFIX: _____   DEFINITION: _____

3. *Gammaglobulins* are found in circulating blood.

   SUFFIX: _____   DEFINITION: _____

4. After reviewing the *renogram*, Dr. Jones noted the patient had an enlarged kidney.

   SUFFIX: _____   DEFINITION: _____

5. The *echograph* is an important diagnostic tool.

   SUFFIX: _____   DEFINITION: _____

6. *Echocardiography* is a noninvasive method for inspecting the heart.

   SUFFIX: _____   DEFINITION: _____

7. Mark's family physician referred him to a *urologist*.

   SUFFIX: _____   DEFINITION: _____

8. *Aphonia* might be the result of a stroke.

   SUFFIX: _____   DEFINITION: _____

9. *Radiology* is one of several medical specialties.

   SUFFIX: _____   DEFINITION: _____

10. *Erythrocytes* are one of the major components of blood.

    SUFFIX: _____   DEFINITION: _____

EXERCISE 17

Match the suffix in Column 1 with the meaning in Column 2.

COLUMN 1	COLUMN 2
_____ 1. -crine	a. cell
_____ 2. -crit	b. digestion
_____ 3. -cyte	c. eating; swallowing

———	4. -genesis; -genic	d.	record; picture
———	5. -globin; -globulin	e.	pertaining to
———	6. –gram	f.	process of recording
———	7. –graphy	g.	protein
———	8. -(o)logist	h.	secrete
———	9. –ous	i.	specialist
———	10. –pepsia	j.	separate
———	11. –phagia	k.	voice; sound
———	12. –phonia	l.	producing

Review the general suffixes and meanings in Table 1-7 and complete the exercises.

TABLE 1-7   GENERAL SUFFIXES

Suffix	Meaning	Example
-phoresis	carrying; transmission	electro**phoresis** (**ee**-lek-troh-for-**EE**-siss) = carrying or transmission of an electrical charge
-phoria	feeling; mental state	dys**phoria** (diss-**FOR**-ee-ah) = bad feeling
-pnea	breathing	dys**pnea** (disp-**NEE**-ah) = difficult breathing
-poiesis	formation	erythro**poiesis** (air-rith-roh-poy-**EE**-siss) = formation of red blood cells
-scope	instrument for viewing	micro**scope** (**MY**-kroh-scope) = instrument for viewing small objects
-scopy	process of viewing	arthro**scopy** (ar-**THROSS**-koh-pee) = viewing joint(s)
-somnia	sleep	in**somnia** (in-**SOM**-nee-ah) = inability to sleep
-stasis	control; stop	hemo**stasis** (hee-moh-**STAY**-siss) = stopping blood flow
-therapy	treatment	chemo**therapy** (**kee**-moh-**THAIR**-ah-pee) = treatment using drugs
-thorax	chest; pleural cavity	hemo**thorax** (hee-moh-**THOR**-acks) = blood in the chest or pleural cavity
-tocia	labor; birth	dys**tocia** (diss-**TOH**-see-ah) = abnormal labor
-tresia	opening	a**tresia** (ah-**TREE**-see-ah) = lack of a normal opening
-trophy	growth; development	dys**trophy** (**DISS**-troh-fee) = abnormal or bad growth
-tropin	nourish; develop; stimulate	somato**tropin** (**soh**-mat-oh-**TROH**-pin) = stimulates body growth
-version	to turn	retro**version** (**reh**-troh-**VER**-zhun) = to turn backward

EXERCISE 18

Read each sentence. Write the suffix and its definition for each italicized medical term. Using your medical dictionary, write a brief definition of the term.

1. Dr. Jefferson used an *otoscope* during Marilyn's annual physical.

   SUFFIX: _____   DEFINITION: _____

2. *Hematopoiesis* takes place in the bone marrow.

   SUFFIX: _____   DEFINITION: _____

3. *Cardioversion* is used to correct heart rhythm problems.

   SUFFIX: _____   DEFINITION: _____

4. Disuse *atrophy* is caused by prolonged confinement to bed.

   SUFFIX: _____   DEFINITION: _____

5. After experiencing a *pneumothorax*, the patient's lung collapsed.

   SUFFIX: _____   DEFINITION: _____

6. *Orthopnea* is sometimes associated with congestive heart failure.

   SUFFIX: _____   DEFINITION: _____

7. After winning the lottery, Robert experienced *euphoria*.

   SUFFIX: _____   DEFINITION: _____

8. *Endoscopy* is an important diagnostic technique.

   SUFFIX: _____   DEFINITION: _____

9. *Cryotherapy* is often used to treat skin problems.

   SUFFIX: _____   DEFINITION: _____

EXERCISE 19

Match the suffix in Column 1 with the meaning in Column 2.

COLUMN 1

_____ 1. –phoresis

_____ 2. –phoria

_____ 3. –pnea

_____ 4. –poiesis

_____ 5. –scopy

_____ 6. –somnia

_____ 7. –stasis

_____ 8. –therapy

_____ 9. –tocia

_____ 10. –tresia

_____ 11. –tropin

COLUMN 2

a. breathing

b. carrying; transmission

c. control; stop

d. feeling; mental state

e. formation

f. labor; birth

g. nourish; develop

h. opening

i. process of viewing

j. sleep

k. treatment

EXERCISE 20

Write the suffix for each meaning.

1. to secrete _____
2. separate _____
3. producing; forming _____
4. cell _____
5. process of recording _____
6. study of _____
7. specialist _____
8. eating; swallowing _____
9. formation _____
10. sleep _____
11. to turn _____
12. development; growth _____
13. like; resembling _____
14. chest; pleural cavity _____

Disease and Abnormal Condition Suffixes

Disease and **abnormal condition suffixes** are used to describe what is wrong with a given body part. Review the suffixes and meanings in Table 1-8 and complete the exercises.

TABLE 1-8 DISEASE AND ABNORMAL CONDITION SUFFIXES

Suffix	Meaning	Example
-algia	pain, painful condition	arthr**algia** (ar-**THRAL**-jee-ah) = joint pain
-cele	hernia; herniation	recto**cele** (**REK**-toh-seel) = herniation into the rectum
-cytosis	condition of cells	leuko**cytosis** (**loo**-koh-sigh-**TOH**-siss) = condition of white blood cells (abnormal increase)
-dynia	pain	gastro**dynia** (**gass**-troh-**DIN**-ee-ah) = pain in the stomach
-emesis	vomiting	hemat**emesis** (hee-mah-**TEM**-eh-siss) = vomiting blood
-emia	blood condition	an**emia** (ah-**NEE**-mee-ah) = lack of quantity or quality of blood
-ia; iasis	abnormal condition	lith**iasis** (lih-**THIGH**-ah-siss) = abnormal presence of stones
-itis	inflammation	gingiv**itis** (jin-jih-**VIGH**-tiss) = inflammation of the gums
-lysis; -lytic	break down; destruction	hemo**lysis** (hee-**MALL**-oh-siss) = destruction of blood or red blood cells

(continues)

TABLE 1-8   DISEASE AND ABNORMAL CONDITION SUFFIXES (continued)

Suffix	Meaning	Example
-malacia	softening	osteo**malacia** (**oss**-tee-oh-mah-**LAY**-she-ah) = softening of bone
-megaly	enlargement	cardio**megaly** (**kar**-dee-oh-**MEG**-ah-lee) = enlarged heart
-oma	tumor	aden**oma** (ad-en-**OH**-mah) = tumor of the gland
-osis	abnormal condition	dermat**osis** (der-mah-**TOH**-siss) = skin condition

© 2016 Cengage Learning®

EXERCISE 21

Read each sentence. Write the suffix and its definition for each italicized medical term. Using your medical dictionary, write a brief definition of the term.

1. Exposure to UV rays is the leading cause of *melanoma*.

   SUFFIX: _____   DEFINITION: _____

2. *Spherocytosis* is often seen in some types of anemia.

   SUFFIX: _____   DEFINITION: _____

3. *Bacteremia* is treated with antibiotics.

   SUFFIX: _____   DEFINITION: _____

4. Health care workers are at risk for *hepatitis*.

   SUFFIX: _____   DEFINITION: _____

5. Inadequate nutrition might contribute to *chondromalacia*.

   SUFFIX: _____   DEFINITION: _____

6. *Halitosis* can be a symptom of dental problems.

   SUFFIX: _____   DEFINITION: _____

7. Muscle spasms of the head and neck may cause *cephalalgia*.

   SUFFIX: _____   DEFINITION: _____

8. A *cystocele* might require surgical intervention.

   SUFFIX: _____   DEFINITION: _____

9. *Nephromegaly* might be visualized with an x-ray.

   SUFFIX: _____   DEFINITION: _____

10. After exercising for several hours, Rhonda experienced *myodynia*.

    SUFFIX: _____   DEFINITION: _____

EXERCISE 22

Write the suffix for each meaning.

1. abnormal condition   _____

2. blood condition   _____

3. break down; destruction   _____

4. enlargement; enlarged   _____

5. hernia; herniation   _____

6. inflammation   _____

7. pain   _____

8. softening   _____

9. tumor   _____

10. vomiting   _____

Review the disease and abnormal condition suffixes and meanings in Table 1-9 and complete the exercises.

TABLE 1-9   DISEASE AND ABNORMAL CONDITION SUFFIXES

Suffix	Meaning	Example
-paresis	slight paralysis	hemi**paresis** (**hem**-ee-pah-**REE**-siss) = slight paralysis of one side of the body
-pathy	disease	neuro**pathy** (noo-**ROP**-ah-thee) = disease of nerves
-penia	decreased number	leukocyto**penia** (**loo**-koh-**sigh**-toh-PEE-nee-ah) = decreased number of white cells (white blood cells)
-phobia	abnormal fear	arachno**phobia** (ah-**rak**-noh-**FOH**-bee-ah) = abnormal fear of spiders
-plegia	paralysis	quadra**plegia** (kwad-rah-**PLEE**-gee-ah) = paralysis of all four limbs
-ptosis	drooping; sagging; prolapse	nephro**ptosis** (**neff**-rop-**TOH**-siss) = drooping kidney
-ptysis	spitting up	hemo**ptysis** (hee-**MOP**-tih-siss) = spitting up blood
-(r)rhage; -(r)rhagia	bursting forth of blood; bleeding; abnormal excessive fluid discharge	hemor**rhage** (**HEM**-oh-rij) = bursting forth of blood
-(r)rhea	flow; discharge	rhinor**rhea** (**righ**-noh-**REE**-ah) = discharge from the nose; runny nose
-(r)rhexis	rupture	uteror**rhexis** (**yoo**-ter-oh-**RECKS**-iss) = rupture of the uterus
-sclerosis	abnormal hardening	arterio**sclerosis** (ar-**teer**-ee-oh-sclair-**ROH**-siss) = hardening of the arteries
-spasm	contraction; twitching	cardio**spasm** (**KAR**-dee-oh-spasm) = twitching of the heart muscle
-stenosis	narrowing; tightening	arterio**stenosis** (ar-**teer**-ree-oh-sten-OH-siss) = narrowing of an artery

EXERCISE 23

Read each sentence. Write the suffix and its definition for each italicized medical term. Using your medical dictionary, write a brief definition of the term.

1. Sara's infection caused her to experience *hemiparesis*.

    SUFFIX: _____   DEFINITION: _____

2. Elizabeth hoped the physician could find the cause of her *menorrhagia*.

    SUFFIX: _____   DEFINITION: _____

3. *Splenorrhexis* might lead to blood in the abdominal cavity.

    SUFFIX: _____   DEFINITION: _____

4. *Neutropenia* is often a side effect of chemotherapy.

    SUFFIX: _____   DEFINITION: _____

5. An acrobat with *acrophobia* might find it difficult to perform.

    SUFFIX: _____   DEFINITION: _____

6. *Nephroptosis* might require surgical intervention.

    SUFFIX: _____   DEFINITION: _____

7. *Atherosclerosis* is associated with heart disease.

    SUFFIX: _____   DEFINITION: _____

8. After the accident, Marilyn was diagnosed with *hemiplegia*.

    SUFFIX: _____   DEFINITION: _____

9. *Neuropathy* is a complication of diabetes.

    SUFFIX: _____   DEFINITION: _____

10. *Otorrhea* is sometimes present with an ear infection.

    SUFFIX: _____   DEFINITION: _____

EXERCISE 24

Match the suffixes in Column 1 with the meanings in Column 2.

COLUMN 1	COLUMN 2
_____ 1. –malacia	a. abnormal condition
_____ 2. –megaly	b. abnormal fear
_____ 3. -osis	c. bursting forth of blood
_____ 4. –paresis	d. contraction; twitching
_____ 5. –pathy	e. drooping; sagging; prolapse
_____ 6. –phobia	f. disease
_____ 7. –plegia	g. enlargement; enlarged
_____ 8. –ptosis	h. flow; discharge
_____ 9. –ptysis	i. hardening
_____ 10. -(r)rhage	j. narrowing; tightening
_____ 11. -(r)rhea	k. paralysis

_____ 12. –sclerosis   l. slight paralysis

_____ 13. –spasm   m. softening

_____ 14. –stenosis   n. spitting up

EXERCISE 25

Write the suffix for each meaning.

1. bursting forth of blood   _____

2. decreased number   _____

3. drooping; sagging   _____

4. hernia   _____

5. inflammation   _____

6. mass; tumor   _____

7. pain   _____

8. rupture   _____

9. slight paralysis   _____

10. vomiting   _____

Treatment and procedure suffixes

Treatment and **procedure suffixes** describe a variety of medical interventions such as the removal or repair of a body part or an organ. Review the suffixes and meanings in Table 1-10 and complete the exercises.

TABLE 1-10   TREATMENT AND PROCEDURE SUFFIXES

Suffix	Meaning	Example
-centesis	surgical puncture	thora**centesis** (**thor**-ah-sen-**TEE**-siss) = surgical puncture into the chest or thoracic cavity
-desis	binding together	arthro**desis** (ar-throh-**DEE**-siss) = binding together of joints
-ectasia; -ectasis	stretching; dilatation	gast**rectasia** (**gass**-trek-**TAY**-zee-ah) = stretching or dilation of the stomach
-ectomy	surgical removal; cutting out; excision	gast**rectomy** (gass-**TREK**-toh-mee) = surgical removal of all or part of the stomach
-(o)stomy	create a new opening	colo**stomy** (koh-**LOSS**-toh-mee) = create a new opening for the colon
-(o)tomy	incision into	laparo**tomy** (**lap**-ah-**ROT**-oh mee) = incision into the abdominal wall
-pexy	surgical fixation	utero**pexy** (**yoo**-ter-oh-**PEK**-see) = surgical fixation of the uterus
-plasty	surgical repair	rhino**plasty** (**RIGH**-noh-plass-tee) = surgical repair of the nose

(continues)

TABLE 1-10   TREATMENT AND PROCEDURE SUFFIXES (continued)

Suffix	Meaning	Example
-(r)rhaphy	suture; surgical suturing	hernior**rhaphy** (**her**-nee-**OR**-ah-fee) = suturing a hernia
-tripsy	crushing; friction	litho**tripsy** (**LITH**-oh-trip-see) = crushing of stones

© 2016 Cengage Learning®

EXERCISE 26

Read each sentence. Write the suffix and its definition for each italicized medical term. Using your medical dictionary, write a brief definition of the term.

1. Erik underwent an *arthrocentesis* to remove the fluid around his knee.

   SUFFIX: _____   DEFINITION: _____

2. Mark sustained internal injuries and underwent a *splenectomy*.

   SUFFIX: _____   DEFINITION: _____

3. An *ileostomy* is often associated with ulcerative colitis.

   SUFFIX: _____   DEFINITION: _____

4. *Septoplasty* might be the treatment of choice for a broken nose.

   SUFFIX: _____   DEFINITION: _____

5. A *tracheotomy* was performed to allow the patient to breathe.

   SUFFIX: _____   DEFINITION: _____

6. After the birth of her seven children, Mrs. Wilde was scheduled for a *colporrhaphy*.

   SUFFIX: _____   DEFINITION: _____

7. An *orchidopexy* was scheduled to correct Roger's problem.

   SUFFIX: _____   DEFINITION: _____

8. Following *esophagectasia*, Victoria was able to swallow with ease.

   SUFFIX: _____   DEFINITION: _____

EXERCISE 27

Match the suffixes in Column 1 with the meanings in Column 2.

COLUMN 1	COLUMN 2
_____ 1. –centesis	a. binding together
_____ 2. –desis	b. create a new opening
_____ 3. -ectasia; ectasis	c. crushing; friction
_____ 4. –ectomy	d. drooping; sagging; prolapse
_____ 5. -(o)stomy	e. incision into
_____ 6. -(o)tomy	f. opening
_____ 7. –pexy	g. rupture
_____ 8. –plasty	h. spitting up

——— 9.	–ptosis	i. stretching; dilatation
——— 10.	–ptysis	j. surgical fixation
——— 11.	-(r)rhaphy	k. surgical removal; excision
——— 12.	-(r)rhexis	l. surgical repair
——— 13.	–tresia	m. surgical puncture
——— 14.	–tripsy	n. suture

SUMMARY

Prefixes and suffixes are word parts that are added to the beginning and end of word roots. These word parts change the meaning of a medical term. Prefixes can signify colors and numbers as well as indicate a negative meaning for a medical term. Suffixes identify a medical term as a noun or an adjective. There are general, disease, and procedure suffixes.

It is important to memorize the commonly used prefixes and suffixes because these word parts are found in the majority of medical terms. Additional prefixes and suffixes will be presented in the body system chapters, along with the word roots associated with each body system.

CHAPTER REVIEW

EXERCISE 28

Read the medical report. The italicized medical terms are listed after the report. Write the prefixes, suffixes, and the meanings for each term. Using your medical dictionary, look up the definition for each term.

PATIENT NAME: **MATTSON, SARA**
PHYSICIAN NAME: **Erik Gervais, MD**
BRIEF HISTORY
The patient is a 28-year-old female who presents with gradual onset of right upper quadrant pain, vomiting, and (1) *diarrhea*. She was recently (2) *postpartum* and had a postpartum tubal ligation.
PHYSICAL EXAMINATION
Exam today revealed that she was (3) *afebrile*. She exhibited (4) *tachycardia* and massive (5) *hepatomegaly*. Pelvic exam revealed no cervical motion tenderness.
HOSPITAL COURSE
The patient was admitted for workup of her hepatomegaly. She was given (6) *intravenous* fluids for her dehydration and was started on iron for her (7) *anemia*. A liver biopsy revealed several (8) *hepatic* lesions and the tissue resembled neutrophils. (9) *Laparoscopy* was scheduled, a larger sample was taken, and a frozen section was sent to the lab. The final (10) *pathology* report confirmed (11) *adenocarcinoma*. (12) *Oncology* was then consulted and a chemotherapy regime was recommended. Further lab and x-ray reports revealed (13) *hypoalbuminemia* and (14) *bilateral* pleural effusion, respectively. Pain control at home will be accomplished with a (15) *subcutaneous* morphine pump.

MEDICAL TERM	PREFIX AND MEANING	SUFFIX AND MEANING
1. diarrhea	_____	_____
2. postpartum	_____	_____
3. afebrile	_____	_____
4. tachycardia	_____	_____
5. hepatomegaly	_____	_____
6. intravenous	_____	_____
7. anemia	_____	_____
8. hepatic	_____	_____
9. laparoscopy	_____	_____
10. pathology	_____	_____
11. adenocarcinoma	_____	_____
12. oncology	_____	_____
13. hypoalbuminemia	_____	_____
14. bilateral	_____	_____
15. subcutaneous	_____	_____

EXERCISE 29

Write the plural form for the singular word endings listed here.

1. -a   _____
2. -ex   _____
3. -is   _____
4. -on   _____
5. -um   _____
6. -us   _____
7. -nx   _____

EXERCISE 30

Write a short answer for each of the following questions.

1. What is the purpose of a combining vowel?

_____

2. When is it necessary to use a combining vowel?

_____

3. How do you know which syllable should be accented when pronouncing medical terms?

_____

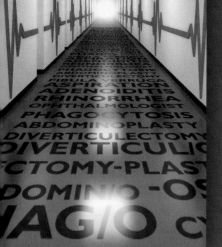

2 General Body Terminology

OBJECTIVES

At the completion of this chapter, the student should be able to:

1. Identify, define, and spell word roots associated with the body structure and organization.
2. Label the five body cavities presented in this chapter.
3. Spell correctly the medical terms related to body structure and organization.
4. Describe the basic components of the 13 body systems.
5. Define the three body planes.
6. Label and define the nine body regions and four body quadrants.
7. Analyze body structure and organization terms by defining the roots, prefixes, and suffixes of these terms.

OVERVIEW

General body terminology includes terms related to structural organization and body cavities, planes, regions, quadrants, and direction. These terms apply to the body as a whole and provide a foundation for understanding the medical terminology related to individual body systems.

General Body Terminology Word Roots

To understand and use general body terminology, it is necessary to acquire a thorough knowledge of the associated word roots. Word roots in Table 2-1 are listed with the combining vowel. Review the word roots and complete the exercises that follow.

TABLE 2-1   BODY TERMINOLOGY WORD ROOTS

Word Root/Combining Form	Meaning
abdomin/o; lapar/o; ceil/o	abdomen
adip/o; lip/o	fat; fatty
anter/o	front
caud/o	lower part of the body; tail
cephal/o	head
chondr/o	cartilage
crani/o	skull
cyt/o	cell
dors/o	back

(continues)

TABLE 2-1   BODY TERMINOLOGY WORD ROOTS (continued)

Word Root/Combining Form	Meaning
gastr/o	stomach
hist/o	tissue
inguin/o	groin
later/o	side; away from the midline
lumb/o	loin
medi/o	middle
nucle/o	nucleus
pelv/i	pelvis
poster/o	back
proxim/o	near
spin/o	spine
thorac/o	chest
umbilic/o	navel
ventr/o	front side; belly
viscer/o	internal organs

© 2016 Cengage Learning®

EXERCISE 1

Write the meaning of each word root.

1. cyt/o _____
2. abdomin/o _____
3. hist/o _____
4. later/o _____
5. ventr/o _____
6. thorac/o _____
7. pelv/i _____
8. chondr/o _____
9. gastr/o _____
10. lapar/o _____

EXERCISE 2

Write the word root with its meaning and a brief definition for each term.

EXAMPLE: laparotomy
ROOT: lapar/o = abdomen   Definition: incision into the abdomen

1. abdominal

   ROOT: _____   DEFINITION: _____

2. cytology

   ROOT: _____   DEFINITION: _____

3. umbilical

ROOT: _____   DEFINITION: _____

4. posterior

ROOT: _____   DEFINITION: _____

5. anterior

ROOT: _____   DEFINITION: _____

6. histology

ROOT: _____   DEFINITION: _____

7. ventral

ROOT: _____   DEFINITION: _____

8. proximal

ROOT: _____   DEFINITION: _____

9. adipose

ROOT: _____   DEFINITION: _____

10. spinal

ROOT: _____   DEFINITION: _____

11. cranial

ROOT: _____   DEFINITION: _____

EXERCISE 3

Write the correct word root(s) for the following definitions.

1. abdomen   _____

2. front   _____

3. internal organs _____

4. navel   _____

5. back   _____

6. front side   _____

7. side   _____

8. near   _____

9. nucleus   _____

10. tissue   _____

11. cartilage   _____

12. stomach   _____

13. loin   _____

14. groin   _____

Structural Organization Terms

Structures of the body are organized into four general categories: cells, tissues, organs, and systems. The categories are described as follows:

- **Cells** are the foundation for all parts of the body.
- **Tissues** are composed of similar cells that come together to perform a common or specialized function. For example, muscle tissue is made up of several types of cells, including muscle cells.
- **Organs** are made up of different types of tissue arranged together to perform a specific function. For example, the heart is an organ with several types of tissue.
- **Systems** include different organs that work together to perform the various functions of the body as a whole. For example, the cardiovascular system consists of the heart, arteries, and veins.

All of the systems come together to form the complete body and enable it to function properly (Figure 2-1).

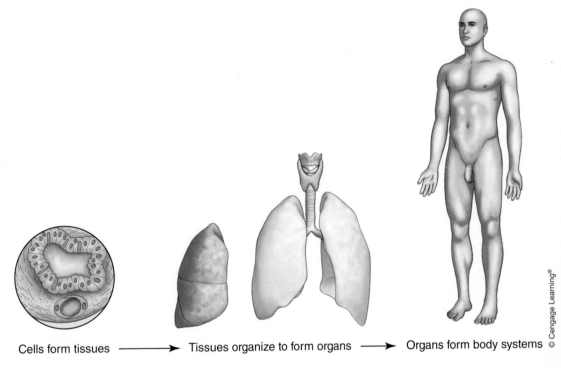

Cells form tissues   ⟶   Tissues organize to form organs   ⟶   Organs form body systems

© Cengage Learning®

Figure 2-1 The human body, from cells to systems.

Cells

The human body is made up of literally trillions of cells that vary in size and shape depending on their function. The study of cells is called **cytology** (sigh-**TALL**-oh-jee). Figure 2-2 illustrates a human cell and some of its structures.

Cells are surrounded by a (1) **cell membrane**, which is the cell's outer covering. The membrane allows materials to pass in and out of the cell so that the cell can receive nutrients and release waste products. The cell's structures are housed in a gel-like substance called (2) **cytoplasm** (**SIGH**-toh-plazm). The (3) **nucleus**

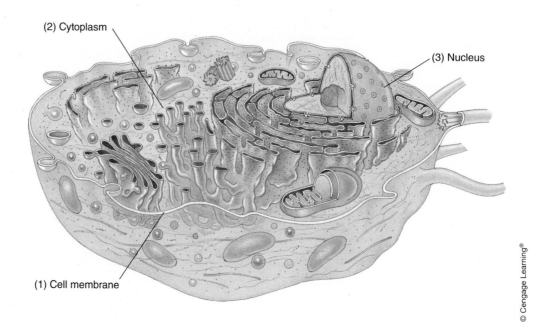

(2) Cytoplasm

(3) Nucleus

(1) Cell membrane

© Cengage Learning®

Figure 2-2 Human cell.

(**NOO**-klee-us) controls cellular functions and is made up of threadlike strands called **chromosomes** (**KROH**-moh-sohms). Chromosomes control the growth, repair, and reproduction functions of the body. Chromosomes contain **deoxyribonucleic** (dee-**ocks**-ee-**right**-boh-noo-**KLAY**-ic) **acid** (**DNA**), which transmits genetic information. The chromosomes also have thousands of segments called **genes**, which are responsible for all hereditary characteristics.

Tissues

Tissues are groups of cells working together to perform a specific function. There are four main types of body tissue: **connective**, **epithelial** (ep-ih-**THEEL**-ee-al), **muscle**, and **nervous**. The study of tissue is called **histology**.

Connective Tissue

Connective tissue functions as the name implies: to connect or support other body tissue or structures. Connective tissue can be liquid, **adipose** (**ADD**-ih-pohs), fibrous, or solid. Bones and cartilage are also called **dense connective tissue**. Table 2-2 lists examples of each type of tissue.

TABLE 2-2   TYPES OF CONNECTIVE TISSUE

Connective Tissue	Example(s)
liquid	blood; lymph
adipose	fat
fibrous	tendons; ligaments
cartilage	nose; ears
solid	bone

© 2016 Cengage Learning®

Epithelial Tissue

Epithelial tissue provides a covering for body organs. It also lines body vessels, cavities, glands, and organs. The skin is an example of epithelial tissue. The lining of the heart, called the **endocardium** (**en**-doh-**KAR**-dee-um), is another example of epithelial tissue.

Muscle Tissue

Muscle tissue functions to produce movement in all parts of the body. Some movement, such as walking, is normally under our control, while other movement, such as the movement of food through the small intestines, is not. There are three types of muscle tissue: skeletal, smooth, and cardiac. Table 2-3 lists each type of muscle tissue and a brief description.

TABLE 2-3   TYPES OF MUSCLE TISSUE

Muscle Tissue	Description
skeletal	attached to bone; moves the skeleton; voluntary muscle
smooth	located in the walls of hollow organs such as the stomach and intestines; produces movement in those organs; involuntary muscle
cardiac	makes up the muscular layer of the heart; involuntary muscle

© 2016 Cengage Learning®

Nervous Tissue

Nervous tissue transmits information throughout the body that allows us to move, think, taste, see, and experience all functions associated with being alive. From blinking the eyes to solving the most complex mathematical equation, nervous tissue is ready to activate the body parts necessary to complete these activities.

Organs

Organs are groups of tissues working together to perform a specific function. Examples of various organs include the heart, stomach, eyes, and skin. The internal organs of the body are known as the **viscera** (**VISS**-er-ah) or **visceral** organs.

Systems

Systems are groups of organs working together to perform the many functions of the body as a whole. Each body system is discussed in the remaining chapters. Table 2-4 lists the body systems and related organs as described in this text.

TABLE 2-4   BODY SYSTEMS AND ORGANS

Body System	Organs
integumentary	skin; hair; nails; glands
skeletal	bones
muscular	muscles; cartilage; ligaments; tendons
cardiovascular	heart; arteries; veins

(continues)

TABLE 2-4   BODY SYSTEMS AND ORGANS (continued)

Body System	Organs
blood/lymph	blood; lymph; lymph glands
respiratory	lungs; trachea; bronchi
digestive	mouth; throat; esophagus; stomach; small and large intestines; liver; gallbladder; and pancreas
urinary	kidneys; ureters; bladder; urethra
endocrine	glands
male reproductive	testes; vas deferens; penis; accessory organs
female reproductive	ovaries; uterus; vagina; fallopian tubes; accessory organs
nervous	nerves; brain; spinal cord
sensory	eyes; ears

© 2016 Cengage Learning®

EXERCISE 4

Write the term for each definition.

1. foundation for all parts of the body   _____

2. organs working together to perform a function   _____

3. cells working together to perform a function   _____

4. tissues working together to perform a function   _____

5. internal organs   _____

6. covering and lining for glands and organs   _____

7. supports and binds other body tissue   _____

8. transmits impulses   _____

9. produces movement   _____

EXERCISE 5

Match the term in Column 1 with the definition in Column 2.

COLUMN 1

_____ 1. chromosome
_____ 2. cytology
_____ 3. cytoplasm
_____ 4. histology
_____ 5. integumentary system
_____ 6. nucleus
_____ 7. proximal
_____ 8. sensory system
_____ 9. ventral
_____ 10. viscera

COLUMN 2

a. eyes; ears
b. study of tissue
c. internal organs
d. pertaining to something near
e. pertaining to the front side
f. contains genes and DNA
g. skin; hair; nails; glands
h. gel-like substance within a cell
i. controls cellular functions
j. study of cells

EXERCISE 6

Write the name of the body system that includes the listed organs.

1. bones; joints   _____
2. muscles; tendons; cartilage   _____
3. lungs; trachea; bronchi   _____
4. kidneys; ureters; urethra; bladder   _____
5. glands; hormones   _____
6. heart; arteries; veins   _____
7. mouth; stomach; large and small intestines   _____
8. brain; spinal cord   _____
9. testes; vas deferens   _____
10. ovaries; uterus   _____

Body Cavities

Body cavities are hollow spaces that contain an orderly arrangement of internal organs. The main body cavities are (1) the **ventral cavity**, located on the front side of the body, and (2) the **dorsal cavity**, located on the back side of the body. Each main body cavity is further subdivided and named for its specific location. Figure 2-3 illustrates the location and name of the main cavities and their subdivisions. Refer to Figure 2-3 as you read about the body cavities.

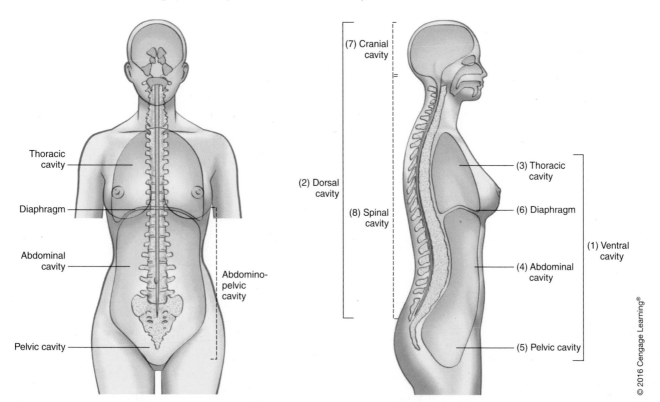

© 2016 Cengage Learning®

Figure 2-3 Frontal and lateral views of the major body cavities. Frontal view on the left; lateral view on the right.

Ventral Cavity

The ventral cavity is divided into the (3) **thoracic** (thoh-**RASS**-ik) **cavity**, the (4) **abdominal cavity**, and the (5) **pelvic cavity**. The thoracic cavity, which is also called the chest cavity, houses the lungs, heart, aorta, esophagus, and trachea. The (6) **diaphragm** (**DIGH**-ah-fram), the muscle that helps us breathe, separates the thoracic cavity from the abdominal cavity.

The abdominal cavity houses the liver, gallbladder, spleen, stomach, pancreas, intestines, and kidneys. There is no specific structure that separates the abdominal cavity from the pelvic cavity. The pelvic cavity houses the urinary bladder and reproductive organs. The abdominal cavity and pelvic cavity are often called the abdominopelvic cavity.

Dorsal Cavity

The dorsal cavity is divided into the (7) **cranial cavity** and the (8) **spinal cavity**. The cranial cavity houses the brain, and the spinal cavity houses the spinal cord.

Body Regions and Quadrants

Body regions are imaginary sections of the abdominopelvic cavity that are located between the diaphragm and pelvis. Physicians use these regions to identify the location of abdominal organs and describe the location of pain. There are nine body regions. Refer to Figure 2-4 as you read the description of each region. The descriptions are presented in Table 2-5.

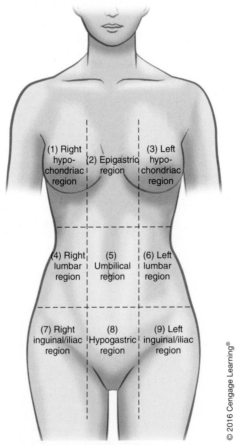

(1) Right hypo-chondriac region
(2) Epigastric region
(3) Left hypo-chondriac region
(4) Right lumbar region
(5) Umbilical region
(6) Left lumbar region
(7) Right inguinal/iliac region
(8) Hypogastric region
(9) Left inguinal/iliac region

© 2016 Cengage Learning®

Figure 2-4 Body regions.

TABLE 2-5 BODY REGIONS

Region	Name and Description
1	**Right hypochondriac (high-poh-KON-dree-ak) region.** Located beneath the cartilage of the lower ribs in the upper-right section of the abdomen.
2	**Epigastric (ep-ee-GASS-trik) region.** Located above the stomach and navel, between the right and left hypochondriac regions.
3	**Left hypochondriac region.** Located beneath the cartilage of the lower ribs in the upper-left section of the abdomen.
4	**Right lumbar region.** Located in the midportion of the abdomen directly below the right hypochondriac region.
5	**Umbilical region.** Located in the midsection of the abdomen at the level of the umbilicus or navel.
6	**Left lumbar region.** Located in the midportion of the abdomen directly below the left hypochondriac region.
7	**Right inguinal (ING-gwih-nal) region.** Located in the lower-right portion of the abdomen, directly below the right lumbar region. Also called the **right iliac region**.
8	**Hypogastric region.** Located in the lower midsection of the abdomen, directly below the umbilical region.
9	**Left inguinal region.** Located in the lower-left portion of the abdomen, directly below the left lumbar region. Also called the **left iliac region**.

© 2016 Cengage Learning®

Body quadrants are four imaginary sections of the abdomen that, like the nine body regions, provide a reference point for locating abdominal organs and pain. The quadrants are named based on their relationship to the umbilicus or navel. Figure 2-5 illustrates the body quadrants. The (1) **right upper quadrant (RUQ)** and (2) **left upper quadrant (LUQ)** are positioned above and to the right and left of the umbilicus. The (3) **right lower quadrant (RLQ)** and (4) **left lower quadrant (LLQ)** are positioned below and to the right and left of the umbilicus.

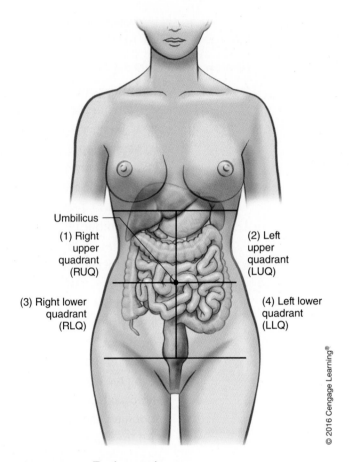

Umbilicus

(1) Right upper quadrant (RUQ)

(2) Left upper quadrant (LUQ)

(3) Right lower quadrant (RLQ)

(4) Left lower quadrant (LLQ)

© 2016 Cengage Learning®

Figure 2-5 Body quadrants.

EXERCISE 7

Analyze the listed body region terms. Identify and define the root, prefix, and suffix for each term. Write the definition for each term.

EXAMPLE:	hemigastrectomy
ROOT:	gastr = stomach
PREFIX:	hemi- = half
SUFFIX:	-ectomy = surgical removal; excision
DEFINITION:	surgical removal of all or part of the stomach

1. hypochondriac

   ROOT: _____

   PREFIX: _____

   SUFFIX: _____

   DEFINITION: _____

2. inguinal

   ROOT: _____

   PREFIX: _____

SUFFIX: _____

DEFINITION: _____

3. epigastric

ROOT: _____

PREFIX: _____

SUFFIX: _____

DEFINITION: _____

4. hypogastric

ROOT: _____

PREFIX: _____

SUFFIX: _____

DEFINITION: _____

5. umbilical

ROOT: _____

PREFIX: _____

SUFFIX: _____

DEFINITION: _____

EXERCISE 8

Write the name of the body cavities shown in Figure 2-6 on the spaces provided.

1. _____

2. _____

3. _____

4. _____

5. _____

6. _____

7. _____

8. _____

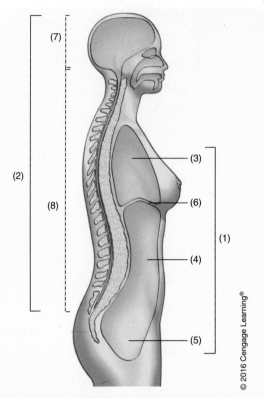

Figure 2-6 Label the body cavities.

EXERCISE 9

Write out the following abbreviations.

1. RUQ _____

2. LLQ _____

3. LUQ _____

4. RLQ _____

EXERCISE 10

Place the abbreviations listed in Exercise 9 in the correct location on Figure 2-7.

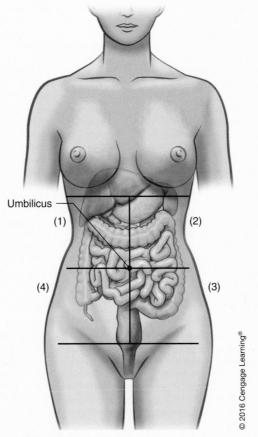

Figure 2-7 Label the body quadrants.

EXERCISE 11

Write the names of the body regions shown in Figure 2-8 on the spaces provided.

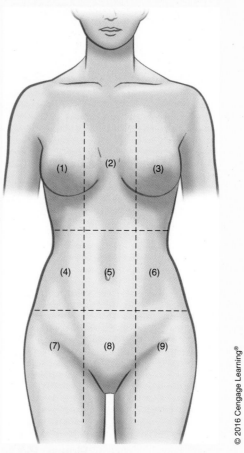

© 2016 Cengage Learning®

Figure 2-8 Label the body regions.

1. _____

2. _____

3. _____

4. _____

5. _____

6. _____

7. _____

8. _____

9. _____

Body Planes

Body planes are imaginary slices, or cuts, that divide the body into right and left, front and back, and upper and lower segments. These slices pass through the body in a specific direction. Table 2-6 lists and describes commonly used body planes. Refer to Figure 2-9 as you review the descriptions of the body planes.

TABLE 2-6   BODY PLANES

Body Plane	Description
(1) midsagittal plane (mid-**SAJ**-ih-tal)	divides the body, starting with the head and continuing through the pelvic region, into equal right and left halves or sides
sagittal plane (**SAJ**-ih-tal)	divides the body into right and left portions or segments
(2) transverse plane	divides the body into upper and lower portions or segments; also called the horizontal plane
(3) frontal plane	divides the body, starting with the head and continuing through the legs and feet, into front and back portions or segments; also called the coronal (koh-**ROH**-nal) plane

© 2016 Cengage Learning®

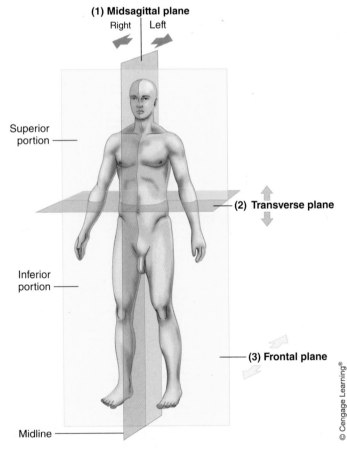

Figure 2-9   Body planes.

Body Direction Terms

Body direction terms are literally the north, south, east, and west of medical terminology. These terms provide health care professionals with a vocabulary that readily describes the location of another body part, an incision, a problem, diagnosis, or disease, and other information related to the human body.

Body direction terms are described in terms of a standard reference position of the body as a whole. This standard reference position is called the **anatomical position**. In the anatomical position, the body is viewed as erect, with the arms at the sides, palms of the hands facing forward, and the head and feet also facing forward. Directional terms keep the same meaning as long as the individual is standing or lying down, face up.

Commonly used directional terms, with pronunciations and meanings, are listed in Table 2-7. Review the pronunciation and meaning of each term and complete the exercises.

TABLE 2-7 DIRECTIONAL TERMS

Term with Pronunciation	Definition
anterior (an-**TEE**-ree-or)	toward the front; pertaining to the front
anteroposterior (AP) (**an**-ter-oh-poss-**TEE**-ree-or)	from the front to the back; pertaining to the front and the back
caudal (**KAWD**-al)	pertaining to the tail; downward
cephalad (**SEFF**-ah-lad)	toward the head; pertaining to the head
cranial (**KRAY**-nee-al)	toward the head; pertaining to the head
deep	away from the surface
distal (**DISS**-tal)	away from the trunk of the body; farthest from the point of origin of a body part (Figure 2-10A)
dorsal (**DOR**-sal)	toward the back; pertaining to the back
inferior (in-**FEER**-ee-or)	below; downward toward the tail or feet
lateral (**LAT**-er-al)	to the side; away from the midline of the body (Figure 2-10B)
medial (**MEE**-dee-al)	toward the midline of the body; pertaining to the middle (Figure 2-10C)
posterior (poss-**TEE**-ree-or)	toward the back; pertaining to the back of the body
posteroanterior (PA) (**poss**-ter-oh-an-**TEE**-ree-or)	from the back to the front; pertaining to the back and front
prone (PROHN)	face down; lying on the abdomen
proximal (**PROCKS**-ih-mal)	toward the trunk of the body; nearest to the point of origin of a body part (see Figure 2-10D)
superficial (soo-per-**FISH**-al)	near the surface; pertaining to the surface
superior (soo-**PEE**-ree-or)	above; upward; toward the head
supine (soo-**PINE**)	face up; lying on the back
ventral (**VEN**-tral)	toward the front; pertaining to the front side

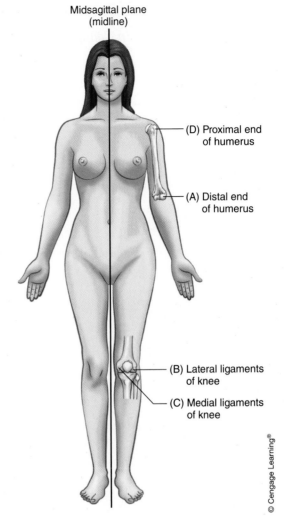

Midsagittal plane
(midline)

(D) Proximal end
of humerus

(A) Distal end
of humerus

(B) Lateral ligaments
of knee

(C) Medial ligaments
of knee

© Cengage Learning®

Figure 2-10   Distal (A), lateral (B), medial (C), and proximal (D) body directions.

EXERCISE 12

Fill in the blanks.

1. The _____ plane divides the body into right and left segments.

2. Horizontal plane is another name for the _____ plane.

3. Coronal plane is also known as the _____ plane.

4. The _____ plane divides the body into right and left halves.

5. A/An _____ wound is near the surface of the body.

6. The _____ position is best for examining the abdomen.

7. The knees are located in a/an _____ position from the ankles.

EXERCISE 13

Match the term in Column 1 with the definition in Column 2.

COLUMN 1

_____ 1. anterior

_____ 2. caudal

_____ 3. distal

_____ 4. lateral

_____ 5. medial

_____ 6. posterior

_____ 7. proximal

_____ 8. supine

_____ 9. midsagittal plane

_____ 10. transverse plane

COLUMN 2

a. toward the tail

b. upper and lower segments

c. face up

d. toward the front

e. farthest away from

f. nearest to

g. toward the side

h. toward the back

i. toward the midline

j. equal right and left segments

EXERCISE 14

Write the directional term that has the opposite meaning of each listed directional term.

EXAMPLE:

	DIRECTIONAL TERM	OPPOSITE MEANING DIRECTIONAL TERM
	deep	superficial

DIRECTIONAL TERM	OPPOSITE MEANING DIRECTIONAL TERM
1. anterior	_____
2. anteroposterior	_____
3. caudal	_____
4. distal	_____
5. lateral	_____
6. prone	_____
7. superficial	_____
8. superior	_____
9. ventral	_____

SUMMARY

General body terminology includes words associated with the organization of the body from cells to body systems; the names of the major body cavities, planes, and organ systems; and the regions and quadrants of the chest and abdomen. The roots and terms presented in this chapter provide a foundation for understanding the medical terminology of the individual body systems.

CHAPTER REVIEW

The Chapter Review can be used as a self-test. Go through each exercise and answer as many questions as you can without referring to previous exercises or earlier discussions within this chapter. Check your answers and fill in any blanks. Practice writing the terms that are misspelled.

EXERCISE 15

Write the meaning of each abbreviation.

1. RLQ   _____
2. LLQ   _____
3. RUQ   _____
4. LUQ   _____
5. AP   _____
6. PA   _____

EXERCISE 16

Select the best answer to each statement.

1. Select the type of tissue that supports other body structures.
   a. connective
   b. muscle
   c. nervous
   d. adipose

2. Which tissue transmits information throughout the body?
   a. adipose
   b. nervous
   c. muscle
   d. connective

3. Choose the tissue that is responsible for body movement.
   a. connective
   b. nervous
   c. adipose
   d. muscle

4. Which tissue is composed of fat?
   a. muscle
   b. nervous
   c. adipose
   d. connective

5. Select the term that means internal body organs.
   a. systems
   b. viscera
   c. ventral
   d. abdominus

6. Which body cavity is **not** a division of the ventral cavity?
   a. thoracic cavity
   b. pelvic cavity
   c. abdominal cavity
   d. cranial cavity

7. Select the group of organs located in the thoracic cavity.
   a. heart; aorta; diaphragm
   b. lungs; esophagus; spleen
   c. lungs; heart; trachea
   d. esophagus; trachea; liver

8. Choose the group of organs located in the pelvic cavity.
   a. kidneys; uterus; ovaries
   b. uterus; ovaries; vas deferens
   c. kidneys; ureters; urinary bladder
   d. urinary bladder; ovaries; spleen

9. Which group of organs is located in the abdominal cavity?
   a. esophagus; liver; stomach
   b. intestines; stomach; urinary bladder
   c. stomach; trachea; spleen
   d. liver; gallbladder; kidneys

10. Select the body cavity that houses the brain.
    a. cranial cavity
    b. dorsal cavity
    c. thoracic cavity
    d. ventral cavity

EXERCISE 17

Match the body system in Column 1 with the components in Column 2.

COLUMN 1
_____ 1. blood/lymph
_____ 2. cardiovascular
_____ 3. digestive
_____ 4. endocrine
_____ 5. female reproductive
_____ 6. integumentary
_____ 7. male reproductive
_____ 8. muscular
_____ 9. nervous
_____ 10. respiratory
_____ 11. sensory
_____ 12. skeletal
_____ 13. urinary

COLUMN 2
a. bones; joints
b. blood; blood cells; lymph glands
c. cartilage; ligaments; tendons
d. eyes; ears
e. glands; hormones
f. heart; arteries; veins
g. kidneys; ureters; bladder
h. lungs; trachea; bronchi
i. mouth; stomach; intestines
j. nerves; brain; spinal cord
k. ovaries; uterus; vagina
l. skin; hair; nails
m. testes; vas deferens; penis

EXERCISE 18

Write a brief definition for each term.

1. cell _____

2. tissue _____

3. organ _____

4. system _____

5. cytology _____

6. sagittal plane _____

7. transverse plane _____

8. supine _____

9. prone _____

10. distal _____

EXERCISE 19

Fill in the blanks.

1. The _____ controls all cellular functions.

2. _____ tissue covers organs and lines vessels.

3. Tendons and ligaments are examples of _____ tissue.

4. The _____ region of the body is at the level of the navel.

5. The _____ region of the body is located above the stomach.

6. A gel-like substance called _____ houses the cell's
   structures.

7. _____ muscle is attached to bones.

8. The _____ region of the body is located below the stomach
   and navel.

9. _____ is defined as the study of tissue.

10. _____ muscle produces movement in hollow organs.

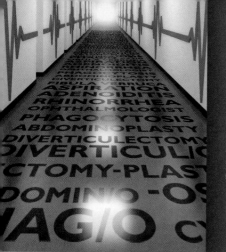

3 Integumentary System

OBJECTIVES

At the completion of this chapter, the student should be able to:

1. Identify, define, and spell word roots associated with the integumentary system.
2. Label the basic structures of the integumentary system.
3. Discuss the functions of the integumentary system.
4. Provide the correct spelling of integumentary terms, given the definition of the term.
5. Analyze integumentary terms by defining the roots, prefixes, and suffixes of these terms.
6. Identify, define, and spell disease, disorder, and procedure terms related to the integumentary system.

OVERVIEW

The integumentary system is made up of the skin, hair, nails, and glands. The structures of the integumentary system function together for the following purposes: (1) to provide a protective covering for the entire body; (2) to regulate body temperature by producing sweat, which cools the body, and oil, which lubricates the body; and (3) to receive sensory information associated with pain, temperature, pressure, and touch. Each integumentary system structure and its unique characteristics are presented individually.

Integumentary System Word Roots

To understand and use integumentary system medical terms, it is necessary to acquire a thorough knowledge of the associated word roots. Integumentary system word roots are listed with the combining vowel. Review the word roots in Table 3-1 and complete the exercises that follow.

TABLE 3-1 INTEGUMENTARY SYSTEM WORD ROOTS

Word Root/Combining Form	Meaning
cut/o; cutane/o	skin
derm/o; dermat/o	skin
hidr/o	sweat
hirsut/o	hairy; rough
kerat/o	horny tissue; hard; thickened

(continues)

54

TABLE 3-1 INTEGUMENTARY SYSTEM WORD ROOTS (continued)

Word Root/Combining Form	Meaning
lip/o	fat; lipid
melan/o	black
myc/o	fungus
onych/o; ungu/o	nail
pachy/o	thick
pil/o	hair
py/o	pus
rhytid/o	wrinkles
seb/o	sebum
squam/o	scale
sud/o; sudor/o	sweat
trich/o	hair
xer/o	dry

© 2016 Cengage Learning®

EXERCISE 1

Write the definitions of the following word roots.

1. melan/o   _____
2. trich/o   _____
3. onych/o   _____
4. cutane/o   _____
5. sud/o; sudor/o   _____
6. hidr/o   _____
7. xer/o   _____
8. myc/o   _____
9. pachy/o   _____
10. rhytid/o   _____

EXERCISE 2

Write the word root and meaning for each of the listed medical terms.

EXAMPLE: cutaneous
ROOT: cutane   MEANING: skin

1. dermatitis

   ROOT: _____   MEANING: _____

2. keratosis

   ROOT: _____   MEANING: _____

3. melanocyte

ROOT: _____   MEANING: _____

4. rhytidoplasty

ROOT: _____   MEANING: _____

5. squamous

ROOT: _____   MEANING: _____

6. sebum

ROOT: _____   MEANING: _____

7. xeroderma

ROOT: _____   MEANING: _____

8. pachyderma

ROOT: _____   MEANING: _____

9. mycosis

ROOT: _____   MEANING: _____

10. onychophagia

ROOT: _____   MEANING: _____

EXERCISE 3

Write the correct word root/combining forms for the following meanings.

EXAMPLE: skin   cut/o; cutane/o; derm/o; dermat/o

1. black   _____

2. fungus   _____

3. hair   _____

4. horny tissue   _____

5. nail   _____

6. scale   _____

7. sebum   _____

8. skin   _____

9. sweat   _____

10. thick   _____

11. wrinkles   _____

12. dry   _____

Structures of the Integumentary System

The basic structures of the integumentary system include the skin, glands, hair, and nails. The skin provides a protective covering for the body and aids in the identification of sensations such as heat, cold, pain, and touch. The glands produce sweat to help cool the body and oil to lubricate the skin. Nails provide protection for the tips of the fingers and toes.

Skin and Glands

The skin is the largest organ of the body and has two distinct layers: the (1) **epidermis** (**ep**-ih-**DERM**-is), the outermost layer of the skin, and the (2) **dermis** (**DERM**-is), the middle or inner layer of the skin. The (3) **subcutaneous** (**sub**-kyoo-**TAYN**-ee-us) tissue, as the name implies, is below the skin. However, this tissue is so closely attached to the dermis it is sometimes called the third layer of the skin. Refer to Figure 3-1 as you read about the layers and glands of the skin.

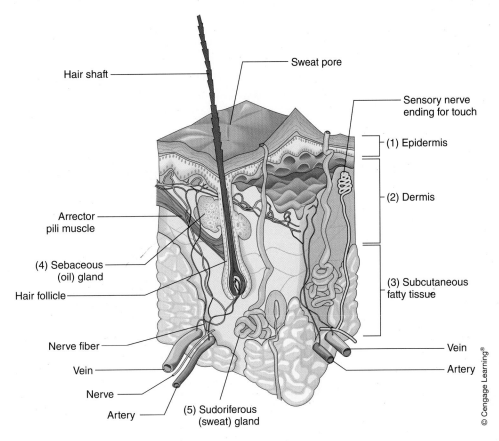

Figure 3-1 Structures of the skin.

Epidermis

The epidermis has several layers. The surface of the epidermis is covered with flat, horny cells that are constantly shed. A deeper epidermal layer contains **melanin** (**MELL**-ah-nin), the substance that gives skin its color. The deepest epidermal layer, called the basal layer, produces new cells to replace those that are being shed.

Dermis

The dermis contains blood vessels, sensory nerve endings, oil and sweat glands, and hair follicles. The dermis is often called the "living" tissue of the skin. (4) **Sebaceous** (seh-**BAY**-shus) glands secrete **sebum** (**SEE**-bum), or oil, into hair follicles. Sweat glands, also called (5) **sudoriferous** (**soo**-dor-**IF**-er-us) glands, emerge through pores to the surface of the skin.

Subcutaneous Tissue

Although the subcutaneous tissue is not a layer of skin per se, it is closely associated with the dermal layer of the skin. The subcutaneous layer is made up of (3) **adipose** (**ADD**-ih-pohs), fatty tissue, and connective tissue. This layer provides insulation and protection for deeper body structures.

Hair and Nails

Hair is defined as a meshwork of cells that contain the protein **keratin** (**KAIR**-ah-tin). Hair originates from the hair (1) **follicles** (**FAH**-lih-kuls), which are located in the dermis of the skin. The hair (2) root is embedded in the hair follicle. The (3) arrector pili muscle provides support for hair follicles. The hair (4) shaft is the visible portion of the hair. The hair shaft is actually dead tissue and does not have nerve endings or a blood supply, which is why it does not hurt when your hair is cut. Figure 3-2 illustrates the major structures of hair.

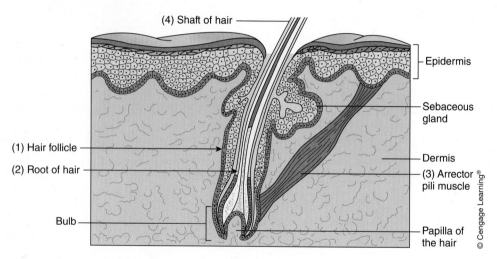

Figure 3-2   Structures of hair.

Fingernails and toenails are also made up of keratin and originate in the epidermis. Although both hair and nails contain keratin, nails are arranged as flat, hard, plate-like coverings located at the ends of toes and fingers. Nails consist of the (1) nail plate, also called the nail body; the (2) **lunula** (**LOO**-noo-lah), a pale or white half-moon-shaped area at the base of the nail plate; and the (3) cuticle, a narrow band of epidermal skin at the base and sides of the nail plate. Figure 3-3 highlights nail structures.

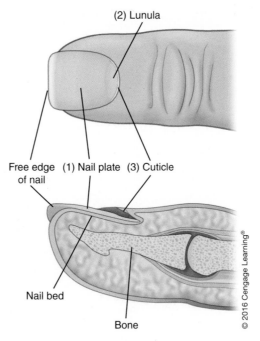

(2) Lunula

Free edge   (1) Nail plate   (3) Cuticle
of nail

Nail bed

Bone

© 2016 Cengage Learning®

Figure 3-3 Structures of nails.

EXERCISE 4

Match the structures in Column 1 with the definitions in Column 2.

COLUMN 1

_____ 1. arrector pili
_____ 2. cuticle
_____ 3. dermis
_____ 4. epidermis
_____ 5. follicle
_____ 6. hair
_____ 7. lunula
_____ 8. melanin
_____ 9. nail
_____ 10. sebaceous gland
_____ 11. sweat gland

COLUMN 2

a. secretes sebum
b. "living" skin tissue
c. produces sweat
d. flat, platelike coverings
e. outermost skin layer
f. contains hair root
g. provides skin color
h. meshwork of cells with protein
i. area at the base of the nail
j. band of skin around the nail plate
k. provides support to the hair
   follicle

EXERCISE 5

On the spaces provided, write the name of the numbered skin structures shown in Figure 3-4.

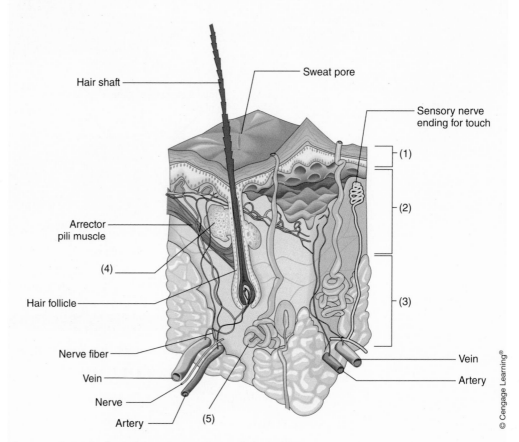

Figure 3-4 Label the structures of the skin.

1. _____

2. _____

3. _____

4. _____

5. _____

On the spaces provided, write the name of the numbered hair structures shown in Figure 3-5.

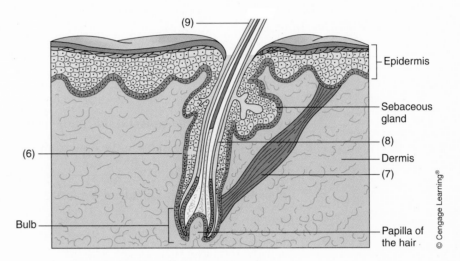

Figure 3-5 Label the structures of the hair.

6. _____

7. _____

8. _____

9. _____

On the spaces provided, write the name of the numbered nail structures shown in Figure 3-6.

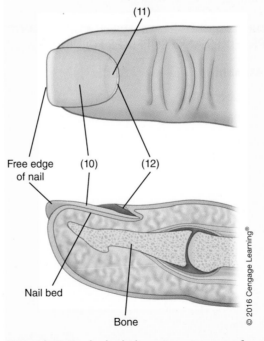

Figure 3-6 Label the structures of nails.

10. _____

11. _____

12. _____

Write the name of the defined integumentary system structure.

1. contains blood vessels, nerve endings, glands _____

2. epidermal skin at the base and side of the nail _____

3. made of keratin; originates in the epidermis _____

4. outermost layer of the skin _____

5. originates in the dermis; made of keratin _____

6. produces sweat _____

7. provides color _____

8. secretes oil _____

9. white, half-moon-shaped area at the nail's base _____

Integumentary System Medical Terminology

Integumenary medical terms are organized into three main categories: (1) general medical terms, (2) diseases and disorders, and (3) procedure and surgery terms. Prefixes and suffixes listed in Table 3-2 are commonly a part of integumentary system medical terms. Review the prefixes and suffixes and complete the related exercises. The exercises are designed to help you learn integumentary system medical terms by recalling the meaning of these word parts.

TABLE 3-2   PREFIXES AND SUFFIXES FOR INTEGUMENTARY SYSTEM TERMS

Prefix	Meaning	Suffix	Meaning
epi-	on; upon; over	-ectomy	excision; surgical removal
hypo-	beneath; below	-ia; -iasis; -osis	abnormal condition of
intra-	within	-itis	inflammation
para-	around; beside	-malacia	softening
per-	through	-(o)logy	study of
sub-	under; below	-(o)logist	specialist in the study of
		-oma	tumor; swelling
		-plasty	surgical repair
		-(r)rhea	flow; excessive discharge
		-tome	cutting instrument

EXERCISE 7

Write the meaning of the prefixes and suffixes for the following terms.

EXAMPLE: subcutaneous
PREFIX sub- = under; below   SUFFIX -ous = pertaining to

1. intramuscular

    PREFIX: _____   SUFFIX: _____

2. percutaneous

    PREFIX: _____   SUFFIX: _____

3. epidermal

    PREFIX: _____   SUFFIX: _____

4. seborrhea

    PREFIX: _____   SUFFIX: _____

5. hypodermic

    PREFIX: _____   SUFFIX: _____

6. melanoma

    PREFIX: _____   SUFFIX: _____

7. keratome

    PREFIX: _____   SUFFIX: _____

8. mycosis

    PREFIX: _____   SUFFIX: _____

9. onychomalacia

    PREFIX: _____   SUFFIX: _____

10. rhytidectomy

    PREFIX: _____   SUFFIX: _____

Integumentary System General Medical Terms

Review the pronunciation and meaning of each term in Table 3-3. Note that some terms are built from word parts and some are not. Complete the exercises for these terms.

TABLE 3-3 INTEGUMENTARY SYSTEM GENERAL MEDICAL TERMS

Term with Pronunciation	Definition
adipose (**ADD**-ih-pohs)	fat
dermatologist (**der**-mah-**TALL**-oh-jist) dermat/o = skin -logist = specialist	physician who specializes in diagnosing and treating disorders of the skin

(continues)

TABLE 3-3 INTEGUMENTARY SYSTEM GENERAL MEDICAL TERMS (continued)

Term with Pronunciation	Definition
dermatology (**der**-mah-**TALL**-oh-jee) dermat/o = skin -logy = study of	study of the skin
epidermal (**ep**-ih-**DER**-mal) epi- = upon derm/o = skin -al = pertaining to	pertaining to the epidermal layer of the skin
hypodermic (**high**-poh-**DER**-mik) hypo- = beneath derm/o = skin -ic = pertaining to	pertaining to beneath the skin
intradermal (**in**-trah-**DER**-mal) intra- = within derm/o = skin -al = pertaining to	pertaining to within the skin
percutaneous (**per**-kyoo-**TAY**-nee-us) per- = through cutane/o = skin -ous = pertaining to	pertaining to through the skin
subcutaneous (**sub**-kyoo-**TAY**-nee-us) sub- = under, below cutane/o = skin -ous = pertaining to	pertaining to under or below the skin

© 2016 Cengage Learning®

EXERCISE 8

Analyze the listed medical terms by separating the root, prefix, suffix, and combining vowel with vertical slashes. Using the word part meanings, write a definition for the term. (Remember that it is often helpful to define a medical term suffix first, prefix second, and word root last.) Check the definition with your medical dictionary.

EXAMPLE: dermatologist

(none)	/ *dermat*	/ *o*	/ *logist*
prefix	*root*	*combining vowel*	*suffix*

DEFINITION: physician who specializes in diagnosing and treating disorders of the skin

1. dermatology

prefix	root	combining vowel	suffix

DEFINITION: _____

2. percutaneous

prefix	root	combining vowel	suffix

DEFINITION: _____

3. intradermal

prefix	root	combining vowel	suffix

DEFINITION: _____

4. hypodermic

prefix	root	combining vowel	suffix

DEFINITION: _____

5. epidermal

prefix	root	combining vowel	suffix

DEFINITION: _____

Integumentary System Disease and Disorder Terms

Integumentary system diseases and disorders include familiar problems such as the common blister as well as other, more complex and less familiar diagnoses. The disease and disorder terms are presented in alphabetical order. Review the pronunciation and definition for each term in Table 3-4 and complete the exercises.

TABLE 3-4   INTEGUMENTARY SYSTEM DISEASE AND DISORDER TERMS

Term with Pronunciation	Definition
abrasion (uh-**BRAY**-zhun)	scraping away of the skin; a scrape
acne (**AK**-nee)	inflammatory disease of the sebaceous glands and hair follicles
actinic keratosis (ak-**TIN**-ik **kair**-ah-**TOH**-sis)	precancerous skin condition related to excessive sunlight exposure
albinism (al-**BYN**-ism)	condition characterized by a lack of skin pigmentation; white
alopecia (**al**-oh-**PEE**-she-ah)	loss of hair; baldness

(continues)

TABLE 3-4   INTEGUMENTARY SYSTEM DISEASE AND DISORDER TERMS
(continued)

Term with Pronunciation	Definition
basal cell carcinoma (**BAY**-zal sell **kar**-sin-**OH**-mah) carcin- = cancer -oma = tumor	cancerous tumor of the basal cell layer of the epidermis
bulla (**BULL**-ah)	a large blister, usually more than 0.5 cm in diameter
burn	injury to body tissue caused by heat, flame, electricity, sun, chemicals, or radiation; severity is measured by the total body skin surface affected and the layers of skin involved (Figure 3-7)

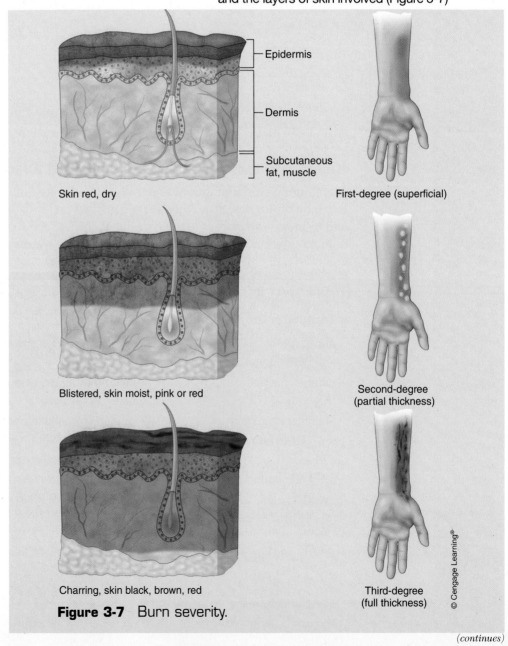

Skin red, dry — First-degree (superficial)

Epidermis

Dermis

Subcutaneous fat, muscle

Blistered, skin moist, pink or red — Second-degree (partial thickness)

Charring, skin black, brown, red — Third-degree (full thickness)

© Cengage Learning®

Figure 3-7 Burn severity.

(continues)

TABLE 3-4 INTEGUMENTARY SYSTEM DISEASE AND DISORDER TERMS (continued)

Term with Pronunciation	Definition
carbuncle (**KAR**-bung-kal)	skin infection characterized by a cluster of boils
cicatrix (**SIH**-kah-triks; or sih-**KAY**-triks)	a scar left by a healed wound
contusion (kon-**TOO**-zhun)	an injury characterized by pain, swelling, and discoloration without a break in the skin; a bruise
cyst (**SIST**)	abnormal, closed sac containing gas, fluid, or semisolid material (Figure 3-8)

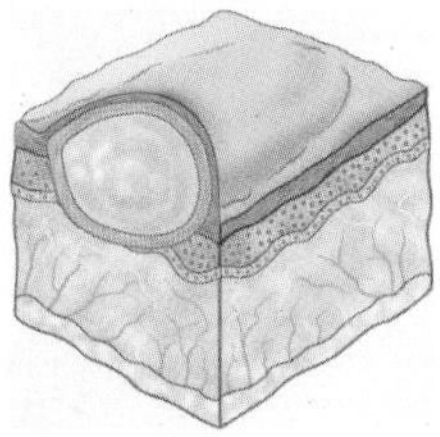

© 2016 Cengage Learning®

Figure 3-8 Cyst.

dermatitis (**der**-mah-**TIGH**-tis) dermat/o = skin -itis = inflammation	inflammation of the skin
diaphoresis (**digh**-ah-for-**EE**-sis)	excessive sweating
ecchymosis (eh-kee-**MOH**-sis)	superficial discoloration caused by blood in the tissue; a bruise
eczema (**EGGS**-ih-mah)	inflammatory skin disorder characterized by redness, itching, vesicles, weeping, oozing, and crusting
edema (eh-**DEE**-mah)	abnormal swelling of tissue
erythema (**air**-ih-**THEEM**-ah)	redness
exanthem (eck-**ZAN**-thum)	widespread rash, usually in children
excoriation (**eks**-kor-ee-**AY**-shun)	a scratch
furuncle (**FIR**-ung-kal)	inflamed hair follicle; a boil
herpes simplex (**HER**-peez **SIM**-pleks)	fever blister; cold sore
herpes varicella (**HER**-peez var-ih-**SELL**-ah)	highly contagious disease usually seen in childhood, commonly called chickenpox

(continues)

TABLE 3-4   INTEGUMENTARY SYSTEM DISEASE AND DISORDER TERMS (continued)

Term with Pronunciation	Definition
herpes zoster (**HER**-peez **ZOSS**-ter)	painful skin eruptions that follow a nerve path; shingles (Figure 3-9)
impetigo (im-peh-**TIGH**-goh)	highly contagious superficial skin infection characterized by pustules

© 2016 Cengage Learning®

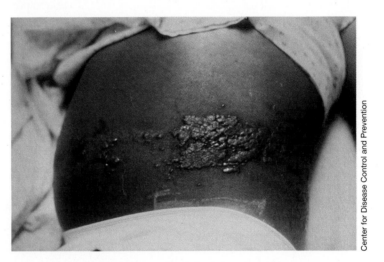

Center for Disease Control and Prevention

Figure 3-9   Herpes zoster (Centers for Disease Control and Prevention).

EXERCISE 9

Replace each italicized definition with the correct medical term.

1. Reggie wanted to try some natural treatments for *baldness*.

   MEDICAL TERM: _____

2. The dermatologist stated it would take several treatments to clear up the *cluster of boils*.

   MEDICAL TERM: _____

3. *Inflammation of the skin* has many causes.

   MEDICAL TERM: _____

4. *Excessive or profuse sweating* can be a symptom of a myocardial infarction.

   MEDICAL TERM: _____

5. A *fever blister* often appears on the lips.

   MEDICAL TERM: _____

6. Joe made an appointment to have a *boil* removed.

MEDICAL TERM: _____

7. Henry's *scratch* became infected.

MEDICAL TERM: _____

8. After sliding across the basketball floor, Jenny had a large *scrape* on her arm.

MEDICAL TERM: _____

9. Rachel's *scar* required surgical intervention.

MEDICAL TERM: _____

EXERCISE 10

Using your medical dictionary, write a brief definition for the italicized medical terms.

1. The *ecchymosis* on Julia's forearm did not prevent her from playing volleyball.

DEFINITION: _____

2. Many over-the-counter lotions claim they can relieve *erythema*.

DEFINITION: _____

3. Standing on your feet for prolonged periods may cause *edema*.

DEFINITION: _____

4. Marlena's dermatologist prescribed a new medication for her *eczema*.

DEFINITION: _____

5. *Actinic keratosis* is related to excessive sunlight exposure.

DEFINITION: _____

6. Jim's *herpes zoster* affected his trunk and back.

DEFINITION: _____

7. *Acne* can affect an individual at any age.

DEFINITION: _____

8. When Lisa was diagnosed with *impetigo*, she avoided contact with her fellow students.

DEFINITION: _____

EXERCISE 11

Match the medical term in Column 1 with the definition in Column 2.

COLUMN 1	COLUMN 2
_____ 1. abrasion	a. shingles
_____ 2. acne	b. cancerous tumor of the epidermis
_____ 3. albinism	c. disease of sebaceous glands and hair follicles

_____ 4. basal cell carcinoma   d. scratch

_____ 5. cicatrix   e. highly contagious superficial skin infection

_____ 6. contusion   f. lack of skin pigmentation

_____ 7. diaphoresis   g. scar

_____ 8. eczema   h. scraping away of the skin; a scrape

_____ 9. excoriation   i. excessive sweating

_____ 10. herpes zoster   j. bruise

_____ 11. impetigo   k. skin disorder; redness, itching, weeping, and crusting

EXERCISE 12

Review the list of medical terms and rewrite the terms that are misspelled.

1. alopecea   _____

2. abrasion   _____

3. exzema   _____

4. furuncle   _____

5. erithema   _____

6. excoriation   _____

7. diaphoresis   _____

8. impatigo   _____

9. basil cell carcinoma   _____

10. carbuncle   _____

Review the pronunciation and definition for each term in Table 3-5 and complete the exercises.

TABLE 3-5 INTEGUMENTARY SYSTEM DISEASE AND DISORDER TERMS

Term with Pronunciation	Definition
jaundice (**JAWN**-dis)	yellow discoloration of the skin
Kaposi's sarcoma (**KAP**-oh-seez sar-**KOH**-mah) sarc/o = flesh -oma = tumor	a cancerous growth that begins as soft, purple-brown papules on the feet and gradually spreads in the skin
keloid (**KEE**-loyd)	abnormally large, raised or thickened scar
keratosis (**kerr**-ah-**TOH**-sis) kerat/o = horny tissue; hard -osis = condition	any condition, such as a wart or callus, characterized by hard, thickened tissue

(continues)

TABLE 3-5 INTEGUMENTARY SYSTEM DISEASE AND DISORDER TERMS
(continued)

Term with Pronunciation	Definition
laceration (lass-er-**AY**-shun)	a cut
lesion (**LEE**-zhun)	any damage to tissue caused by trauma or disease
macule (**MAK**-yool)	small, flat discoloration of skin less than 1 cm in diameter (Figure 3-10)

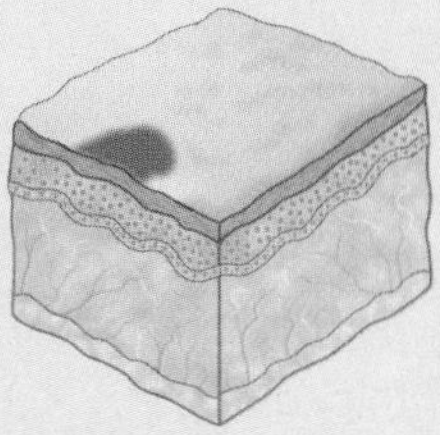

© 2016 Cengage Learning®

Figure 3-10   Macule.

malignant melanoma (mah-**LIG**-nant **mell**-ah-**NOH**-mah) melan/o = black -oma = tumor	cancerous skin tumor originating from the melanocytes of a mole, freckles, or pigmented skin; skin cancer (Figure 3-11)

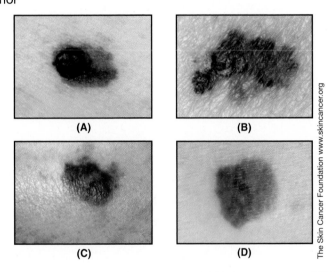

(A)   (B)

(C)   (D)

The Skin Cancer Foundation www.skincancer.org

Figure 3-11   Malignant melanoma signs. [A] Asymmetry, [B] border irregularity, [C] color variation, and [D] diameter larger than a pencil eraser.

nevus (pl. nevi) (**NEE**-vus; pl. **NEE**-vigh)	pigmented area at birth; mole, birthmark
onychocryptosis (**on**-ih-koh-krip-**TOH**-sis) onych/o = nail crypt/o = hidden -osis = condition	literally, hidden condition of the nails; commonly known as an ingrown toenail

(continues)

TABLE 3-5   INTEGUMENTARY SYSTEM DISEASE AND DISORDER TERMS
(continued)

Term with Pronunciation	Definition
onychomalacia (**on**-ee-koh-mah-**LAY**-shee-ah) onych/o = nail -malacia = softening	softening of the nails
onychomycosis (**on**-ee-koh-my-**KOH**-sis) onych/o = nail myc/o = fungus -osis = condition	fungal infection of the nails
pachyderma (pack-ee-**DER**-mah) pachy- = thickening derm/o = skin -a = noun ending	thickening of the skin
pallor (**PAL**-or)	paleness
papule (**PAP**-yool)	small, solid, raised lesion that is less than 0.5 cm in diameter; pimple (Figure 3-12)

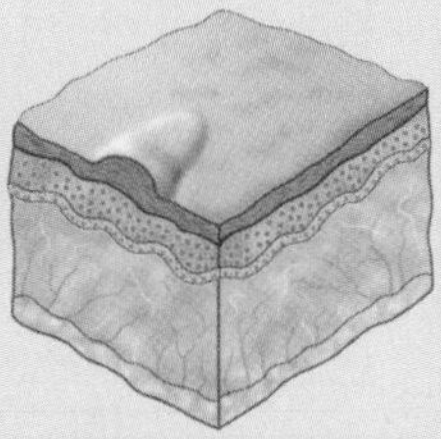

© 2016 Cengage Learning®

Figure 3-12   Papule.

Term with Pronunciation	Definition
pediculosis (peh-**dik**-yoo-**LOH**-sis)	lice infestation associated with skin and hair
petechia (pl. petechiae) (peh-**TEE**-kee-ah; pl. peh-**TEE**-kee-ee)	pinpoint bleeding in the skin
pressure ulcer	open lesion of the skin characterized by a breakdown of skin and underlying tissues as a result of constant pressure to bony prominences under the skin and an inadequate blood supply to the area; also known as a decubitus ulcer

(continues)

TABLE 3-5   INTEGUMENTARY SYSTEM DISEASE AND DISORDER TERMS (continued)

Term with Pronunciation	Definition
psoriasis (soh-**RIGH**-ah-sis)	chronic skin condition characterized by dry, silvery scales covering red lesions (Figure 3-13)

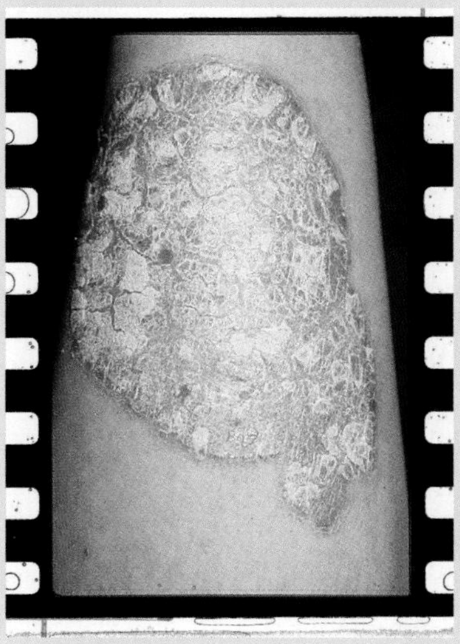

Center for Disease Control and Prevention/Dr. N.J. Fiumara

Figure 3-13   Psoriasis.

pruritus (proo-**RIGH**-tus)	severe itching
purpura (**PER**-pyoo-rah)	large bruises under the skin associated with hemorrhages into tissue
pustule (**PUST**-yool)	circumscribed elevation of the skin containing pus (Figure 3-14)

© 2016 Cengage Learning®

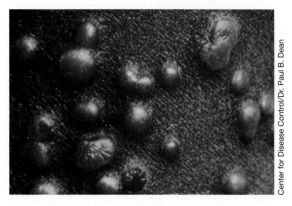

Center for Disease Control/Dr. Paul B. Dean

Figure 3-14   Pustule.

EXERCISE 13

Replace the italicized phrase with the correct medical term. Write the term on the space provided.

1. The treatment for *lice infestation* often includes washing the hair with a special shampoo.

   MEDICAL TERM: _____

2. Rebecca's *cut* required three sutures.

   MEDICAL TERM: _____

3. *Paleness* is a symptom that may be associated with more than one illness.

   MEDICAL TERM: _____

4. Benadryl lotion seemed to relieve Mark's *severe itching*.

   MEDICAL TERM: _____

5. Ron has several *moles* removed from his back.

   MEDICAL TERM: _____

6. *Yellowish discoloration of the skin* may be a sign of hepatitis.

   MEDICAL TERM: _____

7. Carl's poor nutrition resulted in a *softening of his fingernails*.

   MEDICAL TERM: _____

8. Acne is often characterized by *pus-filled elevations of the skin*.

   MEDICAL TERM: _____

9. Marissa's *abnormally large, raised, and thickened scar* was removed.

   MEDICAL TERM: _____

10. Denise consulted her dermatologist when she noticed *pinpoint bleeding* on her forearms.

    MEDICAL TERM: _____

EXERCISE 14

Write a brief definition for each medical term.

1. Kaposi's sarcoma

   DEFINITION: _____

2. lesion

   DEFINITION: _____

3. macule

   DEFINITION: _____

4. malignant melanoma

   DEFINITION: _____

5. onychomycosis

   DEFINITION: _____

6. pachyderma

   DEFINITION: _____

7. papule

   DEFINITION: _____

8. psoriasis

   DEFINITION: _____

9. purpura

   DEFINITION: _____

Review the pronunciation and definition for each term in Table 3-6 and complete the exercises.

TABLE 3-6   INTEGUMENTARY SYSTEM DISEASE AND DISORDERS TERMS

Term with Pronunciation	Definition
scabies (**SKAY**-beez)	skin infection caused by infestation of the itch mite
scleroderma (sklair-oh-**DER**-mah) sclero- = hardening derm/o = skin -a = noun ending	hardening of the skin
seborrhea (seb-oh-**REE**-ah) seb/o = sebum -(r)rhea = flow; discharge	excessive discharge of sebum
squamous cell carcinoma (**SKWAY**-mus sell **kar**-sin-**OH**-mah) squam/o = scale -ous = like; pertaining to carcin- = cancer -oma = tumo	cancer of the squamous or scale-like cells of the skin
tinea (**TIN**-ee-ah)	fungal infection of the skin; ringworm
tinea corporis (**TIN**-ee-ah **KOR**-por-is)	fungal infection of the body
tinea cruris (**TIN**-ee-ah **KROO**-ris)	fungal infection of the groin; jock itch

(continues)

TABLE 3-6 INTEGUMENTARY SYSTEM DISEASE AND DISORDERS TERMS (continued)

Term with Pronunciation	Definition
tinea pedis (**TIN**-ee-ah **PEE**-dis)	fungal infection of the foot; athlete's foot
urticaria (**er**-tih-**KAY**-ree-ah)	skin eruption of wheals; hives
verrucae (ver-**ROO**-kee)	also known as warts; small hard skin lesions caused by the human papilloma virus
vesicle (**VESS**-ih-kul)	small skin elevation filled with clear liquid; a blister (Figure 3-15)

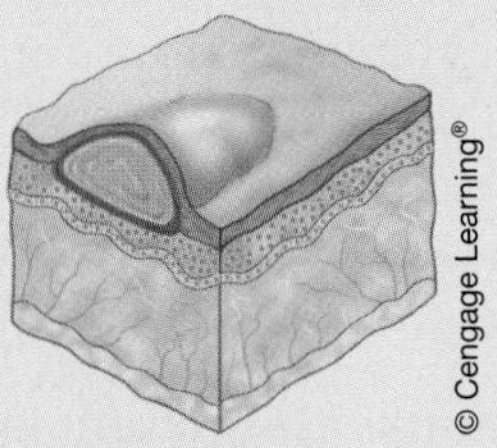

Figure 3-15 Vesicle.

vitiligo (**vih**-tih-**LIE**-goh)	condition characterized by irregular white patches of skin that are totally lacking in pigmentation due to the destruction of melanocytes
wheal (WHEEL)	transient, round, itchy elevation of the skin; one hive (Figure 3-16)

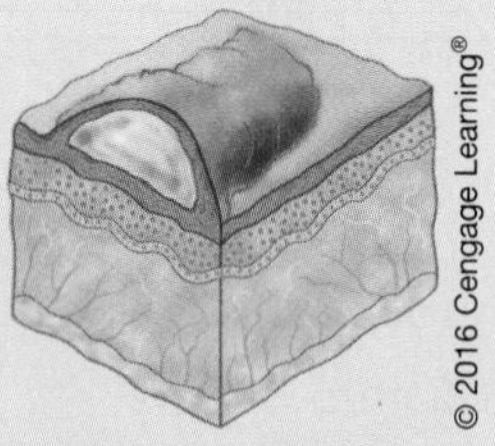

Figure 3-16 Wheal.

xeroderma (**zee**-roh-**DERM**-mah) xer/o = dry derm/o = skin -a = noun ending	dry skin

© 2016 Cengage Learning®

EXERCISE 15

Replace the italicized phrase with the correct medical term. Write the term on the space provided.

1. Martin's *infestation of the itch mite* was highly contagious.

    MEDICAL TERM: _____

2. *Athlete's foot* is a fungal infection of the foot.

    MEDICAL TERM: _____

3. *Hives* can be caused by an allergic reaction to certain foods.

    MEDICAL TERM: _____

4. Tawanda's *dry skin* was relieved with a prescription-strength lotion.

    MEDICAL TERM: _____

5. *Ringworm* is a fungal infection that is treated with oral medication.

    MEDICAL TERM: _____

6. *Cancer of the scalelike cells of the skin* is a slow-growing tumor.

    MEDICAL TERM: _____

7. Liquid nitrogen is often used to remove a *wart*.

    MEDICAL TERM: _____

Integumentary System Procedural and Surgical Terms

Review the pronunciation and definition of the procedural and surgical terms in Table 3-7.

TABLE 3-7   INTEGUMENTARY SYSTEM PROCEDURE AND SURGICAL TERMS

Term with Pronunciation	Definition
biopsy (**BY**-op-see)	removal of living tissue for the purpose of microscopic examination
cryosurgery (**krigh**-oh-**SER**-jer-ee)	use of extreme cold to freeze and destroy unwanted tissue
debridement (dah-**BREED**-mon)	removal of dead or damaged tissue and foreign material from a wound
dermabrasion (derm-ah-**BRAY**-zhun)	removal of skin blemishes and wrinkles using mechanical or chemical methods
dermatome (**DER**-mah-tohm) derm/o = skin -tome = instrument for cutting	instrument for cutting skin

(continues)

TABLE 3-7   INTEGUMENTARY SYSTEM PROCEDURE AND SURGICAL TERMS (continued)

Term with Pronunciation	Definition
dermatoplasty (**DER**-mah-toh-**plass**-tee) dermat/o = skin -plasty = surgical repair	surgical repair of the skin; skin transplant
electrodesiccation (ee-**lek**-troh-**dess**-ih-**KAY**-shun)	destruction of tissue by burning or drying the tissue with an electric spark; primarily used to destroy superficial growths such as warts, but may also be used on deeper tissues
Mohs surgery (mohz)	surgical procedure for malignant skin growths that involves the removal of the visible and root portions of the malignancy in mapped layers
rhytidectomy (**rit**-ih-**DEK**-toh-mee) rhytid/o = wrinkles -ectomy = surgical removal; excision	excision or removal of excess skin for the elimination of wrinkles; also called a face-lift
rhytidoplasty (**RIT**-ih-doh-**plass**-tee) rhytid/o = wrinkles -plasty = surgical repair	surgical repair of wrinkles

© 2016 Cengage Learning®

EXERCISE 16

Write the roots, prefixes, suffixes, and meanings of the listed terms. Based on the meaning of the word parts, write a definition for the term. Use your dictionary to check your definition.

1. dermatoplasty

    ROOT: _____ MEANING: _____

    PREFIX: _____ MEANING: _____

    SUFFIX: _____ MEANING: _____

    DEFINITION: _____

2. rhytidectomy

    ROOT: _____ MEANING: _____

    PREFIX: _____ MEANING: _____

    SUFFIX: _____ MEANING: _____

    DEFINITION: _____

3. rhytidoplasty

ROOT: _____ MEANING: _____

PREFIX: _____ MEANING: _____

SUFFIX: _____ MEANING: _____

DEFINITION: _____

4. dermatome

ROOT: _____ MEANING: _____

PREFIX: _____ MEANING: _____

SUFFIX: _____ MEANING: _____

DEFINITION: _____

Abbreviations

Review the integumentary system abbreviations in Table 3-8. Practice writing out the meaning of each abbreviation.

TABLE 3-8 ABBREVIATIONS

Abbreviation	Meaning
bx; Bx	biopsy
decub	decubitus ulcer
subcu	subcutaneous

© 2016 Cengage Learning®

CHAPTER REVIEW

The Chapter Review can be used as a self-test. Go through each exercise and answer as many questions as you can without referring to previous exercises or earlier discussions within this chapter. Check your answers and fill in any blanks. Practice writing any terms you might have misspelled.

EXERCISE 17

Analyze the listed medical terms by separating the root, prefix, suffix, and combining vowel with vertical slashes. Using the word part meanings, write a definition for the term. Use your medical dictionary to check your definition.

1. dermatitis

| *prefix* | *root* | *combining vowel* | *suffix* |

DEFINITION: _____

2. dermatoplasty

| *prefix* | *root* | *combining vowel* | *suffix* |

DEFINITION: _____

3. onychomalacia

prefix	root	combining vowel	suffix

DEFINITION: _____

4. onychomycosis

prefix	root	combining vowel	suffix

DEFINITION: _____

5. pachyderma

prefix	root	combining vowel	suffix

DEFINITION: _____

6. rhytidectomy

prefix	root	combining vowel	suffix

DEFINITION: _____

7. rhytidoplasty

prefix	root	combining vowel	suffix

DEFINITION: _____

8. scleroderma

prefix	root	combining vowel	suffix

DEFINITION: _____

9. seborrhea

prefix	root	combining vowel	suffix

DEFINITION: _____

10. xeroderma

prefix	root	combining vowel	suffix

DEFINITION: _____

EXERCISE 18

Fill in the blanks.

1. _____ is responsible for skin color.
2. A/An _____ specializes in the study of the skin and related diseases.
3. The medical term for shingles is _____.
4. An infestation of head lice is called _____.
5. _____ is the rubbing or scraping away of skin.
6. _____ is the removal of dead or damaged tissue from a wound.

7. Baldness is the layperson term for _____.

8. Small, pinpoint bleeding of the skin is called _____.

9. The medical term for athlete's foot is _____.

10. A scar left by a healed wound is called a/an _____.

EXERCISE 19

Carefully read the following progress note. Replace each italicized phrase with the correct medical term. For extra practice, rewrite the note using the correct medical terms.

PROGRESS NOTE

Roberto was seen in the office for (1) *an inflammation of the skin.* (2) *Severe itching* has been bothering him and keeping him awake most of the night. After treating the area with a topical cream, I examined his fingertips for signs of (3) *a fungal infection of the nails.* Roberto has been free of (4) *hives* and (5) *boils* for the past year. A follow-up visit was scheduled.

1. _____

2. _____

3. _____

4. _____

5. _____

EXERCISE 20

Read the following patient history and write a brief definition for each italicized medical term.

PATIENT HISTORY

Marian is a 21-year-old female with a history of several skin problems. At age 8 she had a bout of contact dermatitis that initially went untreated due to her severe (1) *psoriasis.* The dermatitis was caused by laundry detergent. With the onset of puberty, she developed (2) *acne,* which was ultimately treated with (3) *dermabrasion.* At the same time, she experienced (4) *eczema* of the scalp, which was attributed to (5) *seborrhea.* She denies any incidence of (6) *pediculosis,* (7) *impetigo,* or (8) *scabies.*

Currently, Marian has noticed changes in several (9) *nevi.* She states that she is a "sun-worshipper" and has never been concerned about exposure and tanning. She uses sunscreen "when I remember to bring it, which is almost never." Marian agreed to a (10) *biopsy* of the suspicious (11) *lesions.* I explained that the biopsy was necessary to rule out (12) *malignant melanoma.*

1. _____

2. _____

3. _____

4. _____

5. _____

6. _____

7. _____

8. _____

9. _____

10. _____

11. _____

12. _____

EXERCISE 21

Label the numbered structures of the integumentary system in Figure 3-17.

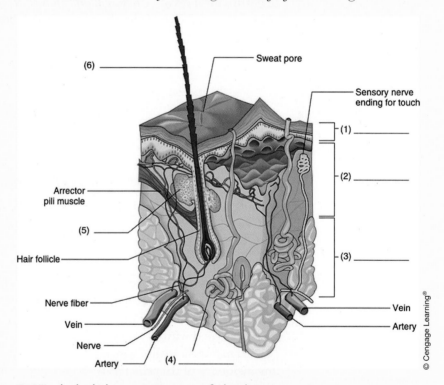

Figure 3-17   Label the structures of the integumentary system.

1. _____

2. _____

3. _____

4. _____

5. _____

6. _____

EXERCISE 22

Select the best answer to each statement.

1. The medical term for bruise is
   a. contusion
   b. melanoma
   c. purulent
   d. verruca

2. A cut or wound is usually called a/an
   a. abrasion
   b. excoriation
   c. laceration
   d. incision

3. Select the medical term for ringworm of the body.
   a. tinea
   b. tinea cruris
   c. tinea pedis
   d. tinea corporis

4. Small pinpoint hemorrhages under the skin are called
   a. petechiae
   b. purpura
   c. erythema
   d. ecchymosis

5. Large bruises under the skin caused by hemorrhage into tissue are known as
   a. petechiae
   b. purpura
   c. erythema
   d. ecchymosis

6. Which term best describes a pus-filled elevation in the skin?
   a. macule
   b. papule
   c. pustule
   d. wheal

7. Which term usually means pimple?
   a. macule
   b. papule
   c. pustule
   d. wheal

8. The medical term for blister is
   a. impetigo
   b. cyst
   c. vesicle
   d. pruritus

9. Which medical term best describes a face-lift?
   a. dermatoplasty
   b. rhytidectomy
   c. rhytidoplasty
   d. dermabrasion

10. A dermatologist would diagnosis shingles with the term
    a. herpes zoster
    b. herpes simplex
    c. scabies
    d. pediculosis

CHALLENGE EXERCISE

Using any Internet search engine, enter the keywords malignant melanoma. Select one of the matches, read the information, and answer the following questions:

1. How many "matches" did your search identify?

   _____

2. Was the information easy to understand? Why or why not?

   _____

3. What was the most valuable piece of information you learned from your search?

   _____

Pronunciation Review

Review the terms from this chapter. Pronounce each term using the phonetic pronunciations. Check off each term when you are comfortable saying it.

TERM	PRONUNCIATION
☐ abrasion	uh-**BRAY**-zhun
☐ acne	**AK**-nee
☐ actinic keratosis	ak-**TIN**-ik **kair**-ah-**TOH**-sis
☐ adipose	**ADD**-ih-pohs
☐ albinism	al-**BYN**-ism
☐ alopecia	**al**-oh-**PEE**-she-ah
☐ basal cell carcinoma	**BAY**-zal sell **kar**-sin-**OH**-ma
☐ biopsy	**BY**-op-see
☐ carbuncle	**KAR**-bung-kal
☐ cicatrix	**SIH**-kay-trix; or sih-**KAY**-trix
☐ contusion	kon-**TOO**-zhun
☐ cryosurgery	**krigh**-oh-**SER**-jer-ee

TERM	PRONUNCIATION
☐ debridement	dah-**BREED**-mon
☐ decubitus ulcer	deh-**KYOO**-bih-tus **ULL**-sir
☐ dermabrasion	derm-ah-**BRAY**-zhun
☐ dermatitis	**der**-mah-**TIGH**-tis
☐ dermatologist	**der**-mah-**TALL**-oh-jist
☐ dermatology	**der**-mah-**TALL**-oh-jee
☐ dermatome	**DER**-mah-tohm
☐ dermatoplasty	**DER**-mat-oh-**plass**-tee
☐ dermis	**DERM**-is
☐ diaphoresis	**digh**-ah-for-**EE**-sis
☐ ecchymosis	eh-kee-**MOH**-sis
☐ eczema	**EGGS**-ih-mah
☐ edema	eh-**DEE**-mah
☐ epidermal	**ep**-ih-**DER**-mal
☐ epidermis	**ep**-ih-**DERM**-is
☐ electrodesiccation	ee-**lek**-troh-**dess**-ih-**KAY**-shun
☐ erythema	**air**-ih-**THEEM**-ah
☐ excoriation	**eks**-kor-ee-**AY**-shun
☐ follicle	**FAH**-lih-kul
☐ furuncle	**FIR**-ung-kal
☐ herpes simplex	**HER**-peez **SIM**-plex
☐ herpes zoster	**HER**-peez **ZOSS**-ter
☐ hypodermic	**high**-poh-**DER**-mik
☐ impetigo	im-peh-**TIGH**-goh
☐ intradermal	**in**-trah-**DER**-mal
☐ jaundice	**JAWN**-dis
☐ Kaposi's sarcoma	**KAP**-oh-seez sar-**KOH**-mah
☐ keloid	**KEE**-loyd
☐ laceration	lass-er-**AY**-shun
☐ lesion	**LEE**-zhun
☐ lunula	**LOO**-noo-lah
☐ macule	**MAK**-yool
☐ malignant melanoma	mah-**LIG**-nant **mell**-ah-**NOH**-mah
☐ melanin	**MELL**-ah-nin
☐ nevus (pl. nevi)	**NEE**-vus (pl. **NEE**-vigh)
☐ onychomalacia	**on**-ee-koh-mah-**LAY**-shee-ah
☐ onychomycosis	**on**-ee-koh-my-**KOH**-sis
☐ pachyderma	pack-ee-**DER**-mah
☐ pallor	**PAL**-or
☐ papule	**PAP**-yool
☐ pediculosis	peh-**dik**-yoo-**LOH**-sis
☐ percutaneous	**per**-kyoo-**TAY**-nee-us
☐ petechia (pl. petechiae)	peh-**TEE**-kee-ah (pl. peh-**TEE**-kee-ee)
☐ pruritus	proo-**RIGH**-tus
☐ psoriasis	soh-**RIGH**-ah-sis
☐ purpura	**PER**-pyoo-rah
☐ pustule	**PUST**-yool
☐ rhytidectomy	**rit**-ih-**DEK**-toh-mee

TERM	PRONUNCIATION
☐ rhytidoplasty	**RIT**-ih-doh-**plass**-tee
☐ scabies	**SKAY**-beez
☐ scleroderma	sklair-oh-**DER**-mah
☐ sebaceous	seh-**BAY**-shus
☐ seborrhea	seb-oh-**REE**-ah
☐ sebum	**SEE**-bum
☐ squamous cell carcinoma	**SKWAY**-mus sell **kar**-sin-**OH**-mah
☐ subcutaneous	**sub**-kyoo-**TAYN**-ee-us
☐ sudoriferous	**soo**-dor-**IF**-er-us
☐ tinea	**TIN**-ee-ah
☐ tinea corporis	**TIN**-ee-ah **KOR**-por-is
☐ tinea cruris	**TIN**-ee-ah **KROO**-ris
☐ tinea pedis	**TIN**-ee-ah **PEE**-dis
☐ urticaria	**er**-tih-**KAY**-ree-ah
☐ vesicle	**VESS**-ih-kul
☐ wheal	WHEEL
☐ xeroderma	**zee**-roh-**DERM**-mah

4 Skeletal System

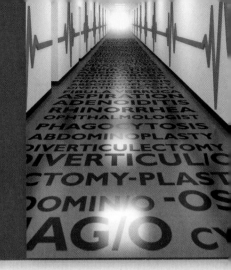

OBJECTIVES

At the completion of this chapter, the student should be able to:

1. Identify, define, and spell word roots associated with the skeletal system.
2. Label the basic structures of the skeletal system.
3. Discuss the functions of the skeletal system.
4. Provide the correct spelling of skeletal terms, given the definition of the term.
5. Analyze skeletal system terms by defining the roots, prefixes, and suffixes of these terms.
6. Identify, define, and spell disease, disorder, and procedure terms related to the skeletal system.

OVERVIEW

The skeletal system is made up of bones and joints that function together for the following purposes: (1) to provide a supporting framework for the body; (2) to protect the internal organs from injury; (3) to provide points of attachment for muscles, ligaments, and tendons; (4) to serve as a storage location for minerals such as calcium and phosphorous; and (5) to play a role in blood cell formation.

Skeletal System Word Roots

To understand and use skeletal system medical terms, it is necessary to acquire a thorough knowledge of the associated word roots. Word roots associated with the skeletal system are listed with the combining vowel. Review the word roots in Table 4-1 and complete the exercises that follow.

TABLE 4-1 SKELETAL SYSTEM WORD ROOTS

Word Root/Combining Form	Meaning
arthr/o	joint
articul/o	joint
burs/o	bursa
carp/o	wrist bones
chondr/o	cartilage
clavicul/o	clavicle; collar bone
coccyg/o	coccyx; tailbone
cost/o	rib

(continues)

TABLE 4-1   SKELETAL SYSTEM WORD ROOTS (continued)

Word Root/Combining Form	Meaning
crani/o	skull
femor/o	femur; thigh bone
fibul/o	fibula; lateral (outer) lower leg bone
humer/o	humerus; upper arm bone
ili/o	ilium; superior (upper) segment of the hip bone
ischi/o	ischium; inferior (lower) segment of the hip bone
lamin/o	lamina; thin, flat plate or layer
lumb/o	lower back
mandibul/o	mandible; lower jaw bone
maxill/o	maxilla; upper jaw bone
metacarp/o	hand bones
metatars/o	foot bones
myel/o	bone marrow
orth/o	straight
oss/e, oss/i, ost/o, oste/o	bone
patell/o	patella; kneecap
pelv/i	pelvis
phalang/o	finger and toe bones
pubi/o; pub/o	pubis; pelvic bone, anterior section
radi/o	radius; lateral (outer) lower arm bone
scapula/o	scapula; shoulder blade
spondyl/o	vertebra; bones of the spine
stern/o	sternum; breastbone
tars/o	ankle bones; bones of the spine
vertebr/o	vertebra

EXERCISE 1

Write the meaning for each word root.

1. carp/o   _____
2. cost/o   _____
3. coccyg/o   _____
4. lumb/o   _____
5. metacarp/o   _____
6. myel/o   _____
7. orth/o   _____
8. phalang/o   _____

9. spondyl/o   _____

10. arthr/o   _____

11. articul/o   _____

12. burs/o   _____

EXERCISE 2

Write the word root and meaning for the following medical terms.

EXAMPLE: costochondritis
ROOT: cost/o   MEANING: rib   ROOT: chondr/o   MEANING: cartilage

1. chondritis

    ROOT: _____   MEANING: _____

2. clavicular

    ROOT: _____   MEANING: _____

3. laminectomy

    ROOT: _____   MEANING: _____

4. osteomalacia

    ROOT: _____   MEANING: _____

5. craniotomy

    ROOT: _____   MEANING: _____

6. costovertebral

    ROOT: _____   MEANING: _____

7. femorocele

    ROOT: _____   MEANING: _____

8. pelvimetry

    ROOT: _____   MEANING: _____

9. pubiotomy

    ROOT: _____   MEANING: _____

10. arthritis

    ROOT: _____   MEANING: _____

EXERCISE 3

Write the correct word root/combining forms for the following bones.

1. fibula   _____

2. humerus   _____

3. ilium   _____

4. ischium   _____

5. mandible   _____

  6. maxilla   _____

  7. metatarsal   _____

  8. patella   _____

  9. radius   _____

10. scapula   _____

11. sternum   _____

12. tarsal   _____

EXERCISE 4

Write the word root/combining form for each meaning.

  1. cartilage   _____

  2. coccyx   _____

  3. bone marrow   _____

  4. straight   _____

  5. vertebra   _____

  6. finger/toe bone   _____

  7. foot bone   _____

  8. hand bone   _____

  9. joint   _____

10. bursa   _____

Bones

Bones are formed by a process called **ossification** (**ah**-sih-fih-**KAY**-shun). The process begins at approximately 3 months of age and continues through adolescence. Ossification is also responsible for repairing minor bone damage that occurs during normal activity and repairing bone fractures.

The bones of the skeleton are often classified according to their shape. According to this classification method, there are five types of bone: long, short, flat, irregular, and sesamoid. Table 4-2 gives a brief description and a few examples of each type of bone.

TABLE 4-2 BONES

Type of Bone	Description	Examples
long bones	longer than wide	femur, radius, ulna, tibia, fibula, phalanges
short bones	nearly as long as wide	carpals, tarsals
flat bones	broad, thin, flat	sternum, ribs, scapula
irregular bones	various sizes	vertebrae, facial bones
sesamoid bones	round; embedded in tendons	patella

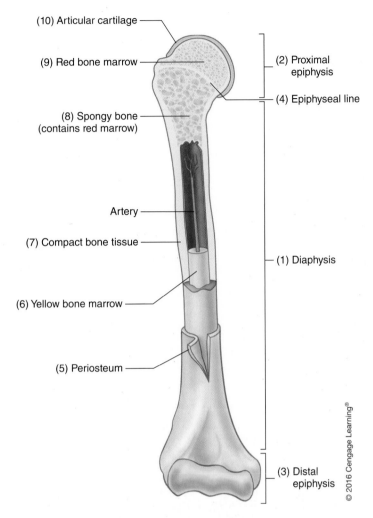

(10) Articular cartilage

(9) Red bone marrow

(2) Proximal epiphysis

(4) Epiphyseal line

(8) Spongy bone (contains red marrow)

Artery

(7) Compact bone tissue

(1) Diaphysis

(6) Yellow bone marrow

(5) Periosteum

(3) Distal epiphysis

© 2016 Cengage Learning®

Figure 4-1 Structures and tissues of a long bone.

Long bones have several structures that have specific functions. Refer to Figure 4-1 as you read the description of the structures.

The shaft of a long bone is called the (1) **diaphysis** (digh-**AFF**-ih-sis). The (2) **proximal epiphysis** (**PROCKS**-ih-mal eh-**PIFF**-ih-sis) is the upper end of a long bone and the (3) **distal epiphysis** is the lower end. The (4) **epiphyseal** (**ep**-ih-**FIZZ**-ee-al) **line** is a layer of cartilage between the diaphysis and epiphysis where bone growth occurs. The (5) **periosteum** (**pair**-ee-**OSS**-tee-um) is a white membrane that covers the shaft of a long bone.

Other long bone structures include (6) **yellow bone marrow**, which stores fat; (7) **compact bone**, which is the hard, outer shell of the bone; (8) **spongy** or **cancellous bone**, which contains the (9) **red bone marrow** that produces red blood cells; and the (10) **articular** (ar-**TIK**-you-lar) **cartilage**, which is a thin layer of cartilage that covers the ends of long bones and the surface of the joints.

Groups of bones are divided into the **axial** (**ACK**-see-al) and **appendicular** (**ap**-en-**DICK**-yoo-lar) skeleton. The axial skeleton includes bones of the skull; middle ear (**ossicles** [**AH**-sih-kls]); rib cage; vertebral column (spine); and the **hyoid** (**HIGH**-oyd) bone, located in the throat between the chin and thyroid gland.

The appendicular skeleton includes bones of the upper extremities (shoulders, arms, wrists, and hands) and the lower extremities (hips, thighs, legs, ankles, and feet). Figure 4-2 illustrates the anterior and posterior views of the skeleton.

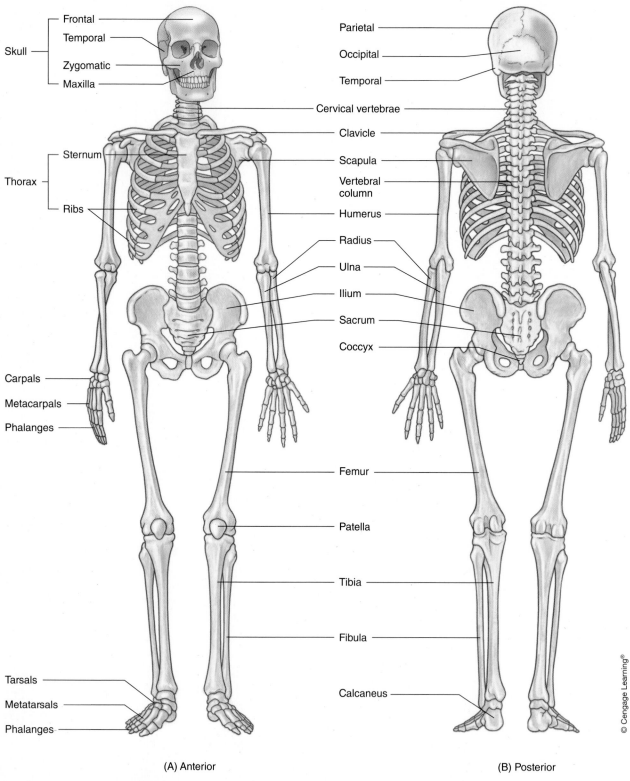

(A) Anterior

(B) Posterior

© Cengage Learning®

Figure 4-2 Anterior and posterior views of the skeleton.

The names and location of selected bones are presented in this chapter as follows:

- bones of the skull
- bones of the shoulders, chest (also called the **bony thorax**), arms, and hands
- bones of the hips, pelvis, legs, and feet
- bones of the vertebral or spinal column

Bone Processes and Depressions

In addition to their shape, bones have other markings called **processes** and **depressions.** Bone processes, also known as projections, help form joints and serve as attachment points for muscles and tendons. Commonly known bone processes include the following:

- **condyle** (**KON**-dill)—round knucklelike projection
- **crest**—prominent ridge along the border of a bone
- **head**—large, rounded end of a long bone set off from the shaft of the bone by a neck
- **spine**—sharp projection from the surface of a bone
- **trochanter** (troh-**KAN**-ter)—large, somewhat rounded projections near the neck of the femur

Bone depressions are holes or indentations that allow nerves and blood vessels to pass through or into the bones. Commonly known bone depressions include the following:

- **fissure**—groove or slitlike opening
- **foramen** (foh-**RAY**-men)—hole or opening in a bone
- **fossa** (**FOSS**-ah)—indentation in the surface of a bone
- **sinus**—air space or opening in the bones of the skull

Bone processes and depressions are noted on the bone illustrations in this chapter.

Bones of the Skull

The **skull** consists of the **cranium** (**KRAY**-nee-um), facial bones, and the ossicles. The cranium is the portion of the skull that encloses and protects the brain. Part of the cranium also protects the eyes. Cranial bones are joined by fibrous joints that are called **sutures**. Facial bones form the face and protect the eyes. The ossicles are three small bones of the middle ear. Ossicles are described in Chapter 15. Major cranial and facial bones are presented here. Refer to Figures 4-3 and 4-4 as you read about the cranial and facial bones.

The (1) **frontal bone** forms the forehead and part of the bony protection for the eyes. Just behind the frontal bone are the (2) **parietal** (pah-**RIGH**-eh-tal) **bones**, one on each side of the head. These bones form the top and upper sides of the cranium. A single (3) **occipital** (ok-**SIP**-ih-tal) **bone** forms the back of the head and the base of the skull. The (4) **temporal** (**TEM**-por-al) **bones**, one on each side of the head, form the lower sides and part of the base of the skull.

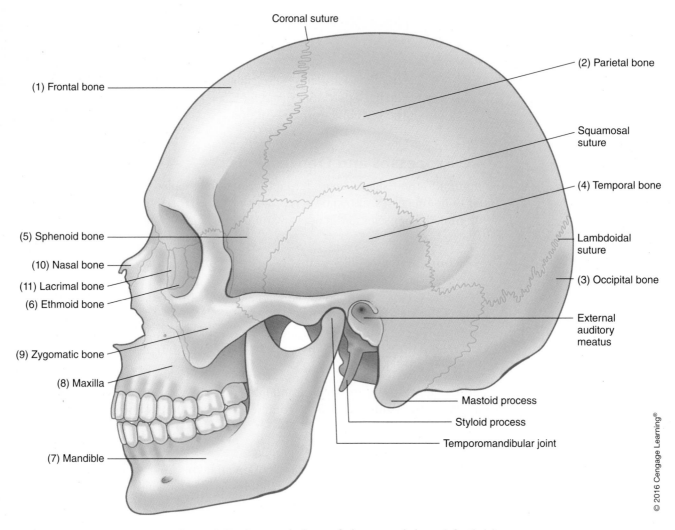

Figure 4-3 Lateral view of the cranial and facial bones.

The (5) **sphenoid** (**SFEE**-noyd) bone is an irregular wedge-shaped bone that helps form the base of the cranium, the sides of the skull, and the floors and sides of the eye socket. The (6) **ethmoid** (**ETH**-moyd) bone is light, spongy bone located at the roof and sides of the nose. It separates the nasal cavity from the brain and forms part of the eye sockets.

The facial bones include the (7) **mandible**, the lower jawbone and the only cranial bone that moves; the (8) **maxilla** or upper jawbone; and the (9) **zygomatic** (**zigh**-goh-**MAT**-ik) **bones**, one on each side of the face, which form the cheekbones and the outer part of the bony protection for the eyes.

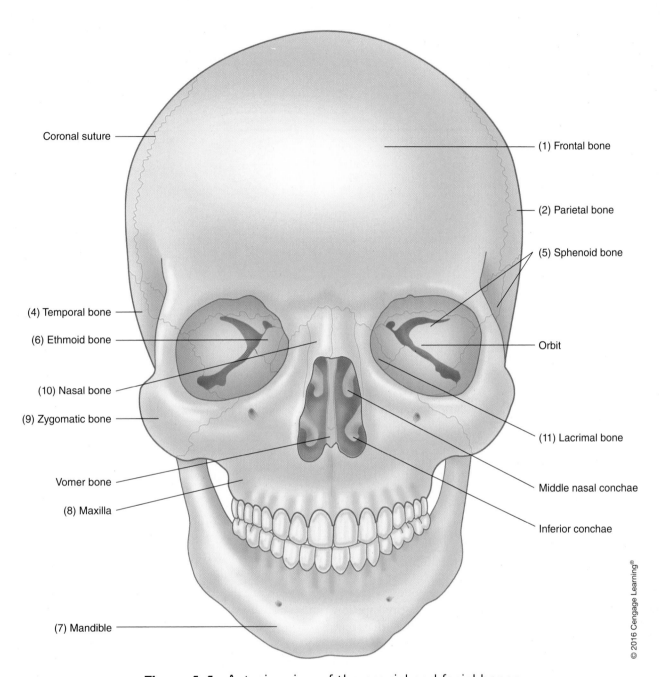

Coronal suture — (1) Frontal bone
(2) Parietal bone
(5) Sphenoid bone
(4) Temporal bone
(6) Ethmoid bone
Orbit
(10) Nasal bone
(9) Zygomatic bone
(11) Lacrimal bone
Middle nasal conchae
Vomer bone
(8) Maxilla
Inferior conchae
(7) Mandible

Figure 4-4 Anterior view of the cranial and facial bones.
(Note: The (3) occipital bone is not visible via the anterior view.)

The (10) **nasal bones** form the upper part of the bridge of the nose; and the (11) **lacrimal** (**LACK**-rih-mal) **bones** are part of the eye socket.

Bones of the Shoulders, Chest, Arms, and Hands

The bones of the shoulders, chest, arms, and hands are illustrated in Figures 4-5 and 4-6. Refer to the figures as you read about these bones.

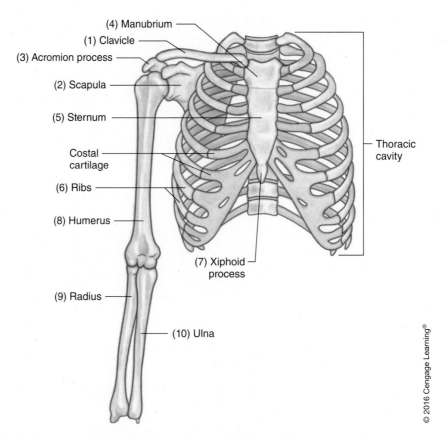

(4) Manubrium

(1) Clavicle

(3) Acromion process

(2) Scapula

(5) Sternum

Costal cartilage

(6) Ribs

(8) Humerus

(7) Xiphoid process

(9) Radius

(10) Ulna

Thoracic cavity

© 2016 Cengage Learning®

Figure 4-5   Anterior view of the bones of the shoulders, chest, and arms. (Cartilaginous structures are shown in blue.)

The bones of the shoulder are the (1) **clavicle**, (**KLAV**-ih-kul), layman's term collar bone; and the (2) **scapula**, (**SKAP**-yoo-lah), layman's term shoulder blade. A section of the scapula, the (3) **acromion** (ah-**KROH**-mee-on) **process**, joins with the clavicle to create the most superior (highest) part of the scapula.

The bones of the chest or thorax are the (4) **manubrium** (mah-**NOO**-bree-um), which forms the superior portion of the (5) **sternum** (**STER**-num). The sternum, layman's term breastbone, is a flat bone located in the middle of the chest. It is joined to the (6) **ribs** and forms the anterior portion of the rib cage. The (7) **xiphoid** (**ZIF**-oyd) **process** is made of cartilage and forms the inferior portion of the sternum.

The bones of the arms are the (8) **humerus** (**HYOO**-mer-us), the upper arm bone; the (9) **radius** (**RAY**-dee-us), the lateral bone of the lower arm; and the (10) **ulna** (**ULL**-nah), the medial bone of the lower arm. The **olecranon** (oh-**LEK**-rah-non) **process**, a large projection on the superior end of the ulna, forms the point of the elbow. The bones of the hands are the (11) **carpals** (**KAR**-palz), the wrist bones; the (12) **metacarpals** (**met**-ah-**KAR**-palz), the bones of the palm; and the (13) **phalanges** (fah-**LAN**-jeez), the finger bones. The bones of the toes are also called phalanges. **Phalanx** (**FAL**-lanx) is the singular form of phalanges. Each of the four fingers consists of the (14) **distal phalanx**, (15) **middle phalanx**, and (16) **proximal phalanx**. The thumb consists of a distal and proximal phalanx.

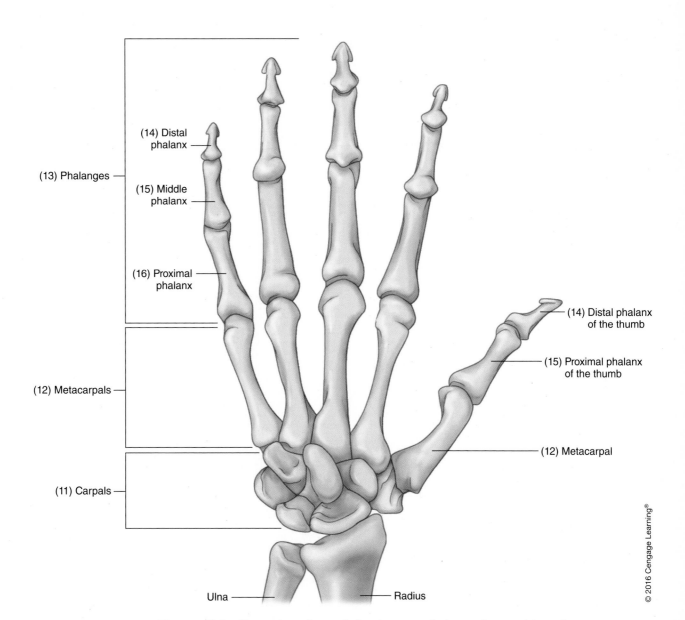

(13) Phalanges

(14) Distal phalanx

(15) Middle phalanx

(16) Proximal phalanx

(12) Metacarpals

(11) Carpals

(14) Distal phalanx of the thumb

(15) Proximal phalanx of the thumb

(12) Metacarpal

Ulna

Radius

Figure 4-6 Superior view of the bones of the wrist and hand.

Using Figure 4-7 as a guide, write the medical term for the structures and tissues of a long bone.

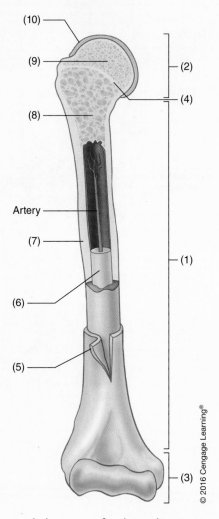

Figure 4-7 Structures and tissues of a long bone.

1. _____

2. _____

3. _____

4. _____

5. _____

6. _____

7. _____

8. _____

9. _____

10. _____

EXERCISE 6

Write the medical term for each definition.

1. breastbone _____
2. cheekbone _____
3. ridge along the border of a bone _____
4. lower jawbone _____
5. upper jawbone _____
6. round, knucklelike projection _____
7. wrist bone(s) _____
8. hole or opening in a bone _____
9. shoulder blade _____
10. indentation in the surface of a bone _____

EXERCISE 7

Match the names of the bones and processes in Column 1 with the descriptions in Column 2.

COLUMN 1

_____ 1. acromion process
_____ 2. clavicle
_____ 3. frontal bone
_____ 4. humerus
_____ 5. metacarpals
_____ 6. occipital bone
_____ 7. parietal bones
_____ 8. radius
_____ 9. sternum
_____ 10. temporal bones
_____ 11. ulna
_____ 12. xiphoid process

COLUMN 2

a. back of the head
b. upper arm bone
c. collarbone
d. breastbone
e. forehead
f. top, upper sides of the cranium
g. highest point of the shoulder
h. lower sides of the cranium
i. lateral lower arm bone
j. palm; hand bones
k. lower end of the sternum
l. medial lower arm bone

EXERCISE 8

Write the names of the following bones next to the correct skeletal structure.

carpals	metacarpals	scapula
clavicle	occipital bone	sternum
frontal bone	parietal bones	temporal bones
humerus	phalanges	ulna
mandible	radius	zygomatic bones
maxilla	ribs	

1. Cranium: _____

2. Shoulders and chest: _____

3. Arms and hands: _____

Bones of the Hips, Pelvis, Legs, and Feet

The bones of the hips and pelvis are formed by three fused bones and two sections of the vertebral column. This group of bones, called the **pelvic girdle**, protects internal organs and supports the lower extremities. Refer to Figure 4-8 as you learn about these bones.

The (1) **ilium** (**ILL**-ee-um) is a broad, flat-shaped bone that forms the back and sides of the pelvic girdle. The (2) **iliac crest** is a long curved ridge along the border of the ilium. The iliac crest forms the prominence of the hips and is a good source of red bone marrow. The (3) **ischium** (**ISH**-ee-um) is the lowest and strongest segment of the pelvis. This is the bone you sit on. The (4) **pubis** (**PYOO**-biss) is the anterior segment of the pelvis. The two bones of the pubis meet in the front and are connected by a cartilage joint called the (5) **symphysis** (**SIM**-fih-siss) **pubis** or pubic symphysis.

Other structures of the hips and pelvis are the (6) **acetabulum** (ass-eh-**TAB**-yoo-lum), the socket for the femur; the (7) **coccyx** (**KOCK**-sicks), which is also known as the tailbone and is the fifth segment of the vertebral column; and the (8) **sacrum** (**SAY**-krum), which is the fourth segment of the vertebral column.

The bones of the legs and feet are collectively known as the bones of the lower extremities. Figures 4-9 through 4-11 illustrate the bones of the lower extremities. Refer to these figures as you learn about the bones.

The (1) **femur**, also called the thigh bone, is the heaviest, longest, and strongest bone in the body. The rounded (2) head of the femur fits into the

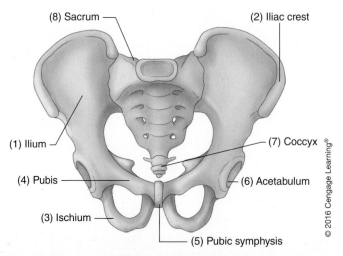

Figure 4-8 Anterior view of the pelvic girdle (pelvis and hips).

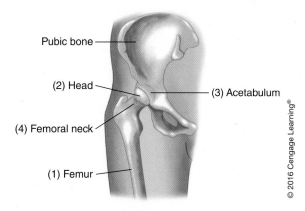

Pubic bone

(2) Head

(3) Acetabulum

(4) Femoral neck

(1) Femur

© 2016 Cengage Learning®

Figure 4-9 Structures of the proximal end of the femur and the acetabulum (hip socket).

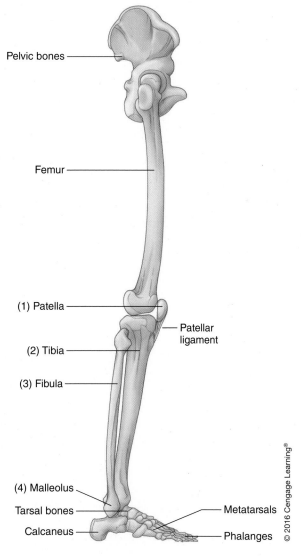

Pelvic bones

Femur

(1) Patella

Patellar ligament

(2) Tibia

(3) Fibula

(4) Malleolus

Tarsal bones

Metatarsals

Calcaneus

Phalanges

© 2016 Cengage Learning®

Figure 4-10 Lateral view of the lower leg bones.

(3) acetabulum to form the hip joint. The (4) **neck** of the femur, also called the **femoral** (**FEM**-oh-ral) **neck**, is the narrow area just below the head. The long segment of the femur is called the shaft. Figure 4-9 illustrates these four structures.

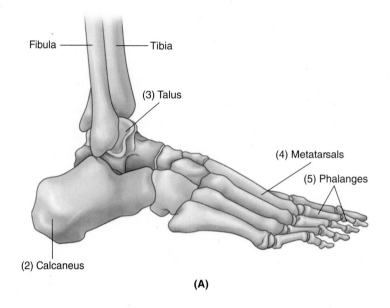

(A)

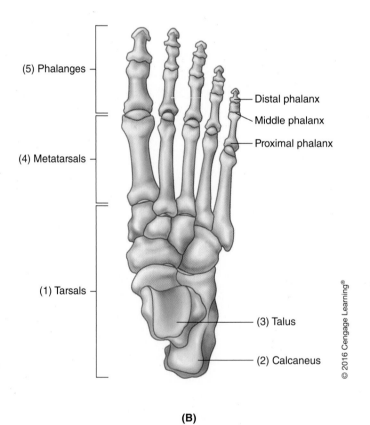

(B)

Figure 4-11   Bones of the ankle and foot. [A] Lateral view. [B] Superior view.

The (1) **patella** (pah-**TELL**-ah), also called the kneecap, is a large sesamoid bone that protects the knee joint. The two lower leg bones are the (2) **tibia** (**TIB**-ee-ah), the larger of the two bones, and the (3) **fibula** (**FIB**-yoo-lah), a slender non-weight-bearing bone. The (4) **malleolus** (**mal**-ee-**OH**-lus) is a round process at the distal end of the fibula. Figure 4-10 illustrates these bones.

The bones of the ankle and foot (Figure 4-11) bear the full weight of our bodies every time we walk, skip, run, or jump. The bones of the ankle are called the (1) **tarsals** (**TAR**-sals), a group of seven irregular bones. The largest ankle bone is the (2) **calcaneus** (kal-**KAY**-nee-us), also called the heel bone. The (3) **talus** (**TAL**-us), located just above the calcaneus, articulates with the tibia and fibula to form the ankle joint. The bones of the foot are called the (4) **metatarsals** (**met**-ah-**TAR**-sals); and the bones of the toes, like the finger bones, are called (5) **phalanges**.

Bones of the Vertebral/Spinal Column

The bones of the vertebral column literally provide each of us with a "backbone." The vertebral column protects the spinal cord. The vertebral column has 24 individual bones called **vertebra** (**VER**-teh-bruh) (plural form is **vertebrae** [**VER**-teh-bray]), the **sacrum** (**SAY**-krum), and **coccyx** (**KOCK**-sicks). Figure 4-12 illustrates the major structures of a vertebra.

The anterior portion of the vertebrae is called the (1) **body**. It is solid and provides strength to the spine. The posterior portion is called the (2) **lamina** (**LAM**-ih-nah). The (3) **spinous** and (4) **transverse** processes serve as attachments for muscles and

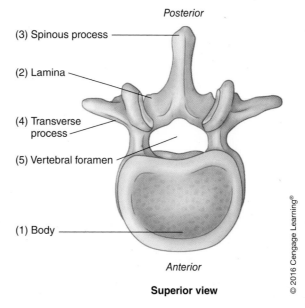

Posterior

(3) Spinous process

(2) Lamina

(4) Transverse process

(5) Vertebral foramen

(1) Body

Anterior

Superior view

© 2016 Cengage Learning®

Figure 4-12   Major structures of a vertebra.

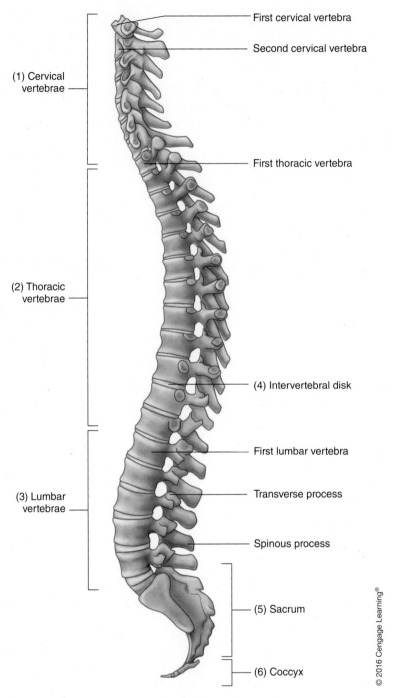

Figure 4-13 Lateral view of the vertebral column illustrating normal curvature.

tendons. The (5) **vertebral foramen** (for-**AY**-men) is the opening that allows the spinal cord to pass through the spinal column.

The vertebrae of the spinal column are divided into three distinct sections: cervical, thoracic, and lumbar. Figure 4-13 illustrates the sections of the spinal column. The first seven vertebrae are the (1) **cervical vertebrae**, which are abbreviated as C1 through C7. The next 12 vertebrae are the (2) **thoracic vertebrae**, which are abbreviated as T1 through T12. The thoracic vertebrae provide the posterior attachments for the ribs. The next five vertebrae are the (3) **lumbar vertebrae**, which are abbreviated as L1 through L5. An (4) **intervertebral disk** sits between each of the 24 vertebrae. The disks are made of cartilage and act as shock absorbers that keep the vertebrae from rubbing against each other and also allow movement of the spine.

The last two segments of the spine are the (5) **sacrum** and the (6) **coccyx**. The adult sacrum is a single, triangular-shaped bone that results from the fusion of the five individual sacral vertebrae during childhood. The adult coccyx is also a single bone that results from the fusion of four individual coccygeal vertebrae.

Joints

The area where two or more bones meet is called a **joint** or an **articulation** (ar-**tik**-yoo-**LAY**-shun). Joints are classified by their construction or by the type of movement they allow. **Fibrous** (**FIGH**-brus) joints are nonmoveable and are located between the cranial bones. Recall that the fibrous joints between cranial bones are called *sutures* (Figure 4-3). **Cartilaginous** (**kar**-tih-**LAJ**-in-us) joints allow limited movement. The pubic symphysis (Figure 4-8) of the pelvis is an example of a cartilaginous joint. The pubic symphysis allows the pelvic bones to expand during childbirth.

Synovial (sin-**OH**-vee-al) joints permit more movement than fibrous or cartilaginous joints. There are six types of synovial joints, each with a characteristic type of movement. Table 4-3 identifies the six types of joints, gives a brief definition of the movement associated with the joint, and lists a few examples of the joint.

It is beyond the scope of this text to give a detailed explanation of each type of joint. The remainder of this section applies to structures and tissues often associated with a ball-and-socket and hinge type synovial joint. The knee joint is used for illustrations and examples.

A synovial joint is enclosed within a **joint capsule** made up of ligaments. Refer to Figure 4-14 as you read about the structures and tissues of a synovial joint. The (1) **synovial membrane** lines the capsule and secretes a lubricating fluid called (2) **synovial fluid**. This fluid circulates in the **synovial cavity**, the space between the bones, and allows the joint to move freely. The ends of the bones in a synovial joint are covered with (3) **articular cartilage** (ar-**TIK**-yoo-lar **KAR**-tih-laj), a protective covering for the bones. Fibrous sacs, called (4) **bursae** (**BER**-see) or bursa (singular), are filled with synovial fluid and provide a cushion for the friction points between tendons and bone. Bursae are located in the elbow, knee, and shoulder joints. The (5) **meniscus** (meh-**NISS**-kus) is a C-shaped piece of cartilage that provides a cushion between the tibia and femur and helps stabilize the knee. The knee joint has two **menisci** (meh-**NISS**-kigh). Figure 4-15 also shows the location of the menisci.

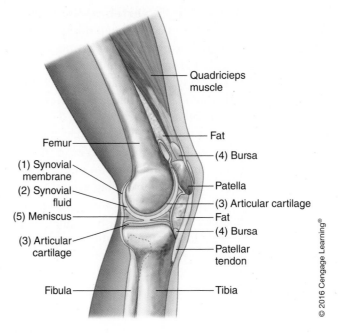

Quadricieps
muscle

Fat

(4) Bursa

Femur

(1) Synovial
membrane

(2) Synovial
fluid

Patella

(5) Meniscus

(3) Articular cartilage

Fat

(3) Articular
cartilage

(4) Bursa

Patellar
tendon

Fibula

Tibia

© 2016 Cengage Learning®

Figure 4-14 A lateral view of the knee showing the structures of a synovial joint and bursa.

TABLE 4-3 SYNOVIAL JOINTS

Joint	Movement	Examples
Gliding joint	sliding, twisting, as two plates sliding around each other; wrist and ankle bone joints, joints between vertebrae; also called *plane* joints	waving hands side to side
Hinge joint	flexion, extension; joints of the elbow, knee, and phalanges (fingers)	kneeling, opening and closing hands
Ball-and-socket joint	all movements except gliding; joints of the shoulder and hip	making circles with arms and legs
Condyloid joint	flexion, abduction, adduction, no rotation; joints between the metacarpals and phalanges, and the mandible and temporal bones	making a fist, chewing

(continues)

TABLE 4-3   SYNOVIAL JOINTS (continued)

Joint	Movement	Examples
Saddle joint	back and forth, side to side, bending motion without sliding; joints of the thumb, joint between the first metacarpal and trapezium (wrist bone)	moving thumb toward and away from fingers
Pivot joint	movement around an axis, rotation, twisting; joint between first and second cervical vertebra, and ulna and radius	moving head side to side; supination (turning hand palm up) pronation (turning hand palm down)

© 2016 Cengage Learning®

Synovial joints also consist of **ligaments** (**LIG**-ah-mentz). The number of ligaments depends on the complexity of the joint. Ligaments are bands of fibrous tissue that help form the joint by connecting one bone to another bone or joining bone to cartilage. Ligaments play an essential role in joint stability and movement. The four major ligaments of the knee are shown in Figure 4-15. These ligaments are often the site of sports-related injuries. The (1) **anterior cruciate** (**KROO**-shee-at) **ligament** and the (2) **posterior cruciate** ligament connect the femur to the tibia. They are located in the center of the knee. The (3) **lateral collateral ligament** connects the femur to the fibula. The (4) **medial collateral ligament** connects the femur to the tibia. The (5) **menisci** cushion the femur and tibia.

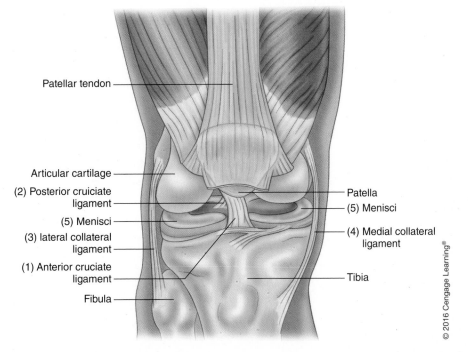

© 2016 Cengage Learning®

Figure 4-15   Anterior view of the major ligaments and menisci of the knee.

EXERCISE 9

Using Figure 4-16 as a guide, write the medical term for the structures of the pelvic girdle (pelvis and hips).

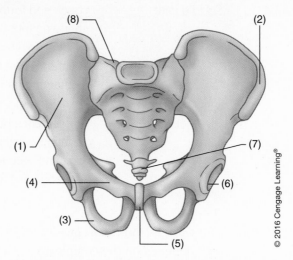

Figure 4-16 Bones of the pelvic girdle (pelvis and hips).

1. _____

2. _____

3. _____

4. _____

5. _____

6. _____

7. _____

8. _____

EXERCISE 10

Write the medical term for each definition.

1. ankle bone(s)   _____

2. kneecap   _____

3. large projection near the neck of the femur   _____

4. heel   _____

5. thighbone   _____

6. toe bone(s)   _____

7. foot bone(s)   _____

8. large, rounded end of the femur   _____

9. anterior segment of the pelvic bones   _____

EXERCISE 11

Match the terms in Column 1 with the descriptions in Column 2.

COLUMN 1

_____ 1. cervical vertebrae

_____ 2. coccyx

_____ 3. fibula

_____ 4. intervertebral disk

_____ 5. lumbar vertebrae

_____ 6. sacrum

_____ 7. talus

_____ 8. thoracic vertebrae

_____ 9. tibia

_____ 10. vertebra

COLUMN 2

a. part of the ankle joint

b. L1–L5

c. T1–T12

d. spinal column bone

e. triangular-shaped bone

f. non-weight-bearing bone

g. larger lower leg bone

h. C1–C7

i. cushions the vertebrae

j. tailbone

EXERCISE 12

Write the joint term for each definition.

1. sac of lubricating fluid   _____

2. freely moveable joint   _____

3. nonmoveable joint   _____

4. slightly moveable joint   _____

5. lubricating fluid in a joint   _____

6. lining of a joint capsule   _____

7. type of joint that permits a wide range of movement   _____

8. type of joint that permits movement in one direction   _____

9. protective covering for the end of bones in
   a freely moveable joint   _____

10. alternate term for joint   _____

Skeletal System Medical Terminology

Skeletal system medical terms are organized into three main categories: (1) general medical terms; (2) diseases and conditions; and (3) diagnostic procedure, surgery, and laboratory test terms. Roots, prefixes, and suffixes listed in Table 4-4 are commonly a part of skeletal system medical terms. Review these word parts and complete the related exercises. The exercises are designed to help you learn skeletal system medical terms by recalling the meaning of the word parts.

TABLE 4-4 ROOTS, PREFIXES, AND SUFFIXES FOR SKELETAL SYSTEM TERMS

Root	Meaning	Prefix	Meaning	Suffix	Meaning
ankyl/o	crooked; bent; stiff; immobile	sub-	below; under	-blast	immature
kyph/o	bent; hump	supra-	above	-clasis -desis -malacia	surgical fracture surgical fixation; to bind; to tie together softening
lord/o	curve; swayback; bent			-oma	tumor
scoli/o	curved; crooked; bent			-osis	abnormal condition

© 2016 Cengage Learning®

EXERCISE 13

Write the word root, prefix, suffix, and meanings for the following medical terms. Using the meanings, write a definition for the medical term. Use a medical dictionary to check your definition.

EXAMPLE: osteoblast
ROOT: oste/o = bone   PREFIX: none   SUFFIX: -blast = immature
DEFINITION: immature bone

1. osteoma

   ROOT: _____ PREFIX: _____ SUFFIX: _____

   DEFINITION: _____

2. scoliosis

   ROOT: _____ PREFIX: _____ SUFFIX: _____

   DEFINITION: _____

3. subcostal

   ROOT: _____ PREFIX: _____ SUFFIX: _____

   DEFINITION: _____

4. lordosis

   ROOT: _____ PREFIX: _____ SUFFIX: _____

   DEFINITION: _____

5. suprapubic

   ROOT: _____ PREFIX: _____ SUFFIX: _____

   DEFINITION: _____

6. osteoclasis

   ROOT: _____ PREFIX: _____ SUFFIX: _____

   DEFINITION: _____

7. kyphosis

    ROOT: _____   PREFIX: _____   SUFFIX: _____

    DEFINITION: _____

8. chondromalacia

    ROOT: _____   PREFIX: _____   SUFFIX: _____

    DEFINITION: _____

9. ankylosis

    ROOT: _____   PREFIX: _____   SUFFIX: _____

    DEFINITION: _____

Skeletal System General Medical Terms

Review the pronunciation and meaning of each term in Table 4-5. Note that some terms are built from word parts and some are not. Complete the exercises for these terms.

TABLE 4-5   SKELETAL SYSTEM GENERAL MEDICAL TERMS

Term with Pronunciation	Definition
articulation (ar-**tik**-yoo-**LAY**-shun) articul/o = joint	area where two or more bones meet; a joint
chiropractor (**KIGH**-roh-prak-tor)	practitioner who uses mechanical manipulation of the spinal column as a primary treatment method
cranial (**KRAY**-nee-al) crani/o = cranium; skull -al = pertaining to	pertaining to the cranium or skull
femoral (**FEM**-or-al) femor/o = femur -al = pertaining to	pertaining to the femur
humeral (**HYOO**-mor-al) humer/o = humerus -al = pertaining to	pertaining to the humerus
intercostal (**in**-ter-**KOSS**-tal) inter- = between cost/o = ribs -al = pertaining to	pertaining to between the ribs

(continues)

TABLE 4-5   SKELETAL SYSTEM GENERAL MEDICAL TERMS (continued)

Term with Pronunciation	Definition
intervertebral (**in**-ter-**VER**-teh-bral) inter- = between vertebr/o = vertebra -al = pertaining to	pertaining to between the vertebrae
ischiopubic (**ih**-shee-oh-**PYOO**-bik) ischi/o = ischium pub/o = pubis -ic = pertaining to	pertaining to the ischium and pubis
lumbar (**LUM**-bar) lumb/o = lower back -ar = pertaining to	pertaining to the lower back
lumbosacral (**lum**-boh-**SAY**-kral) lumb/o = lower back sacr/o = sacrum -al = pertaining to	pertaining to the lower back or lumbar region and sacrum
orthopedics (**or**-thoh-**PEE**-diks) orth/o = straight ped/o = foot -ic = pertaining to	branch of medicine pertaining to the study and treatment of diseases and abnormalities of the skeletal and muscular systems
orthopedist (**or**-thoh-**PEE**-dist) orth/o = straight ped/o = foot -ist = specialist	physician who specializes in orthopedics
osteoblast (**OSS**-tee-oh-blast) oste/o = bone -blast = immature	immature bone or bone cell
osteocyte (**OSS**-tee-oh-sight) oste/o = bone -cyte = cell	mature bone cell
submandibular (**sub**-man-**DIB**-yoo-lar) sub- = below; under mandibul/o = mandible -ar = pertaining to	pertaining to under or below the mandible

(continues)

TABLE 4-5 SKELETAL SYSTEM GENERAL MEDICAL TERMS (continued)

Term with Pronunciation	Definition
submaxillary (sub-**MACKS**-ih-lair-ee) sub- = under; below maxill/o = maxilla -ary = pertaining	pertaining to under or below the maxilla
substernal (sub-**STERN**-al) sub- = under; below stern/o = sternum -al = pertaining to	pertaining to under or below the sternum
supraclavicular (**soo**-prah-klah-**VIK**-yoo-lar) supra- = above clavicul/o = clavicle -ar = pertaining to	pertaining to above the sternum and clavicle

© 2016 Cengage Learning®

EXERCISE 14

Analyze each term by writing the root, prefix, suffix, and combining vowel separated by vertical slashes.

EXAMPLE: subclavicular

sub	/ *clavicul*	*(none)*	/ *ar*
prefix	*root*	*combining vowel*	*suffix*

1. cranial

prefix	*root*	*combining vowel*	*suffix*

2. femoral

prefix	*root*	*combining vowel*	*suffix*

3. humeral

prefix	*root*	*combining vowel*	*suffix*

4. intercostal

prefix	*root*	*combining vowel*	*suffix*

5. intervertebral

prefix	*root*	*combining vowel*	*suffix*

6. ischiopubic

prefix	*root*	*combining vowel*	*suffix*

7. lumbosacral

prefix	*root*	*combining vowel*	*suffix*

8. osteocyte

prefix	root	combining vowel	suffix

9. substernal

prefix	root	combining vowel	suffix

10. supraclavicular

prefix	root	combining vowel	suffix

Skeletal System Disease and Disorder Terms

Skeletal system disease and disorder terms are presented in alphabetical order in Table 4-6. All fractures are listed under the main term *fracture*. Review the pronunciation and definition for each term and complete the exercises.

TABLE 4-6 SKELETAL SYSTEM DISEASE AND DISORDER TERMS

Term with Pronunciation	Definition
ankylosing spondylitis (**ang**-kih-**LOH**-sing **spon**-dih-**LIGH**-tiss) ankyl/o = stiff spondyl/o = spinal column -itis = inflammation	inflammation of one or more vertebrae characterized by joint stiffness or immobility; rheumatoid arthritis of the spine
ankylosis (ang-kih-**LOH**-sis) ankyl/o = stiff -osis = condition	immobility of a joint
arthralgia (ar-**THRAL**-jee-ah) arthr/o = joint -algia = pain	joint pain
arthritis (ar-**THRIGH**-tis) arthr/o = joint -itis = inflammation	inflammation of a joint
arthrochondritis (**ar**-throh-kon-**DRIGH**-tis) arthr/o = joint chondr/o = cartilage -itis = inflammation	inflammation of an articular cartilage
Baker's cyst	accumulation of synovial fluid in the knee joint
bunion	inflammation and enlargement of the bursa of the joint of the great (big) toe; also known as hallux valgus

(continues)

TABLE 4-6 SKELETAL SYSTEM DISEASE AND DISORDER TERMS (continued)

Term with Pronunciation	Definition
bursitis (ber-**SIGH**-tis) burs/o = bursa -itis = inflammation of	inflammation of the bursa
chondromalacia (**kon**-droh-mah-**LAY**-she-ah) chondr/o = cartilage -malacia = softening	softening of cartilage
crepitation (**crep**-ih-**TAY**-shun)	crackling or clicking sound present during joint movement
dislocation (**diss**-loh-**KAY**-shun)	temporary displacement of a bone from its joint
fracture (Figure 4-17 illustrates four types of fractures.)	breaking of a bone; broken bone

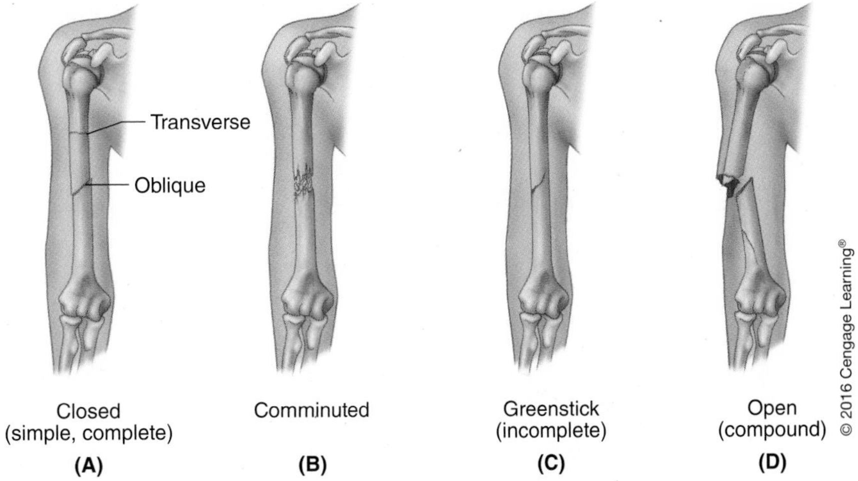

Figure 4-17 Types of fractures. (A) Closed (simple, complete). (B) Comminuted. (C) Greenstick (incomplete). (D) Open (compound).

Term with Pronunciation	Definition
fracture, closed	break in a bone without interrupting the skin; simple, complete fracture (Figure 4-17A)
fracture, Colles'	fracture of the distal end of the radius, just above the wrist (Figure 4-18)
fracture, comminuted	fracture in which the bone is broken or splintered into pieces (Figure 4-17B)

(continues)

TABLE 4-6   SKELETAL SYSTEM DISEASE AND DISORDER TERMS (continued)

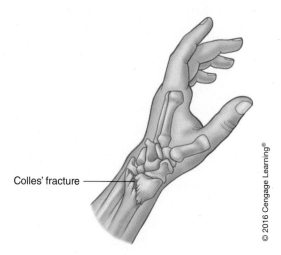

Colles' fracture

© 2016 Cengage Learning®

Figure 4-18   Colles' fracture of the distal radius.

Term with Pronunciation	Definition
fracture, greenstick	fracture in which the bone is partially bent and partially broken; incomplete fracture (Figure 4-17C)
fracture, impacted	fracture in which the bone is broken and wedged into the interior of another bone
fracture, open	fracture in which the bone is broken and bone fragments protrude through the skin; compound fracture (Figure 4-17D)
fracture, pathological	fracture associated or caused by an underlying disease

© 2016 Cengage Learning®

EXERCISE 15

Analyze each term. Identify and define the root(s), prefix, and suffix. Use your medical dictionary and write a brief definition.

1. chondromalacia

   ROOT: _____   PREFIX: _____   SUFFIX: _____

   DEFINITION: _____

2. ankylosing spondylitis

   ROOT: _____   PREFIX: _____   SUFFIX: _____

   ROOT: _____   PREFIX: _____   SUFFIX: _____

   DEFINITION: _____

3. arthralgia

   ROOT: _____   PREFIX: _____   SUFFIX: _____

   DEFINITION: _____

4. arthritis

   ROOT: ____________ PREFIX: ____________ SUFFIX: ____________

   DEFINITION: ____

5. arthrochondritis

   ROOT: ____________ PREFIX: ____________ SUFFIX: ____________

   ROOT: ____________ PREFIX: ____________ SUFFIX: ____________

   DEFINITION: ____

6. bursitis

   ROOT: ____________ PREFIX: ____________ SUFFIX: ____________

   DEFINITION: ____

EXERCISE 16

Identify each type of fracture shown in Figure 4-19.

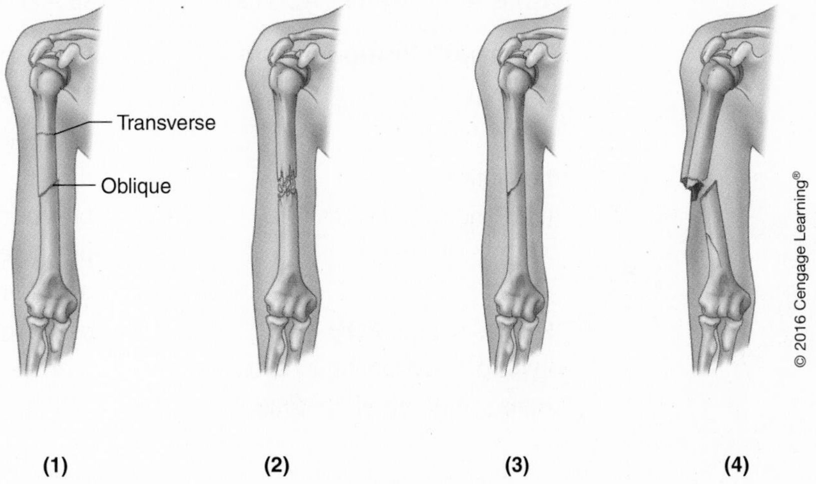
Transverse
Oblique
© 2016 Cengage Learning®
(1)
(2)
(3)
(4)

Figure 4-19 Label the types of fractures.

1. ____________________
2. ____________________
3. ____________________
4. ____________________

EXERCISE 17

Replace the italicized phrase with the correct medical term.

1. Rodney fell off his skateboard and sustained a *broken radius just above his wrist.*

   ____

2. Angelo experienced pain when he walked because of the *accumulation of synovial fluid in the knee joint* in his left leg.

   ____

3. Ling was scheduled for surgery to remove the *inflamed and enlarged joint bursa of her great toe* of her right foot.

   _____

4. A *crackling sound during joint movement* may indicate a fracture of the joint bones.

   _____

5. During gymnastic practice, Quo needed medical attention for the *temporary displacement* of his shoulder joint.

   _____

6. Dion was hospitalized for a *partially bent and partially broken bone.*

   _____

Review the pronunciation and definition for each term in Table 4-7 and complete the exercises.

TABLE 4-7   SKELETAL SYSTEM DISEASE AND DISORDER TERMS

Term with Pronunciation	Definition
gout	acute arthritis characterized by inflammation of the first joint of the great toe
herniated disk (**HER**-nee-ay-ted disk)	rupture of the intervertebral disk, which protrudes between the vertebra and puts pressure on the spinal nerve root; also called a *ruptured* or *slipped disk* (Figure 4-20)
kyphosis (kigh-**FOH**-sis) kyph/o = pertaining to a hump -osis = abnormal condition	outward (posterior) curvature of the thoracic spine; humpback (Figure 4-21)

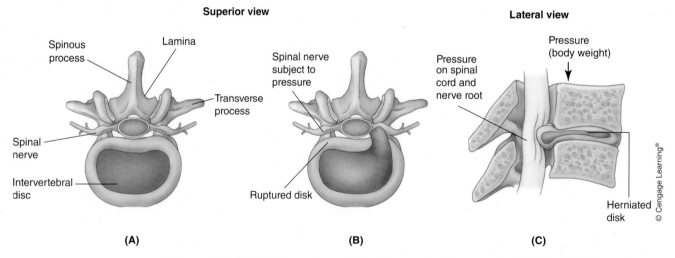

Figure 4-20 (A) Superior view of a normal invertebral disk. (B) Superior and (C) lateral views of a ruptured disk causing pressure on a spinal nerve.

(continues)

TABLE 4-7   SKELETAL SYSTEM DISEASE AND DISORDER TERMS (continued)

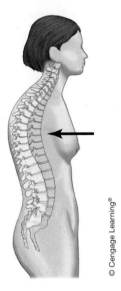

Figure 4-21   Kyphosis (normal curvature is shown in shadow.)

Term with Pronunciation	Definition
lordosis (lor-**DOH**-sis) lord/o = swayback -osis = abnormal condition	forward (anterior) curvature of the lumbar spine; swayback (Figure 4-22)
myeloma (**my**-eh-**LOH**-mah) myel/o = bone marrow -oma = tumor	tumor originating from the bone marrow

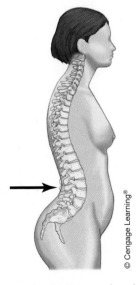

Figure 4-22   Lordosis (normal curvature is shown in shadow.)

(continues)

TABLE 4-7   SKELETAL SYSTEM DISEASE AND DISORDER TERMS (continued)

Term with Pronunciation	Definition
osteitis (**oss**-tee-**EYE**-tis) oste/o = bone -itis = inflammation	inflammation of the bone
osteochondritis (**oss**-tee-oh-kon-**DRIGH**-tis) oste/o = bone chondr/o = cartilage -itis = inflammation	inflammation of bone and cartilage
osteofibroma (**oss**-tee-oh-fih-**BROH**-mah) oste/o = bone fibr/o = fibrous tissue -oma = tumor	tumor of bony and fibrous tissue
osteomalacia (**oss**-tee-oh-mah-**LAY**-she-ah) oste/o = bone -malacia = softening	softening of the bone in adults
osteomyelitis (**oss**-tee-oh-my-eh-**LIGH**-tis) oste/o = bone myel/o = bone marrow -itis = inflammation	inflammation of the bone and bone marrow
osteoporosis (**oss**-tee-oh-poh-**ROH**-sis) oste/o = bone -porosis = porous condition	decreased bone density or loss of bone mass
osteosarcoma (**oss**-tee-oh-sar-**KOH**-mah) oste/o = bone sarc/o = flesh -oma = tumor	malignant tumor of bone
rheumatoid arthritis (RA) (**ROO**-mah-toyd ar-**THRIGH**-tis) arthr/o = joint -itis = inflammation	chronic, systemic inflammatory disease of the joints, especially the joints of the hands and feet
scoliosis (skoh-lee-**OH**-sis) scoli/o = crooked, bent -osis = abnormal condition	abnormal lateral curvature of the spine (Figure 4-23)
spondylitis (spon-dih-**LIGH**-tiss) spondyl/o = spinal column; vertebra -itis = inflammation	inflammation of one or more vertebrae

(continues)

TABLE 4-7   SKELETAL SYSTEM DISEASE AND DISORDER TERMS (continued)

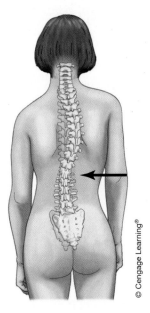

Figure 4-23   Scoliosis. (normal curvature is shown in shadow.)

Term with Pronunciation	Definition
spur	bony growth arising from the surface of the bone
subluxation (sub-luks-**AY**-shun)	partial dislocation of a bone from its joint
talipes (**TAL**-ih-peez)	congenital deformity characterized by an abnormal alignment of the bones of the feet; layman's term clubfoot

© 2016 Cengage Learning®

EXERCISE 18

Analyze each term. Identify and define the root(s), prefix, and suffix. Use your medical dictionary and write a brief definition for each term.

1. osteomalacia

   ROOT: _____   PREFIX: _____   SUFFIX: _____

   DEFINITION: _____

2. osteomyelitis

   ROOT: _____   PREFIX: _____   SUFFIX: _____

   DEFINITION: _____

3. osteoporosis

ROOT: _____   PREFIX: _____   SUFFIX: _____

DEFINITION: _____

4. osteosarcoma

ROOT: _____   PREFIX: _____   SUFFIX: _____

DEFINITION: _____

5. spondylitis

ROOT: _____   PREFIX: _____   SUFFIX: _____

DEFINITION: _____

6. myeloma

ROOT: _____   PREFIX: _____   SUFFIX: _____

DEFINITION: _____

7. osteochondritis

ROOT: _____   PREFIX: _____   SUFFIX: _____

DEFINITION: _____

8. osteitis

ROOT: _____   PREFIX: _____   SUFFIX: _____

DEFINITION: _____

9. osteofibroma

ROOT: _____   PREFIX: _____   SUFFIX: _____

DEFINITION: _____

EXERCISE 19

Write the medical term for each definition.

1. clubfoot   _____

2. abnormal lateral curvature of the spine   _____

3. acute arthritis and inflammation of the first joint of the great toe   _____

4. slipped disk   _____

5. abnormal outward curvature of the spine   _____

6. incomplete dislocation of a bone from its joint   _____

7. decreased bone density   _____

8. abnormal forward curvature of the spine   _____

9. chronic, systemic inflammatory disease of the joints   _____

10. bony growth from the surface of a bone   _____

Skeletal System Diagnostic, Treatment, and Surgical Terms

Review the pronunciation and definition of the diagnostic and treatment terms in Table 4-8. Complete the exercises for each set of terms.

TABLE 4-8   SKELETAL SYSTEM DIAGNOSTIC, TREATMENT, AND SURGICAL TERMS

Term with Pronunciation	Definition
arthrocentesis (**ar**-throh-sen-**TEE**-sis) arthr/o = joint -centesis = surgical puncture to withdraw fluid	surgical puncture of a joint to withdraw fluid
arthroclasis (**ar**-throh-**CLAY**-sis) arthr/o = joint -clasis = therapeutic or surgical breaking	therapeutic breaking of a joint or adhesions of a joint
arthrodesis (**ar**-throh-**DEE**-sis) arthr/o = joint -desis = surgical fixation	surgical fixation, binding, or immobilization of a joint
arthrogram (**AR**-throh-gram) arthr/o = joint -gram = picture or record of a joint	picture or record of a joint
arthrography (ar-**THROG**-rah-fee) arthr/o = joint -graphy = process of recording	process of obtaining a radiograph of the internal structures of a joint aided by the injection of a contrast medium
arthroplasty (**AR**-throh-**plass**-tee) arthr/o = joint -plasty = surgical repair	surgical repair of a joint
arthroscopy (ar-**THROSS**-koh-pee) arthr/o = joint -scopy = process of viewing; visualization	visualization of the internal structures of a joint using an endoscope
arthrotomy (ar-**THROT**-oh-mee) arthr/o = joint -tomy = incision into	incision into a joint

(continues)

TABLE 4-8 SKELETAL SYSTEM DIAGNOSTIC, TREATMENT, AND SURGICAL TERMS (continued)

Term with Pronunciation	Definition
bone marrow aspiration (ass-per-**AY**-shun)	removing a sample of bone marrow using an aspiration needle
bone scan	visualization of the structure of the bone using a radioisotope; a nuclear medicine examination
bunionectomy (bun-yun-**ECK**-toh-mee) -ectomy = surgical removal	surgical removal of a bunion
bursectomy (ber-**SEK**-toh-mee) burs/o = bursa -ectomy = surgical removal	surgical removal of a bursa
bursotomy (ber-**SOT**-oh-mee) burs/o = bursa -tomy = incision into	incision into a bursa
closed reduction	process of aligning fractured bones through manual manipulation or traction
craniotomy (**kray**-nee-**OT**-oh-mee) crani/o = skull -tomy = incision into	incision into the cranium or bones of the skull
diskectomy (disk-**EK**-toh-mee) -ectomy = surgical removal	surgical removal of a herniated intervertebral disk
dual-energy x-ray absorptiometry (DEXA) (ab-**sorp**-she-**AH**-meh-tree)	noninvasive x-ray procedure that measures bone density
dual-photon absorptiometry (**FOH**-ton ab-**sorp**-she-**AH**-meh-tree)	noninvasive procedure using a small amount of radiation to measure bone density
external fixation	fracture treatment procedure in which pins (or other fixation devices) are placed through the soft tissues and bone and an external appliance is used to hold the bone in alignment; the external fixation appliance is removed after healing occurs (Figure 4-24)

(continues)

TABLE 4-8   SKELETAL SYSTEM DIAGNOSTIC, TREATMENT, AND SURGICAL TERMS (continued)

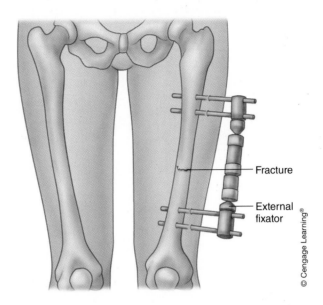

Figure 4-24   External fixation of the femur stabilizes the bone and is removed after the bone has healed.

Term with Pronunciation	Definition
laminectomy (lam-in-**EK**-toh-mee) lamin/o = lamina -ectomy = surgical removal	surgical removal of the posterior arch of the vertebra
open reduction	alignment of fractured bones through a surgically opened wound
open reduction and internal fixation (ORIF)	surgical alignment of fractured bones using screws, pins, wires, or nails to maintain bone alignment; internal fixation devices are not removed after the bone is healed (Figure 4-25)
osteoclasis (**oss**-tee-oh-**KLAY**-sis) oste/o = bone -clasis = surgical fracture	surgical fracture of a bone
osteoplasty (**OSS**-tee-oh-plass-tee) oste/o = bone -plasty = surgical repair	surgical repair of a bone
osteotomy (**oss**-tee-**OT**-oh-mee) oste/o = bone -tomy = incision into	incision into a bone

(continues)

TABLE 4-8   SKELETAL SYSTEM DIAGNOSTIC, TREATMENT, AND SURGICAL TERMS (continued)

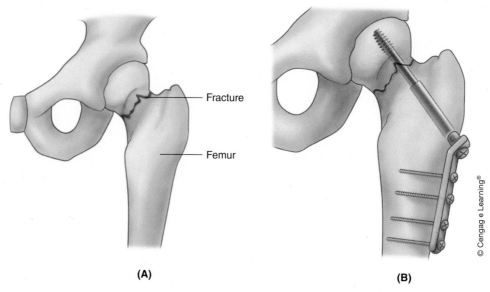

Figure 4-25 Internal fixation of fractured hip. (A) Fracture of the femoral neck. (B) Internal fixation pins are placed to stabilize the bone. These pins are not removed after the bone has healed.

Term with Pronunciation	Definition
spinal fusion	permanent joining of two or more vertebrae
synovectomy (**sin**-oh-**VEK**-toh-mee) -ectomy = surgical removal	surgical removal of a synovial membrane
total hip replacement (THR)	surgical replacement of the head and neck of the femur and the acetabulum with synthetic components; a synthetic stem (shaft) is placed in the shaft of the femur (Figure 4-26)
total knee replacement (TKR)	surgical replacement of the knee with synthetic components (Figure 4-27)

(continues)

TABLE 4-8   SKELETAL SYSTEM DIAGNOSTIC, TREATMENT,
AND SURGICAL TERMS (continued)

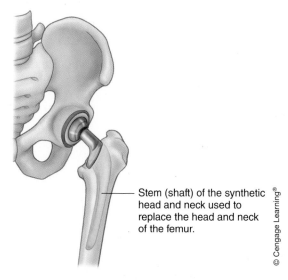

Stem (shaft) of the synthetic
head and neck used to
replace the head and neck
of the femur.

© Cengage Learning®

Figure 4-26   Total hip replacement (THR).

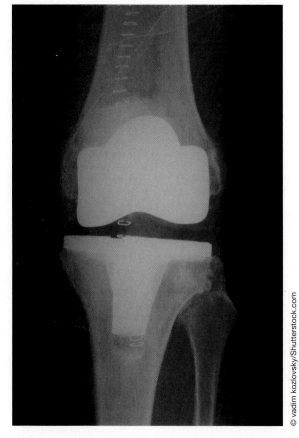

© vadim kozlovsky/Shutterstock.com

Figure 4-27   Radiograph of a total knee replacement. Metallic
components appear brighter than the surrounding bone.

EXERCISE 20

Analyze each term. Identify and define the root, prefix, and suffix. Use your medical dictionary and write a brief definition for each term.

1. craniotomy

   ROOT: _____   PREFIX: _____   SUFFIX: _____

   DEFINITION: _____

2. diskectomy

   ROOT: _____   PREFIX: _____   SUFFIX: _____

   DEFINITION: _____

3. laminectomy

   ROOT: _____   PREFIX: _____   SUFFIX: _____

   DEFINITION: _____

4. osteoclasis

   ROOT: _____   PREFIX: _____   SUFFIX: _____

   DEFINITION: _____

5. osteoplasty

   ROOT: _____   PREFIX: _____   SUFFIX: _____

   DEFINITION: _____

6. osteotomy

   ROOT: _____   PREFIX: _____   SUFFIX: _____

   DEFINITION: _____

7. arthrocentesis

   ROOT: _____   PREFIX: _____   SUFFIX: _____

   DEFINITION: _____

8. arthroclasis

   ROOT: _____   PREFIX: _____   SUFFIX: _____

   DEFINITION: _____

9. arthrodesis

   ROOT: _____   PREFIX: _____   SUFFIX: _____

   DEFINITION: _____

10. arthroscopy

   ROOT: _____   PREFIX: _____   SUFFIX: _____

   DEFINITION: _____

11. arthrotomy

   ROOT: _____   PREFIX: _____   SUFFIX: _____

   DEFINITION: _____

EXERCISE 21

Write the medical term for the italicized phrase.

1. Quentin's fractured humerus was aligned via *manual manipulation*.

   _____

2. Dr. Rodriguez ordered a *bone density measurement* scan to assess the patient's osteoporosis.

   _____

3. Darrell's crushed calcaneus was repaired by *surgical alignment with pins and screws*.

   _____

4. Degenerative disk disease might be corrected by *permanent joining of vertebrae*.

   _____

5. *Surgical repair of a joint* might be accomplished as an open or closed procedure.

   _____

Abbreviations

Review the skeletal system abbreviations in Table 4-9. Practice writing the meaning of each abbreviation.

TABLE 4-9 ABBREVIATIONS

Abbreviation	Meaning
fx	fracture
C1–C7	cervical vertebrae, 1 through 7
DEXA	dual-energy x-ray absorptiometry
L1–L5	lumbar vertebrae, 1 through 5
ORIF	open reduction and internal fixation
T1–T12	thoracic vertebrae, 1 through 12
THR	total hip replacement
TKR	total knee replacement

© 2016 Cengage Learning®

CHAPTER REVIEW

The Chapter Review can be used as a self-test. Go through each exercise and answer as many questions as you can without referring to previous exercises or earlier discussions within this chapter. Check your answers and fill in any blanks. Practice writing any terms that you might have misspelled.

EXERCISE 22

Analyze the listed medical terms by separating the root, prefix, suffix, and combining vowel with vertical slashes. Using the word part meanings, write a definition for the term. Use a medical dictionary to verify your definitions.

EXAMPLE: subclavicular

sub	/ clavicul	(none)	/ ar
prefix	root	combining vowel	suffix

1. intercostal

prefix	root	combining vowel	suffix

DEFINITION: _____

2. osteoblast

prefix	root	combining vowel	suffix

DEFINITION: _____

3. submandibular

prefix	root	combining vowel	suffix

DEFINITION: _____

4. supraclavicular

prefix	root	combining vowel	suffix

DEFINITION: _____

5. chondromalacia

prefix	root	combining vowel	suffix

DEFINITION: _____

6. kyphosis

prefix	root	combining vowel	suffix

DEFINITION: _____

7. myeloma

prefix	root	combining vowel	suffix

DEFINITION: _____

8. osteoporosis

prefix	root	combining vowel	suffix

DEFINITION: _____

9. craniotomy

prefix	root	combining vowel	suffix

DEFINITION: _____

10. osteoclasis

prefix	root	combining vowel	suffix

DEFINITION: _____

11. arthralgia

prefix	root	combining vowel	suffix

DEFINITION: _____

12. intervertebral

prefix	root	combining vowel	suffix

DEFINITION: _____

13. submaxillary

prefix	root	combining vowel	suffix

DEFINITION: _____

14. osteomyelitis

prefix	root	combining vowel	suffix

DEFINITION: _____

15. arthroscopy

prefix	root	combining vowel	suffix

DEFINITION: _____

16. lumbosacral

prefix	root	combining vowel	suffix

DEFINITION: _____

17. arthrocentesis

prefix	root	combining vowel	suffix

DEFINITION: _____

18. humeral

prefix	root	combining vowel	suffix

DEFINITION: _____

19. ischiopubic

prefix	root	combining vowel	suffix

DEFINITION: _____

20. laminectomy

prefix	root	combining vowel	suffix

DEFINITION: _____

EXERCISE 23

Fill in the blanks.

1. A/An _____ is a mature bone cell.

2. A/An _____ is a physician who specializes in disorders and treatments of the skeletal system.

3. The medical term for the sudden breaking of a bone is

   _____.

4. A/An _____ is commonly called a slipped disk.

5. Forward curvature of the lumbar spine is called _____.

6. The diagnosis _____ is a malignant bone tumor.

7. _____ is commonly known as clubfoot.

8. A/An _____ is an incision into the bones of the skull.

9. The medical term for surgical fracture of a bone is _____.

10. Lateral curvature of the spine is called _____.

11. _____ is also known as rheumatoid arthritis of the spine.

12. The medical term for softening of the bone is _____.

13. A/An _____ specializes in the manipulation of the spine as a primary treatment method.

14. _____ is an incomplete dislocation of a bone from its joint.

15. Crackling and clicking sounds during joint movement is called

    _____.

16. A(n) _____ of a fracture includes surgical intervention.

17. A _____ is a bony growth on the surface of a bone.

18. Surgical fixation of a joint is called _____.

19. A(n) _____ fracture occurs at the distal end of the radius.

20. Tennis elbow is one example of _____, an inflammation of the bursa.

EXERCISE 24

Read the following discharge note. Write the definition for each italicized medical term.

DISCHARGE NOTE
DISCHARGE DIAGNOSES: 1. (1) *Herniated disk*; 2. Status post anterior (2) *cervical diskectomy*
PROCEDURE(S) PERFORMED: Anterior cervical diskectomy
BRIEF HISTORY: This 27-year-old male fell 12 feet from a ladder. He complained of pain radiating to the (3) *occipital* region of the skull. Cervical x-rays were suspicious for a compression (4) *fracture* at the level of (5) *C-5*. A (6) *myelogram* and CT scan of the cervical spine confirmed a herniated disk at the (7) *C5–6* level.

DISPOSITION: The patient was discharged home on the third post-operative day. He will wear a cervical collar at all times and will be seen at the (8) *orthopedic* clinic in 2 weeks.

1. _____
2. _____
3. _____
4. _____
5. _____
6. _____
7. _____
8. _____

EXERCISE 25

Select the best answer to each statement.

1. The area where two or more bones meet is called a(n)
   a. joint capsule
   b. hinge joint
   c. articulation
   d. fibrous joint

2. Select the alternative term for a closed fracture.
   a. Colles' fracture
   b. incomplete fracture
   c. complete fracture
   d. greenstick fracture

3. Which type of fracture is characterized by splintered pieces of bone?
   a. greenstick fracture
   b. comminuted fracture
   c. impacted fracture
   d. pathological fracture

4. Select the term that best describes a fracture caused by an underlying disease.
   a. comminuted fracture
   b. greenstick fracture
   c. impacted fracture
   d. pathological fracture

5. Which term means the same as a compound fracture?
   a. impacted fracture
   b. greenstick fracture
   c. open fracture
   d. pathological fracture

6. An accumulation of synovial fluid in the knee joint is known as a(n)
   a. Baker's cyst
   b. bursal cyst
   c. synovial cyst
   d. articular cyst

7. _____ is the incomplete dislocation of a bone from its joint.
   a. Crepitation
   b. Claudication
   c. Articulation
   d. Subluxation

8. _____ is the temporary displacement of a bone from its joint.
   a. Articulation
   b. Dislocation
   c. Claudication
   d. Subluxation

9. Select the medical term for softening of the bone.
   a. osteoporosis
   b. osteofibroma
   c. osteomegaly
   d. osteomalacia

10. Choose the medical term for therapeutic breaking of joint adhesions.
    a. arthrectomy
    b. arthroplasty
    c. arthroclasis
    d. arthrocentesis

11. Which abbreviation represents a treatment for an open fracture?
    a. DEXA
    b. ORIF
    c. THR
    d. CRIF

12. Choose the diagnostic procedure that includes a radioisotope.
    a. bone scan
    b. DEXA
    c. dual-photon absorptiometry
    d. bone marrow aspiration

13. Select the phrase that is represented with the abbreviation THR.
    a. tibia and hip repair
    b. total hip radiography
    c. tarsal hinge replacement
    d. total hip replacement

14. Which type of fracture is also called an incomplete fracture?
    a. comminuted fracture
    b. open fracture
    c. greenstick fracture
    d. impacted fracture

15. Select the type of fracture characterized by a bone wedged into another bone.
    a. open fracture
    b. impacted fracture
    c. greenstick fracture
    d. comminuted fracture

16. Select the medical term that means incision into a joint.
    a. arthrectomy
    b. arthrotomy
    c. arthroplasty
    d. arthrocentesis

17. Which medical term best describes an x-ray picture of a joint?
    a. arthroscopy
    b. arthrography
    c. arthrogram
    d. arthroplasty

18. The medical term for joint immobility is
    a. arthrodesis
    b. arthroplasty
    c. arthrocentesis
    d. ankylosis

19. A physician specialist for the skeletal system is called a(n)
    a. orthopedist
    b. orthoarthropedist
    c. chiropractor
    d. osteologist

20. Which treatment is usually associated with a simple fracture?
    a. closed reduction
    b. THR
    c. DEXA
    d. open reduction

CHALLENGE EXERCISE

Search the Internet using the keyword osteoporosis. Using the information you find, create a one-page handout that summarizes the cause, prevention, and treatment aspects of this common condition. Share the handout with your instructor and/or other students in your class.

Pronunciation Review

Review the terms from this chapter. Pronounce each term using the following phonetic pronunciations. Check off each term when you are comfortable saying it.

TERM	PRONUNCIATION
☐ ankylosing spondylitis	**ang**-kih-**LOH**-sing **spon**-dih-**LIGH**-tis
☐ ankylosis	ang-kih-**LOH**-sis
☐ arthralgia	ar-**THRAL**-jee-ah
☐ arthritis	ar-**THRIGH**-tis
☐ arthrocentesis	**ar**-throh-sen-**TEE**-sis
☐ arthrochondritis	**ar**-throh-kon-**DRIGH**-tis
☐ arthroclasis	**ar**-throh-**CLAY**-sis
☐ arthrodesis	**ar**-throh-**DEE**-sis
☐ arthrogram	**AR**-throh-gram
☐ arthrography	ar-**THROG**-rah-fee
☐ arthroplasty	**AR**-throh-**PLASS**-tee
☐ arthroscopy	ar-**THROSS**-koh-pee
☐ arthrotomy	ar-**THROT**-toh-mee
☐ articulation	ar-**tik**-yoo-**LAY**-shun
☐ Baker's cyst	Baker's cyst
☐ bone marrow aspiration	bone marrow **ass**-per-**AY**-shun
☐ bunion	**BUN**-yun
☐ bunionectomy	bun-yun-**ECK**-toh-mee
☐ bursectomy	ber-**SEK**-toh-mee
☐ bursitis	ber-**SIGH**-tis
☐ bursotomy	ber-**SOT**-oh-mee
☐ chiropractor	**KIGH**-roh-prak-tor
☐ chondromalacia	**kon**-droh-mah-**LAY**-she-ah
☐ Colles' fracture	**KALL**-eez fracture
☐ comminuted fracture	**KOM**-ih-noo-ted
☐ condyle	**KON**-dill
☐ cranial	**KRAY**-nee-al
☐ craniotomy	**kray**-nee-**OT**-oh-mee
☐ crepitation	**crep**-ih-**TAY**-shun
☐ diskectomy	disk-**EK**-toh-mee
☐ dislocation	**diss**-loh-**KAY**-shun
☐ dual-energy x-ray absorptiometry	dual-energy x-ray ab-**sorp**-she-**AH**-meh-tree
☐ femoral	**FEM**-or-al
☐ fissure	**FIH**-sher
☐ foramen	foh-**RAY**-men

☐ fossa	**FOSS**-ah
☐ gout	GOWT
☐ herniated disk	**HER**-nee-ay-ted disk
☐ humeral	**HYOO**-mor-al
☐ intercostal	**in**-ter-**KOSS**-tal
☐ intervertebral	**in**-ter-**VER**-teh-bral
☐ ischiopubic	**ih**-shee-oh-**PYOO**-bik
☐ kyphosis	kigh-**FOH**-sis
☐ laminectomy	lam-in-**EK**-toh-mee
☐ lordosis	lor-**DOH**-sis
☐ lumbar	**LUM**-bar
☐ lumbosacral	**lum**-boh-**SAY**-kral
☐ myeloma	**my**-eh-**LOH**-mah
☐ orthopedics	**or**-thoh-**PEE**-diks
☐ orthopedist	**or**-thoh-**PEE**-dist
☐ osteitis	**oss**-tee-**EYE**-tis
☐ osteoblast	**OSS**-tee-oh-blast
☐ osteochondritis	**oss**-tee-oh-kon-**DRIGH**-tis
☐ osteoclasis	**oss**-tee-oh-**KLAY**-sis
☐ osteocyte	**OSS**-tee-oh-sight
☐ osteofibroma	**oss**-tee-oh-fih-**BROH**-mah
☐ osteomalacia	**oss**-tee-oh-mah-**LAY**-she-ah
☐ osteomyelitis	**oss**-tee-oh-my-eh-**LIGH**-tis
☐ osteoplasty	**OSS**-tee-oh-plass-tee
☐ osteoporosis	**oss**-tee-oh-poh-**ROH**-sis
☐ osteosarcoma	**oss**-tee-oh-sar-**KOH**-mah
☐ osteotomy	**oss**-tee-**OT**-oh-mee
☐ rheumatoid arthritis	**ROO**-may-toyd ar-**THRIGH**-tis
☐ scoliosis	skoh-lee-**OH**-sis
☐ spondylitis	spon-dih-**LIGH**-tiss
☐ subluxation	sub-luks-**AY**-shun
☐ submandibular	**sub**-man-**DIB**-yoo-lar
☐ submaxillary	sub-**MACKS**-ih-lair-ee
☐ substernal	sub-**STER**-nal
☐ supraclavicular	**soo**-prah-klah-**VIK**-yoo-lar
☐ synovectomy	sin-oh-**VEK**-toh-mee
☐ talipes	**TAL**-ih-peez
☐ trochanter	troh-**KAN**-ter

5 Muscular System

OBJECTIVES

At the completion of this chapter, the student should be able to:

1. Identify, define, and spell word roots associated with the muscular system.
2. Label the basic structures of the muscular system.
3. Discuss the functions of the muscular system.
4. Provide the correct spelling of muscular system terms, given the definition of the term.
5. Analyze the muscular system terms by defining the roots, prefixes, and suffixes of these terms.
6. Identify, define, and spell disease, disorder, and procedure terms related to the muscular system.

OVERVIEW

The muscular system consists of muscles, tendons, fascia, and ligaments. The structures of this system function together to support and maintain body posture and to permit movement. Each structure and its unique characteristics are presented individually.

Muscular System Word Roots

To understand and use muscular system medical terms, it is necessary to acquire a thorough knowledge of the associated word roots. Word roots associated with this system are listed with the combining vowel. Review the word roots in Table 5-1 and complete the exercises that follow.

TABLE 5-1 MUSCULAR SYSTEM ROOT WORDS

Word Root/Combining Form	Meaning
bucc/o	cheek
electr/o	electricity
fasci/o	fascia; band of fibrous tissue
fibr/o	fiber; fibrous tissue
kines/o; kinesi/o	movement
leiomy/o	smooth muscle
ligament/o	ligament
my/o	muscle

(continues)

TABLE 5-1   MUSCULAR SYSTEM ROOT WORDS (continued)

Word Root/Combining Form	Meaning
pector/o	chest
rhabdomy/o	skeletal muscle; striated muscle
ten/o; tend/o; tendin/o	tendon
tenosynov/o	tendon sheath
ton/o	tone; stretching; tension

© 2016 Cengage Learning®

EXERCISE 1

Write the definitions of the following word roots.

1. bucc/o   _____

2. my/o   _____

3. rhabdomy/o   _____

4. fibr/o   _____

5. ten/o   _____

6. leiomy/o   _____

7. fasci/o   _____

8. pector/o   _____

9. ligament/o   _____

EXERCISE 2

Write the word root and meaning of the following medical terms.

1. myalgia

   ROOT: _____   MEANING: _____

2. fibroma

   ROOT: _____   MEANING: _____

3. tendinitis

   ROOT: _____   MEANING: _____

4. pectoral

   ROOT: _____   MEANING: _____

5. fasciotomy

   ROOT: _____   MEANING: _____

6. electromyogram

   ROOT: _____   MEANING: _____

EXERCISE 3

Write the correct word root(s) for the following meanings.

1. smooth muscle   _____

2. fiber   _____

3. ligament   _____

4. muscle   _____

5. fibrous tissue band   _____

6. skeletal muscle   _____

7. chest   _____

8. cheek   _____

9. tendon   _____

10. tendon sheath   _____

Structures of the Muscular System

The major structures of the muscular system include muscles, fascia, tendons, and ligaments. Muscles are named for many reasons, such as the direction of the muscle fibers and the muscle action. Table 5-2 lists the ways muscles are named with examples. Figure 5-1 illustrates some of the major muscles of the body, showing both anterior and posterior views.

The body has more than 600 muscles and many tendons. Fortunately, you will not have to learn the names of all of them. Table 5-3 lists and describes some of the more commonly known muscles and one tendon. The numbers in parentheses correspond to the enumerated muscles in Figure 5-1. Refer to the figure as you read the description of the selected muscles. Complete the exercises that follow Table 5-3.

TABLE 5-2   MUSCLE NAMES

Direction of the muscle fiber
- rectus (straight); muscle is parallel to the midline of the body; *rectus abdominis*
- oblique (angle); muscle at an angle to the midline of the body; *external oblique*
Location in the body
- tibialis (tiabia; shin bone); *tibialis anterior*; muscle on the front of the tibia
- abdominis (abdomen); *rectus abdominis*; parallel muscle of the abdomen
Number of origins*
- biceps (bi = two; ceps = head); *biceps*; two attachments (heads) at the origin
- triceps (tri = three; ceps = head); *triceps*; three attachments (heads) at the origin

*Muscle origins are the part of the body where the muscle attaches, usually to a bone. This part of the muscle does not move when the muscle contracts.

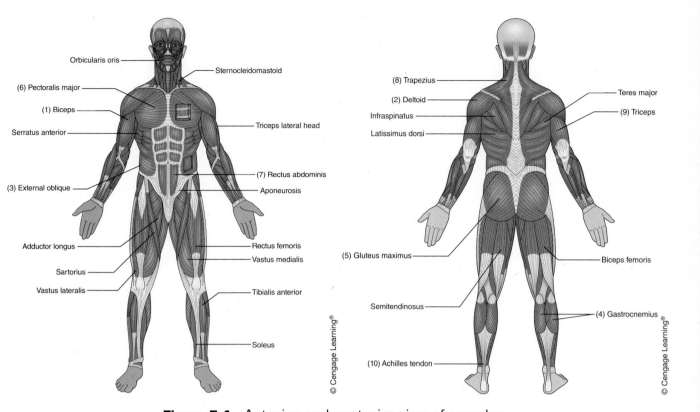

Figure 5-1 Anterior and posterior view of muscles.

TABLE 5-3 MUSCLES AND TENDONS

Muscle/Tendon	Description
biceps (1) (**BIGH**-seps)	located on the anterior surface of the humerus; movements include bending and extending the arms
buccinators (**BUCK**-sin-ay-tor) bucc/o = cheek	cheek muscle; allows actions such as sucking, whistling, blowing, and smiling
deltoid (2) (**DELL**-toyd)	covers the shoulder joint; common site for medication injections
external oblique (3)	muscles of the sides of the upper body; movements include turning or twisting the upper body
gastrocnemius (4) (**gass**-trok-**NEE**-mee-us)	calf muscle; movements include pointing the toes and standing on tiptoe
gluteus maximus (5) (**GLOO**-tee-us **MACKS**-ih-mus)	buttock muscle; moves the thigh (you sit on your gluteus maximus)
hamstring muscles	located on the posterior part of the thigh; a group of three individual muscles; movements include flexing or bending the thigh, squatting

(continues)

TABLE 5-3   MUSCLES AND TENDONS (continued)

Muscle/Tendon	Description
masseter	located at the angle of the jaw; allows actions such as biting and chewing, mastication
pectoralis major (6) (peck-toh-**RAY**-lis)	chest muscle; large, fan-shaped muscle that crosses the upper part of the chest; moves the arms
quadriceps femoris (**KWAHD**-rih-seps **FEM**-or-iss)	anterior thigh muscle; a group of four individual muscles; movements include extending the thigh, kicking
rectus abdominis (7) (**RECK**-tus ab-**DOM**-in-iss)	abdominal muscles; commonly called "abs"; movements include raising the upper body
sternomastoid, sternocleidomastoid (stir-noh-**MASS**-toyd, stir-noh-**KLIGH**-doh-mass-toyd) stern/o = sternum	extends from the sternum up the side of the neck to the mastoid process; moves the head and neck
temporal (**TEMP**-or-al)	located above and near the ear; movements include biting and chewing
tibialis anterior (tib-ee-**AY**-lis)	located on the front lower part of the leg; movements include pulling the foot toward the leg
trapezius (8) (trah-**PEE**-zee-us)	trianglular-shaped muscle that extends across the back of the shoulder, back of the neck, and connects to the clavicle and scapula; moves the shoulders
triceps (9) (**TRIGH**-seps)	located on the posterior surface of the humerus; movements include bending and extending the arms
Achilles tendon (10) (ah-**KILL**-eez)	tendon that attaches the gastrocnemius muscle to the calcaneus

© 2016 Cengage Learning®

EXERCISE 4

Write the name of the muscle for each description.

1. "abs"   _____

2. buttock muscle   _____

3. calf muscle   _____

4. cheek muscle   _____

5. chest muscle   _____

6. mastication or chewing muscle   _____

7. tendon attached to the calcaneus   _____

EXERCISE 5

Match the muscle in Column 1 with the description in Column 2.

COLUMN 1	**COLUMN 2**
_____ 1. biceps	a. above and near the ear; chewing
_____ 2. deltoid	b. anterior surface of the humerus
_____ 3. external oblique	c. anterior thigh muscle
_____ 4. hamstring muscles	d. covers the shoulder; injection site
_____ 5. quadriceps femoris	e. moves the head and neck
_____ 6. sternomastoid	f. moves the shoulders
_____ 7. temporal muscle	g. posterior surface of the humerus
_____ 8. tibialis anterior	h. posterior thigh muscles
_____ 9. trapezius	i. side of the upper body; twisting
_____ 10. triceps	j. walking on the heels

Muscles

Muscles are actually groups of muscle cells called *fibers*. The body contains three types of muscles: **skeletal muscle**, **smooth muscle**, and **cardiac muscle**. Skeletal muscles, also known as **striated** (**STRIGH**-ay-ted) or voluntary muscles, are usually attached to bones. The term *striated* refers to the striped appearance of skeletal muscles when viewed under a microscope. Skeletal muscles are voluntary because the individual must make a conscious choice to move them. Figure 5-2A illustrates skeletal, or striated, muscles.

Smooth muscles, also known as involuntary muscles, are located in the walls of organs such as blood vessels, glands, intestines, stomach, and parts of the respiratory system. Smooth muscles are not under the voluntary control of the individual. Figure 5-2B illustrates smooth, or involuntary, muscles.

Cardiac muscles form the walls of the heart, are striated in appearance, and are classified as involuntary muscles. These tough muscles are arranged in branching fiber bundles and are able to withstand a great deal of stress. Figure 5-2C illustrates cardiac muscle.

Fascia, Tendons, and Ligaments

Muscle fibers are held together by fibrous connective tissue called **fascia** (**FASH**-ee-ah). Muscle fascia extends to form strong fibrous bands of tissue called (1) **tendons**. Tendons attach muscle to the bone. **Ligaments** (2) are connective tissue bands that attach bones to bones and support the joints. Figure 5-3 illustrates a muscle with its associated tendons and ligament.

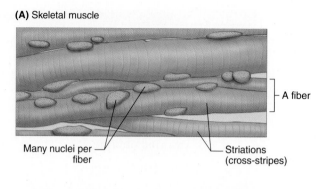

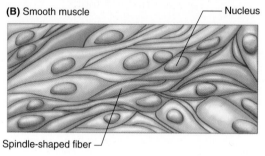

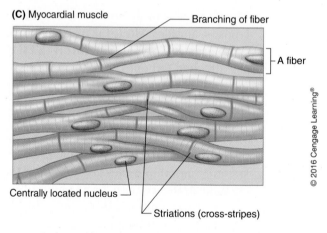

(A) Skeletal muscle

Many nuclei per fiber

Striations (cross-stripes)

A fiber

(B) Smooth muscle

Nucleus

Spindle-shaped fiber

(C) Myocardial muscle

Branching of fiber

A fiber

Centrally located nucleus

Striations (cross-stripes)

© 2016 Cengage Learning®

Figure 5-2 Types of muscle tissue. (A) Skeletal muscle. (B) Smooth muscle. (C) Myocardial muscle.

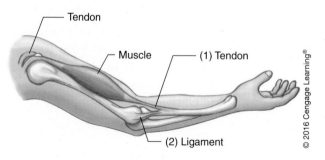

Tendon

Muscle

(1) Tendon

(2) Ligament

© 2016 Cengage Learning®

Figure 5-3 Tendons (1) attach muscle to bone. Ligaments (2) join bone to bone.

EXERCISE 6

Label the muscular system structures shown in Figure 5-4. Write your answers in the spaces provided.

1. _____   4. _____

2. _____   5. _____

3. _____

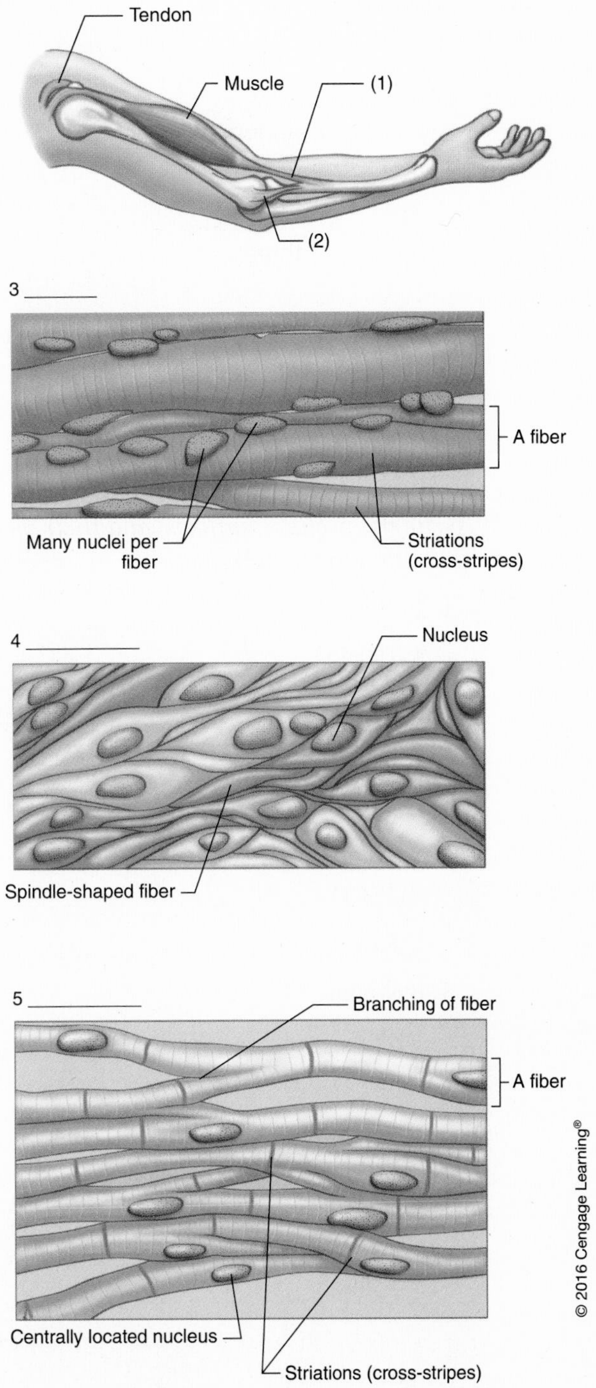

Figure 5-4   Types of muscles and related structures.

Muscular System Medical Terminology

Muscular system medical terms are organized into three main categories: (1) general medical terms; (2) diseases and conditions; and (3) diagnostic procedure, surgery, and laboratory test terms. The prefixes and suffixes associated with this system are listed in Table 5-4. Review these word parts and complete the related exercises.

TABLE 5-4   PREFIXES, AND SUFFIXES FOR MUSCULAR SYSTEM TERMS

Prefix	Meaning	Suffix	Meaning
bi-	twice; double; two	-algia	pain
brady-	slow	-asthenia	without feeling or sensation
dys-	abnormal; difficult	-dynia	pain
intra-	within	-kinesia	movement
poly-	many	-lysis	destruction; breakdown
tri-	three	-oma	tumor
		-tonia	muscle tone
		-trophy	growth; development

© 2016 Cengage Learning®

EXERCISE 7

Write the prefixes, suffixes, and their meanings. Based on the meanings, write a definition for each term.

1. bradykinesia

   PREFIX: _____   MEANING: _____

   SUFFIX: _____   MEANING: _____

   DEFINITION: _____

2. dystrophy

   PREFIX: _____   MEANING: _____

   SUFFIX: _____   MEANING: _____

   DEFINITION: _____

3. dystonia

   PREFIX: _____   MEANING: _____

   SUFFIX: _____   MEANING: _____

   DEFINITION: _____

4. hyperkinesia

PREFIX: _____   MEANING: _____

SUFFIX: _____   MEANING: _____

DEFINITION: _____

5. intramuscular

PREFIX: _____   MEANING: _____

SUFFIX: _____   MEANING: _____

DEFINITION: _____

6. myasthenia

PREFIX: _____   MEANING: _____

SUFFIX: _____   MEANING: _____

DEFINITION: _____

7. myoma

PREFIX: _____   MEANING: _____

SUFFIX: _____   MEANING: _____

DEFINITION: _____

8. polymyositis

PREFIX: _____   MEANING: _____

SUFFIX: _____   MEANING: _____

DEFINITION: _____

9. polymyalgia

PREFIX: _____   MEANING: _____

SUFFIX: _____   MEANING: _____

DEFINITION: _____

Muscular System General Medical Terms

Review the pronunciation and meaning of each term in Table 5-5. Note that most of the terms describe body movement. When one muscle, or set of muscles, flexes, the opposing muscle or set extends and movement occurs. Many of the movement terms can be paired. For example, abduction is movement away from the midline and body, and adduction is movement toward the midline and body. Review the terms in Table 5-5 and complete the exercises.

TABLE 5-5   MUSCULAR SYSTEM GENERAL MEDICAL TERMS

Pronunciation	Meaning
abduction (ab-**DUCK**-shun)	movement away from the midline of the body (Figure 5-5)
adduction (ad-**DUCK**-shun)	movement toward the midline of the body (Figure 5-5)

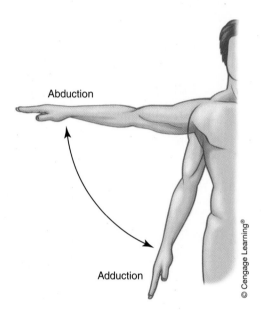

Abduction

Adduction

© Cengage Learning®

Figure 5-5   Abduction moves the arm away from the body. Adduction moves the arm toward the body.

circumduction (**sir**-kum-**DUCK**-shun)	movement in a circular motion (Figure 5-6)
dorsiflexion (**dor**-see-**FLEX**-shun)	moving the foot upward toward the leg (Figure 5-7)
extension (ecks-**TEN**-shun)	straightening motion; movement to increase the angle between bones (Figure 5-8)
flexion (**FLEK**-shun)	bending motion; movement to decrease the angle between bones (Figure 5-8)
intramuscular (**in**-trah-**MUSS**-kyoo-lar) intra- = within muscul/o = muscle -ar = pertaining to	pertaining to within the muscle or muscle tissue
plantar flexion (**PLAN**-tar **FLEK**-shun)	moving the foot in a downward position away from the leg; pointing the toes downward (Figure 5-9)

(continues)

TABLE 5-5   MUSCULAR SYSTEM GENERAL MEDICAL TERMS (continued)

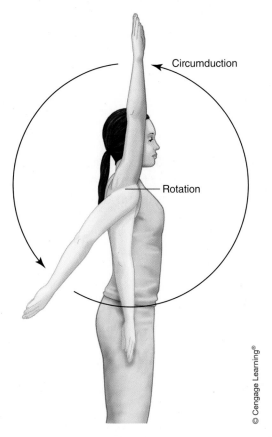

Figure 5-6 Circumduction is the circular movement at the end of a limb. Rotation is a circular movement around an axis, such as the shoulder joint.

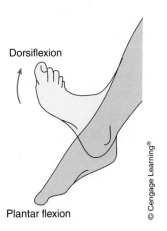

Figure 5-7 Dorsiflexiion.

(continues)

TABLE 5-5   MUSCULAR SYSTEM GENERAL MEDICAL TERMS (continued)

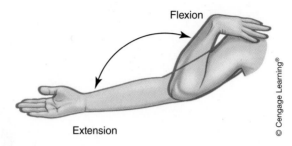

Figure 5-8 Extension increases the angle of the elbow and moves the hand away from the body. Flexion decreases the angle of the elbow and moves the hand toward the body.

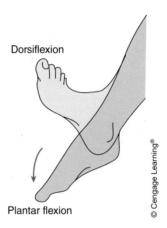

Figure 5-9 Plantar flexion.

Pronunciation	Meaning
pronation (proh-**NAY**-shun)	rotating the arm so that the palm of the hand is turned downward or backward; palms down
rotation (roh-**TAY**-shun)	moving or turning on an axis or pivot point (See Figure 5-6)
supination (**soo**-pih-**NAY**-shun)	rotating the arm so that the palm of the hand is turned forward or upward; palms up

© 2016 Cengage Learning®

EXERCISE 8

Write the term that describes the "paired" or opposite movement of the listed term.

1. adduction   _____

2. dorsiflexion   _____

3. extension   _____

4. pronation   _____

EXERCISE 9

Replace the italicized word or phrase with the correct muscular term.

1. Jorge received a *within the muscle tissue* injection of a potent antibiotic.

   _____

2. *Pointing the toes downward* shortens the Achilles tendon.

   _____

3. *Palms up* allow(s) us to take change from the cashier.

   _____

4. Because of a reaction to her prescription, Neesha was unable to accomplish *moving her head from left to right*.

   _____

5. *Movement in a circular motion* is often used as a warm-up exercise before a tennis match.

   _____

6. *Moving the foot upward toward the leg* stretches the Achilles tendon.

   _____

Muscular System Disease and Disorder Terms

Muscular system diseases include common aches and pains due to overexertion and obscure diagnoses such as Werdnig-Hoffman disease, also known as floppy infant syndrome. Review the pronunciation and definition for each term in Table 5-6 and complete the exercises.

TABLE 5-6   MUSCULAR SYSTEM DISEASE AND DISORDER TERMS

Term with Pronunciation	Definition
atrophy (**AT**-troh-fee) a- = without -trophy = growth; development	wasting or decrease in size of an organ or tissue
bradykinesia (**brad**-ee-kih-**NEE**-see-ah) brady- = slow -kinesia = movement	extremely slow movement

(continues)

TABLE 5-6 MUSCULAR SYSTEM DISEASE AND DISORDER TERMS (continued)

Term with Pronunciation	Definition
carpal tunnel syndrome	Inflamation and swelling of the tendons and median nerve that pass under the carpal ligament; also called repetitive stress syndrome or disease (Figure 5-10)

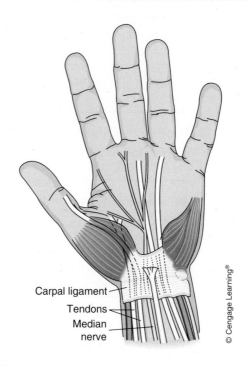

Carpal ligament
Tendons
Median nerve

© Cengage Learning®

Figure 5-10 Carpal tunnel syndrome.

Charcot-Marie-Tooth disease (shar-**KOO**)	hereditary condition characterized by progressive degeneration of the muscles of the lower leg, specifically those associated with the fibula
contraction (con-**TRACK**-shun)	shortening or tightening of a muscle
contracture (kon-**TRAK**-cher)	abnormal and often permanent flexion at a joint caused by atrophy and shortening of muscle fibers
dermatomyositis (der-**mat**-oh-**my**-oh-**SIGH**-tis) dermat/o = skin my/o = muscle -itis = inflammation	connective tissue disease characterized by the destruction of muscle tissue and puritic inflammation of the skin

(continues)

TABLE 5-6 MUSCULAR SYSTEM DISEASE AND DISORDER TERMS (continued)

Term with Pronunciation	Definition
dyskinesia (**diss**-kih-**NEE**-see-ah) dys- = abnormal; difficult -kinesia = movement	abnormal or difficult movement
dystonia (diss-**TOH**-nee-ah) dys- = abnormal; difficult -tonia = muscle tone	abnormal muscle tone; prolonged muscle contractions
dystrophy (**DISS**-troh-fee) dys- = abnormal; difficult -trophy = growth; development	abnormal development
fasciitis (**fash**-ee-**EYE**-tis) fasci/o = fascia -itis = inflammation	inflammation of the fascia
fibroma (fih-**BROH**-mah) fibr/o = fiber -oma = tumor	tumor of connective tissue
fibromyalgia (FM) (**figh**-broh-my-**AL**-jee-ah) fibr/o =fiber my/o = muscle -algia = pain	chronic pain illness characterized by widespread muscular aches, pains, and stiffness
ganglion cyst (**GANG**-lee-on)	noncancerous lump filled with a jellylike fluid; commonly develops along the tendons or joints of the hands; may also occur in the ankles or feet (Figure 5-11)

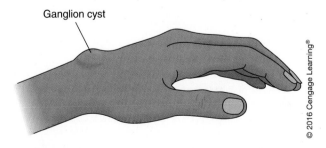

Ganglion cyst

© 2016 Cengage Learning®

Figure 5-11 Ganglion cyst.

(continues)

TABLE 5-6   MUSCULAR SYSTEM DISEASE AND DISORDER TERMS (continued)

Term with Pronunciation	Definition
hyperkinesia (**high**-per-kih-**NEE**-see-ah) hyper- = excessive; increase -kinesia = movement	increased muscular movement and physical activity
hypertrophy (high-**PER**-troh-fee) hyper- = excessive; increase -trophy = growth; development	increased growth or development of an organ or tissue not related to a tumor
leiomyofibroma (**ligh**-oh-**my**-oh-fih-**BROH**-mah) leiomy/o = smooth muscle fibr/o = fiber -oma = tumor	benign tumor of smooth muscle and fibrous connective tissue

© 2016 Cengage Learning®

EXERCISE 10

Analyze each term. Write the root, prefix, suffix, and their meanings in the spaces provided.

1. atrophy

   ROOT: _____ MEANING: _____

   PREFIX: _____ MEANING: _____

   SUFFIX: _____ MEANING: _____

2. bradykinesia

   ROOT: _____ MEANING: _____

   PREFIX: _____ MEANING: _____

   SUFFIX: _____ MEANING: _____

3. dermatomyositis

   ROOT: _____ MEANING: _____

   PREFIX: _____ MEANING: _____

   SUFFIX: _____ MEANING: _____

4. dyskinesia

   ROOT: _____ MEANING: _____

   PREFIX: _____ MEANING: _____

   SUFFIX: _____ MEANING: _____

5. dystonia

ROOT: _____ MEANING: _____

PREFIX: _____ MEANING: _____

SUFFIX: _____ MEANING: _____

6. dystrophy

ROOT: _____ MEANING: _____

PREFIX: _____ MEANING: _____

SUFFIX: _____ MEANING: _____

7. fibroma

ROOT: _____ MEANING: _____

PREFIX: _____ MEANING: _____

SUFFIX: _____ MEANING: _____

8. fibromyalgia

ROOT: _____ MEANING: _____

PREFIX: _____ MEANING: _____

SUFFIX: _____ MEANING: _____

9. hyperkinesia

ROOT: _____ MEANING: _____

PREFIX: _____ MEANING: _____

SUFFIX: _____ MEANING: _____

10. hypertrophy

ROOT: _____ MEANING: _____

PREFIX: _____ MEANING: _____

SUFFIX: _____ MEANING: _____

11. leiomyofibroma

ROOT: _____ MEANING: _____

PREFIX: _____ MEANING: _____

SUFFIX: _____ MEANING: _____

EXERCISE 11

Circle the medical term that completes each statement.

1. Muscular *atrophy/dystrophy* is characterized by abnormal growth and development.

2. Marquisha was treated for *dystonia/dyskinesia* because she experienced prolonged muscle contractions.

3. *Fibroma/Ganglion cyst* is a noncancerous lump of jellylike fluid.

4. *Hyperkinesia/Bradykinesia* is often associated with attention deficit disorder (ADD).

5. A *contraction/contracture* is defined as an abnormal shortening of a muscle.

EXERCISE 12

Match the medical terms in Column 1 with the definitions in Column 2.

COLUMN 1

_____ 1. cystic tumor of a tendon

_____ 2. tumor of connective tissue

_____ 3. benign tumor of smooth muscle

_____ 4. widespread muscle aches, pains, and stiffness

_____ 5. extremely slow movement

_____ 6. repetitive stress disease

_____ 7. prolonged muscle contractions

_____ 8. increased growth of an organ or tissue

_____ 9. disease characterized by muscle tissue destruction

_____ 10. hereditary degeneration of lower leg muscles

COLUMN 2

a. bradykinesia

b. Carcot-Marie-Tooth disease

c. carpal tunnel syndrome

d. dermatomyositis

e. dystonia

f. fibroma

g. fibromyalgia

h. ganglion

i. hypertrophy

j. leiomyofibroma

Review the pronunciation and definition for each term in Table 5-7 and complete the exercises.

TABLE 5-7 MUSCULAR SYSTEM DISEASE AND DISORDER TERMS

Term with Pronunciation	Definition
muscular dystrophy (MD) (**MUSS**-kyoo-lar **DIS**-troh-fee) muscul/o = muscle -ar = pertaining to dys- = bad, painful, abnormal -trophy = growth	progressive weakness and degeneration of muscle fiber; genetically inherited
myalgia (my-**AL**-jee-ah) my/o = muscle -algia = pain	muscle pain
myasthenia (**my**-ass-**THEE**-nee-ah) my/o = muscle -asthenia = without feeling or sensation	muscle weakness and abnormal fatigue

(continues)

TABLE 5-7   MUSCULAR SYSTEM DISEASE AND DISORDER TERMS (continued)

Term with Pronunciation	Definition
myasthenia gravis (**my**-ass-**THEE**-nee-ah **GRAV**-is) my/o = muscle -asthenia = without feeling or sensation	serious, generalized muscle weakness and abnormal fatigue without atrophy
myositis (**my**-oh-**SIGH**-tis) my/o = muscle -itis = inflammation	inflammation of muscle tissue
plantar fasciitis (**PLAN**-tar **fash**-ee-**EYE**-tis) fasci/o = fascia -itis = inflamation	inflammation of the plantar fascia, located on the sole of the foot (Figure 5-12)

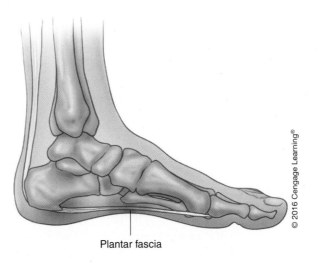

Plantar fascia

© 2016 Cengage Learning®

Figure 5-12   Plantar fasciitis.

polymyositis (**pall**-ee-**my**-oh-**SIGH**-tis) poly- = many my/o = muscle -itis = inflammation	chronic, progressive inflammation of skeletal muscles with muscle weakness and atrophy
rhabdomyolysis (**rab**-doh-**my**-oh-**LIGH**-sis) rhabdomy/o = skeletal muscle -lysis = destruction; break down	hereditary or acquired condition characterized by the destruction of skeletal muscle fibers and the release of muscle cell contents into the bloodstream

(continues)

TABLE 5-7   MUSCULAR SYSTEM DISEASE AND DISORDER TERMS (continued)

Term with Pronunciation	Definition
rhabdomyosarcoma (**rab**-doh-**my**-oh-sar-**KOH**-mah) rhabdomy/o = skeletal muscle sarc/o = flesh -oma = tumor	highly malignant neoplasm or tumor of the skeletal muscle
sprain	injury of the ligaments of a joint caused by wrenching or twisting
tendinitis, tenditis (ten-din-**EYE**-tis, ten-**DIGH**-tis) tendin/o, ten/o = tendon -itis = inflammation	inflammation of a tendon
tenodynia (ten-oh-**DIN**-ee-ah) ten/o = tendon -dynia = pain	tendon pain
tenosynovitis (**ten**-oh-**sin**-oh-**VIGH**-tis)	inflammation of a tendon sheath
torticollis (tor-tih-**KALL**-lis)	shortening of the muscles on one side of the neck; wryneck
Werdnig-Hoffman disease	genetic disorder characterized by progressive atrophy of skeletal muscles; also known as familial spinal muscle atrophy and floppy infant syndrome

© 2016 Cengage Learning®

EXERCISE 13

Analyze each term. Write the root, prefix, suffix, and their meanings in the spaces provided. Note that for ease in pronunciation, an "s" is placed between the combining form my/o and the suffix -itis.

1. myalgia

   ROOT: _____ MEANING: _____

   PREFIX: _____ MEANING: _____

   SUFFIX: _____ MEANING: _____

2. myasthenia

   ROOT: _____ MEANING: _____

   PREFIX: _____ MEANING: _____

   SUFFIX: _____ MEANING: _____

3. myositis

ROOT: _____   MEANING: _____

PREFIX: _____   MEANING: _____

SUFFIX: _____   MEANING: _____

4. polymyositis

ROOT: _____   MEANING: _____

PREFIX: _____   MEANING: _____

SUFFIX: _____   MEANING: _____

5. rhabdomyolysis

ROOT: _____   MEANING: _____

PREFIX: _____   MEANING: _____

SUFFIX: _____   MEANING: _____

6. rhabdomyosarcoma

ROOT: _____   MEANING: _____

PREFIX: _____   MEANING: _____

SUFFIX: _____   MEANING: _____

7. tendonitis

ROOT: _____   MEANING: _____

PREFIX: _____   MEANING: _____

SUFFIX: _____   MEANING: _____

8. tenodynia

ROOT: _____   MEANING: _____

PREFIX: _____   MEANING: _____

SUFFIX: _____   MEANING: _____

9. tenosynovitis

ROOT: _____   MEANING: _____

PREFIX: _____   MEANING: _____

SUFFIX: _____   MEANING: _____

EXERCISE 14

Circle the medical term that best fits the definition.

1. Genetic disorder characterized by degeneration of muscle fiber: *muscular dystrophy* or *Werdnig-Hoffman disease*

2. Malignant neoplasm of skeletal muscle: *rhabdomyolysis* or *rhabdomyosarcoma*

3. Familial spinal muscle atrophy: *Werdnig-Hoffman disease* or *myasthenia gravis*

4. Hereditary condition characterized by skeletal muscle destruction: *muscular dystrophy* or *rhabdomyolysis*

5. Muscle weakness and abnormal fatigue: *myalgia* or *myasthenia*

EXERCISE 15

Match the medical terms in Column 1 with the definitions in Column 2.

COLUMN 1   **COLUMN 2**

_____ 1. muscle cell contents released into   a. muscular dystrophy
         the bloodstream

_____ 2. malignant tumor of skeletal muscle   b. myasthenia gravis

_____ 3. floppy infant syndrome   c. myositis

_____ 4. wryneck   d. polymyositis

_____ 5. serious generalized muscle weakness   e. rhabdomyolysis
         and fatigue

_____ 6. chronic, progressive inflammation of   f. rhabdomyosarcoma
         skeletal muscle

_____ 7. genetic, progressive degeneration of   g. sprain
         muscle fiber

_____ 8. inflammation of a tendon sheath   h. tenodynia

_____ 9. tendon pain   i. tenosynovitis

_____ 10. inflammation of muscle tissue   j. torticollis

_____ 11. wrenching or twisting of a ligament   k. Werdnig-Hoffman disease

Review the pronunciation and definition of the diagnostic, surgical, and treatment terms in Table 5-8 and complete the following exercises.

TABLE 5-8   MUSCULAR SYSTEM DIAGNOSTIC, SURGICAL,
              AND TREATMENT TERMS

Term with Pronunciation	Definition
electromyogram (ee-**lek**-troh-**MY**-oh-gram) electr/o = electricity my/o = muscle -gram = graphic record	graphic record of muscle contraction as a result of electrical stimulation
electromyography (EMG) (ee-**lek**-troh-my-**OG**-rah-fee) electr/o = electricity my/o = muscle -graphy = process of recording	process of recording muscle contraction when receiving electrical stimulation
fasciotomy (fash-ee-**OTT**-oh-mee) fasci/o = fascia -tomy = incision into	surgical incision and division into a fascia

(continues)

TABLE 5-8   MUSCULAR SYSTEM DIAGNOSTIC, SURGICAL, AND TREATMENT TERMS (continued)

Term with Pronunciation	Definition
ganglionectomy (**gang**-lee-oh-**NEK**-toh-mee) -ectomy = surgical removal	excision of a ganglion
myoplasty **MY**-oh-plass-tee) my/o = muscle -plasty = surgical repair	surgical repair or plastic surgery of muscle tissue
myorrhaphy (my-**OR**-ah-fee) my/o = muscle -(r)rhaphy = suture; suturing	suture of muscle tissue or a muscle wound
Range-of-motion testing (**ROM**)	manipulation of a joint to evaluate joint mobility and muscle strength (Figure 5-13)

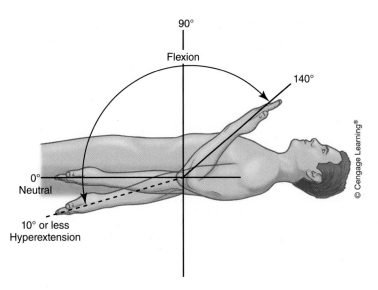

Figure 5-13 Range-of-motion testing is used to evaluate joint mobility. The results are expressed in degrees.

Rest, **I**ce, **C**ompression, and **E**levation (**RICE**)	commonly used first aid treatment for muscular injuries; rest and ice ease pain; compression and elevation help minimize swelling

(continues)

TABLE 5-8 MUSCULAR SYSTEM DIAGNOSTIC, SURGICAL, AND TREATMENT TERMS (continued)

Term with Pronunciation	Definition
tenomyoplasty (**ten**-oh-**MY**-oh-plass-tee) ten/o = tendon my/o = muscle -plasty = surgical repair	surgical repair of muscles and tendons
tenorrhaphy (ten-**OR**-ah-fee) ten/o = tendon -(r)rhaphy = suture, suturing	suturing of a tendon
tenosynovectomy (**ten**-oh-**sin**-oh-**VEK**-toh-mee) tenosynov/o = tendon sheath -ectomy = surgical removal	surgical removal of a tendon sheath

© 2016 Cengage Learning®

EXERCISE 16

Analyze the following terms by separating the roots, combining vowels, and suffixes with vertical slashes. Note that electr/o is the word root for electricity or electrical stimulation.

1. electromyography

    _____
    root   *combining vowel*   *suffix*

2. myoplasty

    _____
    root   *combining vowel*   *suffix*

3. myorrhaphy

    _____
    root   *combining vowel*   *suffix*

4. tenomyoplasty

    _____
    root   *combining vowel*   *suffix*

5. tenorrhaphy

    _____
    root   *combining vowel*   *suffix*

6. tenosynovectomy

    _____
    root   *combining vowel*   *suffix*

7. electromyogram

    _____
    root   *combining vowel*   *suffix*

8. fasciotomy

root	*combining vowel*	*suffix*

9. ganglionectomy

root	*combining vowel*	*suffix*

Abbreviations

Review the muscular system abbreviations in Table 5-9. Practice writing the meaning of each abbreviation.

TABLE 5-9 ABBREVIATIONS

Abbreviation	Meaning
DTR	deep tendon reflexes
EMG	electromyography
FM	fibromyalgia
IM	intramuscular
MD	muscular dystrophy
RICE	rest, ice, compression, and elevation
ROM	range of motion

© 2016 Cengage Learning®

CHAPTER REVIEW

The Chapter Review can be used as a self-test. Go through each exercise and answer as many questions as you can without referring to previous exercises or earlier discussions within this chapter. Check your answers and fill in any blanks. Practice writing any terms you might have misspelled.

EXERCISE 17

Analyze each term. Separate the root, combining vowel, and suffix with vertical slashes. Write a definition for each term.

1. bradykinesia

root	*combining vowel*	*suffix*

DEFINITION: _____

2. dyskinesia

root	*combining vowel*	*suffix*

DEFINITION: _____

3. dystonia

root	*combining vowel*	*suffix*

DEFINITION: _____

4. electromyogram

root	combining vowel	suffix

DEFINITION: _____

5. electromyography

root	combining vowel	suffix

DEFINITION: _____

6. hyperkinesia

root	combining vowel	suffix

DEFINITION: _____

7. leiomyofibroma

root	combining vowel	suffix

DEFINITION: _____

8. myasthenia

root	combining vowel	suffix

DEFINITION: _____

9. polymyositis

root	combining vowel	suffix

DEFINITION: _____

10. rhabdomyosarcoma

root	combining vowel	suffix

DEFINITION: _____

11. tenodynia

root	combining vowel	suffix

DEFINITION: _____

12. tenosynovitis

root	combining vowel	suffix

DEFINITION: _____

13. rhabdomyolysis

root	combining vowel	suffix

DEFINITION: _____

14. fibromyalgia

root	combining vowel	suffix

DEFINITION: _____

15. dermatomyositis

_____

root   _combining vowel_   _suffix_

DEFINITION: _____

EXERCISE 18

Write the medical term for each definition.

1. extremely slow movement   _____

2. abnormal development   _____

3. tumor of connective tissue   _____

4. surgical repair of muscle tissue   _____

5. tendon pain   _____

6. increased muscle movement and physical activity   _____

7. genetic disorder characterized by progressive
   atrophy of skeletal muscles   _____

8. hereditary or acquired condition characterized by
   destruction of skeletal muscle fibers   _____

9. hereditary condition characterized by
   degeneration of lower leg muscles   _____

10. genetic disorder characterized by progressive
    weakness and degeneration of muscles   _____

11. process of recording muscle contractions   _____

12. muscle weakness and abnormal fatigue   _____

13. malignant tumor of skeletal muscle   _____

14. benign tumor of smooth muscle   _____

15. destruction of muscle tissue and puritic
    inflammation of the skin   _____

EXERCISE 19

Read the following progress note and spell out each boldface abbreviation.

PATIENT NAME: GERVAIS, SARA M. **DOB:** 08/05/1978
Ms. Gervais is a 28-year-old female who presents today with flaccid
(1) **DTR**s. She states that she stepped on a rusty nail yesterday and
received an (2) **IM** tetanus injection. After a complete history and physical
examination, an (3) **EMG** was scheduled. Differential diagnoses at this
time include (4) **MD** and (5) **FM**. Treatment and prognosis will be decided
by test results.
SIGNED: Marilyn Shaski, MD

1. _____

2. _____

3. _____

4. _____

5. _____

EXERCISE 20

Select the best answer for each statement or question.

1. Select the term that means muscle pain.
   a. dyskinesia
   b. myositis
   c. myasthenia
   d. myalgia

2. Choose the term for tissue that connects muscle to bones.
   a. fascia
   b. ligament
   c. tendon
   d. suture

3. Which tissue connects bone to bone?
   a. tendon
   b. fascia
   c. ligament
   d. suture

4. Which tissue holds muscle fibers together?
   a. tendon
   b. ligament
   c. suture
   d. fascia

5. Select the term for suturing a muscle.
   a. myoplasty
   b. myopexy
   c. myorrhaphy
   d. myorrhexis

6. Choose the medical term for recording the electrical activity of muscles.
   a. electromyogram
   b. electromyograph
   c. electrocardiography
   d. electromyography

7. Select the genetic/hereditary disease known as floppy infant syndrome.
    a. muscular dystrophy
    b. Werdnig-Hoffman disease
    c. Charcot-Marie-Tooth disease
    d. rhabdomyolitis

8. Which disease is categorized as a chronic pain illness with widespread muscle aches?
    a. Charcot-Marie-Tooth disease
    b. myasthenia gravis
    c. myodynia
    d. fibromyalgia

9. A malignant tumor of skeletal muscle is called
    a. rhabdomyolitis
    b. leiomyofibroma
    c. rhabdosarcoma
    d. myoma

10. Select the medical term for repetitive stress syndrome.
    a. carpal tunnel syndrome
    b. contracture
    c. hypertrophy
    d. dystonia

11. Which medical term has the opposite meaning of abduction?
    a. circumduction
    b. adduction
    c. pronation
    d. suppination

12. The muscle movement that opposes extension is called
    a. dorsiflexion
    b. plantar flexion
    c. rotation
    d. flexion

13. Moving the foot and toes upward toward the leg is called
    a. dorsiflexion
    b. plantar flexion
    c. rotation
    d. flexion

14. Left-to-right movement on an axis or pivot point is called
    a. circumduction
    b. rotation
    c. supination
    d. pronation

15. Moving the palms forward or upward is called
    a. rotation
    b. pronation
    c. supination
    d. flexion

Pronunciation Review

Review the terms in the chapter. Pronounce each term using the following phonetic pronunciations. Check off each term when you are comfortable saying it.

TERM	PRONUNCIATION
☐ abduction	ab-**DUCK**-shun
☐ adduction	ad-**DUCK**-shun
☐ atrophy	**AT**-troh-fee
☐ bradykinesia	**brad**-ee-kih-**NEE**-see-ah
☐ circumduction	**sir**-kum-**DUCK**-shun
☐ contraction	con-**TRACK**-shun
☐ contracture	con-**TRACK**-cher
☐ disuse atrophy	**DISS**-yoos **AT**-troh-fee
☐ dorsiflexion	**dor**-see-**FLEX**-shun
☐ dyskinesia	**diss**-kih-**NEE**-see-ah
☐ dystonia	dis-**TOH**-nee-ah
☐ dystrophy	**DIS**-troh-fee
☐ electromyogram	ee-**lek**-troh-**MY**-oh-gram
☐ electromyography	ee-**lek**-troh-my-**OG**-rah-fee
☐ extension	ecks-**TEN**-shun
☐ fascia	**FASH**-ee-ah
☐ fasciitis	**fash**-ee-**EYE**-tis
☐ fasciotomy	fash-ee-**OTT**-oh-mee
☐ fibroma	fih-**BROH**-mah
☐ fibromyalgia	**figh**-broh-my-**AL**-jee-ah
☐ flexion	**FLEK**-shun
☐ ganglion cyst	**GANG**-lee-on **SIST**
☐ ganglionectomy	**gang**-lee-oh-**NEK**-toh-mee
☐ hyperkinesia	**high**-per-kih-**NEE**-see-ah
☐ hypertrophy	high-**PER**-troh-fee
☐ intramuscular	**in**-trah-**MUSS**-kyoo-lar
☐ leiomyofibroma	**ligh**-oh-**my**-oh-fih-**BROH**-mah
☐ ligament	**LIG**-ah-ment
☐ muscular dystrophy	**MUSS**-kyoo-lar **DIS**-troh-fee
☐ myalgia	my-**AL**-jee-ah
☐ myasthenia	**my**-ass-**THEE**-nee-ah
☐ myasthenia gravis	**my**-ass-**THEE**-nee-ah **GRAV**-is
☐ myoplasty	**MY**-oh-plass-tee
☐ myorrhaphy	my-**OR**-ah-fee
☐ myositis	**my**-oh-**SIGH**-tis
☐ plantar flexion	**PLAN**-tar **FLEK**-shun

☐ polymyositis **pall**-ee-**my**-oh-**SIGH**-tis
☐ pronation proh-**NAY**-shun
☐ rhabdomyosarcoma **rab**-doh-**my**-oh-sar-**KOH**-mah
☐ rotation roh-**TAY**-shun
☐ striated muscle **STRIGH**-ay-ted muscle
☐ supination **soo**-pin-**AY**-shun
☐ tendinitis, tenditis **ten**-din-**EYE**-tis, ten-**DIGH**-tis
☐ tendon **TEN**-don
☐ tenodynia ten-oh-**DIN**-ee-ah
☐ tenomyoplasty **ten**-oh-**MY**-oh-plass-tee
☐ tenorrhaphy ten-**OR**-ah-fee
☐ tenosynovectomy **ten**-oh-**sin**-oh-**VEK**-toh-mee
☐ tenosynovitis **ten**-oh-**sin**-oh-**VIGH**-tis
☐ torticollis tor-tih-**KALL**-lis

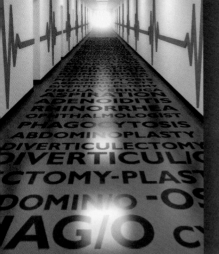

6 Cardiovascular System

OBJECTIVES

At the completion of this chapter, the student should be able to:

1. Identify, define, and spell word roots associated with the cardiovascular system.
2. Label the basic structures of the cardiovascular system.
3. Discuss the functions of the cardiovascular system.
4. Provide the correct spelling of cardiovascular terms, given the definition of the terms.
5. Analyze cardiovascular terms by defining the roots, prefixes, and suffixes of these terms.
6. Identify, define, and spell disease, disorder, and procedure terms related to the cardiovascular system.

OVERVIEW

The cardiovascular system is made up of the heart and blood vessels. The blood vessels include arteries, arterioles, veins, venules, and capillaries. The structures of the cardiovascular system function together for the following purposes: (1) to pump blood to the tissues and cells of the body; (2) to distribute oxygen and nutrients to the tissues and cells; and (3) to remove carbon dioxide and other waste products from the tissues and cells.

Cardiovascular System Word Roots

To understand and use the cardiovascular system medical terms, it is necessary to acquire a thorough knowledge of the associated word roots. Word roots associated with the cardiovascular system are listed with the combining vowel in Table 6-1. Review the word roots and complete the exercises that follow.

TABLE 6-1 CARDIOVASCULAR SYSTEM ROOT WORDS

Word Root/Combining Form	Meaning
aneurysm/o	aneurysm
angi/o	blood or lymph vessel
aort/o	aorta
arter/o; arteri/o	artery
arteriol/o	arteriole
ather/o	fatty, yellowish plaque

(continues)

TABLE 6-1 CARDIOVASCULAR SYSTEM ROOT WORDS (continued)

Word Root/Combining Form	Meaning
cardi/o	heart
coron/o	heart; heart vessel; coronary artery
ech/o	sound
electr/o	electrical
my/o	muscle
phleb/o	vein
ven/o	vein
ventricul/o	ventricle of the heart

© 2016 Cengage Learning®

EXERCISE 1

Write the definitions of the following word roots.

1. cardi/o   _____

2. my/o   _____

3. angi/o   _____

4. arter/o   _____

5. coron/o   _____

6. ventricul/o   _____

7. arteriol/o   _____

8. ech/o   _____

9. ather/o   _____

10. phleb/o   _____

EXERCISE 2

Write and define the word root in each medical term.

1. cardiologist

    ROOT: _____ MEANING: _____

2. myocardium

    ROOT: _____ MEANING: _____

3. angiography

    ROOT: _____ MEANING: _____

4. endocarditis

    ROOT: _____ MEANING: _____

5. electrocardiography

    ROOT: _____ MEANING: _____

6. coronary

ROOT: _____   MEANING: _____

7. arteriole

ROOT: _____   MEANING: _____

8. cardiomegaly

ROOT: _____   MEANING: _____

9. tachycardia

ROOT: _____   MEANING: _____

10. phlebitis

ROOT: _____   MEANING: _____

EXERCISE 3

Write the correct word root(s) for the following definitions.

1. electrical   _____

2. artery   _____

3. fatty, yellowish plaque   _____

4. muscle   _____

5. heart   _____

6. sound   _____

7. vessel   _____

8. aneurysm   _____

9. vein   _____

Structures of the Cardiovascular System

The major structures of the cardiovascular system are the heart and blood vessels, which include arteries, capillaries, and veins. The unique characteristics of cardiovascular system structures are presented individually.

Heart

The heart is about the size of a fist and is located in the **mediastinum** (**mee**-dee-ah-**STIGH**-num), the space between the lungs. Figure 6-1 shows the position of the heart. Figure 6-2 illustrates the chambers of the heart, and septum. Figure 6-3 illustrates the coronary arteries and coronary veins. Refer to these figures as you read about the structures of the heart.

The heart is divided into four chambers. The right and left upper chambers are the (1) **atria** (**atrium**, singular), and the right and left lower chambers are the (2) **ventricles**. A wall called the (3) **septum** separates the chambers. (4) **Coronary arteries** bring oxygen and nutrients to the heart tissue, and (5) **coronary veins** take waste-filled blood away from heart tissue.

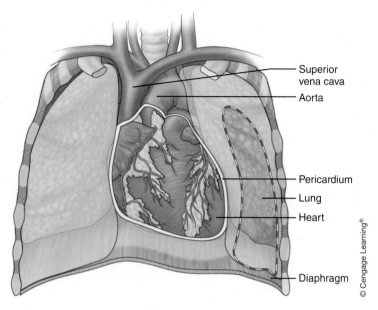

Figure 6-1 Position of the heart in the mediastinum.

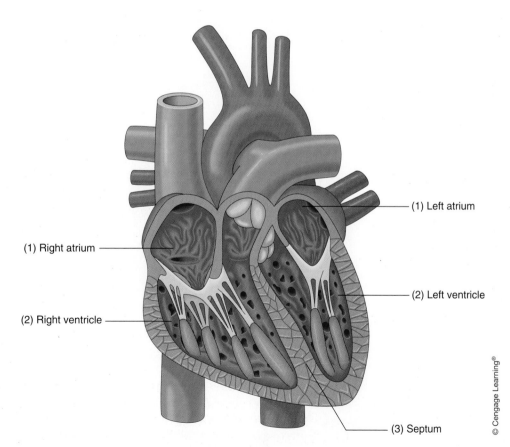

Figure 6-2 Atria, ventricles, and septum of the heart.

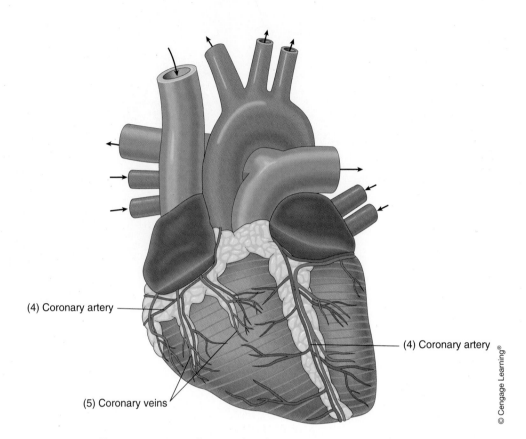

Figure 6-3 Coronary arteries and veins.

(4) Coronary artery

(4) Coronary artery

(5) Coronary veins

© Cengage Learning®

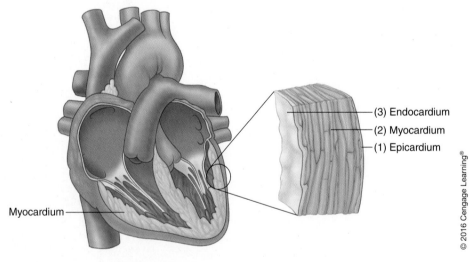

Figure 6-4 A simplified view of the tissues of the heart wall.

(3) Endocardium
(2) Myocardium
(1) Epicardium

Myocardium

© 2016 Cengage Learning®

The heart wall has three layers of tissue as shown in Figure 6-4. Refer to this figure as you read about the layers of the heart wall.

The (1) **epicardium** (**ep**-ih-**KAR**-dee-um) is the outer layer of the heart wall. The (2) **myocardium** (my-oh-**KAR**-dee-um) is the thick, muscular, middle layer of

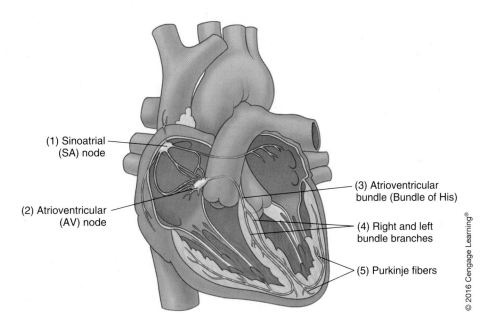

(1) Sinoatrial (SA) node

(2) Atrioventricular (AV) node

(3) Atrioventricular bundle (Bundle of His)

(4) Right and left bundle branches

(5) Purkinje fibers

© 2016 Cengage Learning®

Figure 6-5 Electrical system of the heart.

the heart wall. The (3) **endocardium** (en-doh-**KAR**-dee-um) is the inner layer of the heart wall. A membrane sac, the **pericardium** (pair-ih-**KAR**-dee-um), surrounds and encloses the heart. The pericardium is double-folded membrane that covers the heart and lines the mediastinum. The space between the two folds is called the **pericardial cavity**, and this space is filled with **pericardial fluid**.

Electrical System of the Heart

The pumping action of the heart is controlled by a complex electrical system. The heart's electrical system consists of specialized cardiac muscle tissue that generates the electric impulses, which cause the heart to contract and relax. Figure 6-5 illustrates the key structures of the heart's electrical system. Refer to this figure as you read about the heart's electrical system.

The (1) **sinoatrial** (**sigh**-noh-**AY**-tree-al) **node** (**SA node**) is located in the right atrium. The sinoatrial node is often called the pacemaker because it starts the electrical impulse. The (2) **atrioventricular** (ay-tree-oh-ven-**TRIK**-yoo-lar) **node** (**AV node**) is located between the right atrium and right ventricle. The AV node carries the impulse to the (3) **atrioventricular bundle**. The atrioventricular bundle, also called the **bundle of His**, is located in the septum between the atria and ventricles.

The atrioventricular bundle divides into the right and left (4) **bundle branches**, which are located in the septum between the ventricles. The bundle branches carry the electrical impulse to the (5) **Purkinje** (per-**KIN**-jee) fibers located in the right and left ventricles. These fibers relay the electrical impulses to the cells of the ventricles. This stimulation causes the ventricles to contract. Blood is pushed out of the heart into the **aorta** (ay-**OR**-tah) and **pulmonary** (**PUHL**-mon-**air**-ee) arteries. The aorta sends blood to the body, and the pulmonary arteries send blood to the lungs.

Blood Vessels

Blood vessels carry blood to and from the heart as the blood circulates through the body. The blood vessels include arteries, arterioles, capillaries, veins, and venules. Figure 6-6 illustrates some of the major arteries, and Figure 6-7 illustrates some of the major veins.

(1) **Arteries** are large, thick-walled vessels that carry the blood away from the heart. (2) **Veins** have thinner walls and carry blood to the heart. Arteries branch into smaller vessels called (3) **arterioles**. Arterioles branch into minute vessels called (4) **capillaries**. Oxygen and nutrients pass through the capillaries into the cells. Carbon dioxide and waste products from the cells pass into the (5) **venules** (**VEN**-yoolz). Venules are the smallest veins. Figure 6-8 is a simplified illustration of the relationship between arteries, arterioles, capillaries, venules, and veins.

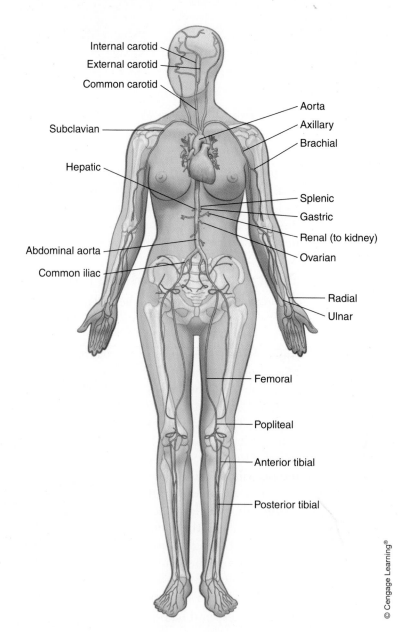

© Cengage Learning®

Figure 6-6 Anterior view, major arteries.

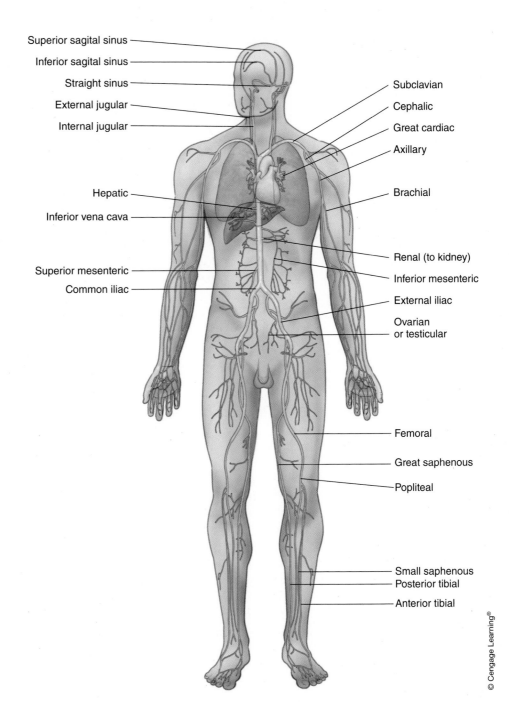

Figure 6-7 Anterior view, major veins.

Circulation

Circulation is the movement of blood to and from the heart. Oxygen-rich blood must be delivered to the cells. Waste-filled (oxygen-poor) blood must be removed from the cells. Refer to Figure 6-9 as you read the description of the circulation process.

- Waste-filled blood is carried to the right atrium by way of the (1) **superior vena cava** and the (2) **inferior vena cava**, the largest veins in the body.

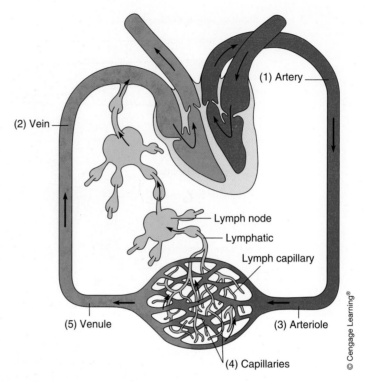

Figure 6-8 Relationship between arteries, arterioles, capillaries, venules, and veins.

- When the right atrium contracts, the waste-filled blood is pushed through the (3) **tricuspid valve** into the right ventricle.
- The right ventricle contracts and pushes the waste-filled blood through the (4) **pulmonary valve** into the right and left (5) **pulmonary arteries**, which lead to the lungs.
- In the lungs, waste products are removed from the blood and the blood picks up oxygen and becomes **oxygenated**.
- The oxygenated blood is sent to the left atrium by way of the right and left (6) **pulmonary veins**.
- When the left atrium contracts, the blood is pushed through the (7) **bicuspid** or **mitral valve** into the left ventricle.
- The left ventricle contracts and sends the blood through the (8) **aortic valve** into the (9) **aorta**, the largest artery in the body.
- The aorta branches into arteries and arteries branch into arterioles so the oxygenated blood can be distributed to the cells.

The circulation of blood from the heart to the lungs and back to the heart is called **pulmonary circulation**. The circulation of blood from the heart to the rest of the body and back to the heart is called **systemic circulation**. Figure 6-10 is a simplified illustration of systemic and pulmonary circulation.

Blood Pressure

Blood pressure is defined as the pressure that circulating blood exerts on the walls of arteries, the veins, and the chambers of the heart. A routine blood pressure check

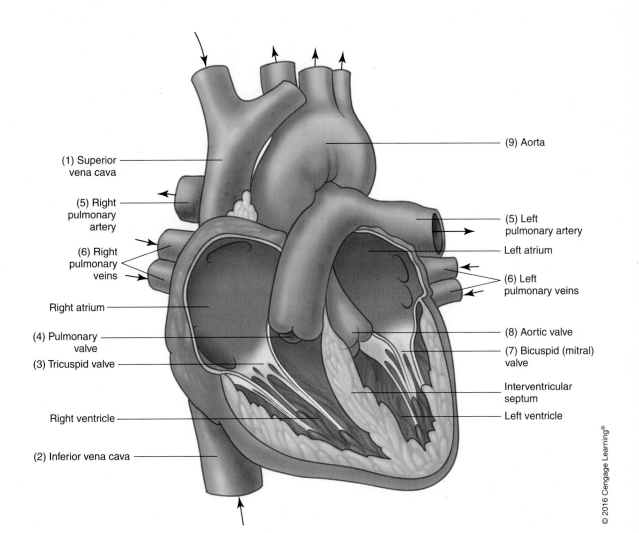

(1) Superior vena cava

(5) Right pulmonary artery

(6) Right pulmonary veins

Right atrium

(4) Pulmonary valve

(3) Tricuspid valve

Right ventricle

(2) Inferior vena cava

(9) Aorta

(5) Left pulmonary artery

Left atrium

(6) Left pulmonary veins

(8) Aortic valve

(7) Bicuspid (mitral) valve

Interventricular septum

Left ventricle

© 2016 Cengage Learning®

Figure 6-9 Circulation of blood to and from the heart.

identifies the pressure exerted on arterial walls. The instrument used to measure this pressure is called a **sphygmomanometer** (**sfig**-moh-man-**AH**-meh-ter), commonly known as a blood pressure cuff. This instrument measures two pressures: (1) **systolic** (sis-**TALL**-ik) pressure; and (2) **diastolic** (**digh**-ah-**STALL**-ik) pressure. Systolic pressure is defined as arterial wall pressure during heart muscle contraction. Diastolic pressure is defined as arterial wall pressure during heart muscle relaxation, or rest period.

Blood pressure measurements are recorded as millimeters (mm) of mercury (Hg). The systolic pressure is given first and the diastolic pressure is given second, as in 120/80 mmHg. In this example, the systolic pressure is 120 and the diastolic pressure is 80. Many factors, such as age, gender, weight, physical health, and emotional state, might affect your blood pressure. In general, a normal systolic pressure ranges from 90 to less than 140 mmHg, and a normal diastolic pressure ranges from 50 to less than 90 mmHg.

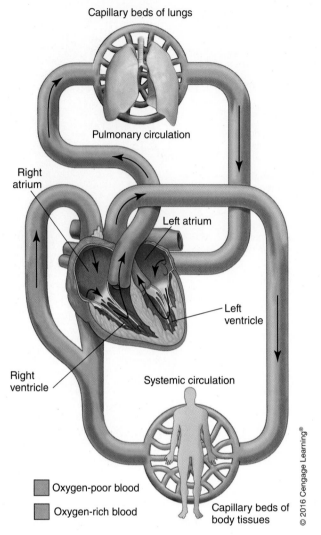

Capillary beds of lungs

Pulmonary circulation

Right atrium

Left atrium

Left ventricle

Right ventricle

Systemic circulation

☐ Oxygen-poor blood

☐ Oxygen-rich blood

Capillary beds of body tissues

© 2016 Cengage Learning®

Figure 6-10 Systemic and pulmonary circulation.

EXERCISE 4

Match the cardiovascular system structures in Column 1 with the correct definition in Column 2.

COLUMN 1

_____ 1. aorta

_____ 2. arteries

_____ 3. atria

_____ 4. capillaries

_____ 5. endocardium

_____ 6. epicardium

_____ 7. myocardium

COLUMN 2

a. carry blood away from the heart

b. carry blood from the lungs to the left atrium

c. inner layer of the heart

d. largest artery in the body

e. carry blood from the right ventricle to the lungs

f. carry blood to the heart

g. largest vein in the body

COLUMN 1	COLUMN 2
____ 8. pulmonary arteries	h. lower chambers of the heart
____ 9. pulmonary veins	i. muscle layer of the heart wall
____ 10. septum	j. outer layer of the heart wall
____ 11. veins	k. smallest, minute blood vessels
____ 12. vena cava	l. upper chambers of the heart
____ 13. ventricles	m. wall between the heart chambers

EXERCISE 5

Circle the term that best fits the definition.

DEFINITION	CIRCLE ONE TERM
1. cause ventricular contraction	*bundle branches* OR *sinoatrial node*
2. between the right atrium and right ventricle	*sinoatrial node* OR *atrioventricular node*
3. located in the septum between the atria and ventricles	*atrioventricular bundle* OR *sinoatrial node*
4. pacemaker of the heart	*sinoatrial node* OR *bundle branches*
5. between the left atrium and left ventricle	*aortic valve* OR *bicuspid valve*
6. between the left ventricle and the aorta	*aortic valve* OR *bicuspid valve*
7. between the right atrium and right ventricle	*pulmonary valve* OR *tricuspid valve*
8. between the right ventricle and pulmonary arteries	*pulmonary valve* OR *tricuspid valve*

EXERCISE 6

Label the heart and related structures in Figure 6-11. Write your answers on the spaces provided.

1. _____

2. _____

3. _____

4. _____

5. _____

6. _____

7. _____

8. _____

9. _____

10. _____

11. _____

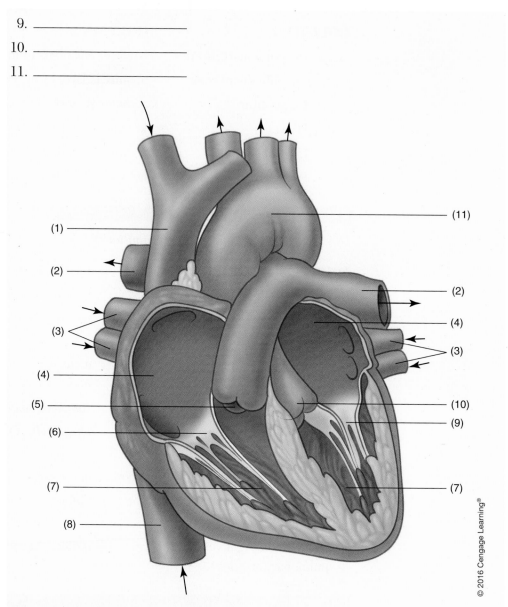

Figure 6-11 Heart and related structures.

© 2016 Cengage Learning®

Cardiovascular System Medical Terminology

Cardiovascular medical terms are organized into three main categories: (1) general medical terms; (2) disease and condition terms; and (3) diagnostic procedure, surgery, and laboratory test terms. There are several roots, prefixes, and suffixes commonly used in many cardiovascular terms. The roots, with the combining vowel, prefixes, and suffixes, are listed in Table 6-2. Review these word parts and complete the related exercises.

TABLE 6-2   ROOTS, PREFIXES, AND SUFFIXES FOR CARDIOVASCULAR SYSTEM TERMS

Word Root	Meaning	Prefix	Meaning	Suffix	Meaning
ischi/o	deficiency, blockage	brady-	slow	-graph	instrument to record
sphygm/o	pulse	poly-	many	-graphy	process of recording
steth/o	chest	tachy-	fast	-gram	record picture
thromb/o	clot			-megaly	enlarged
				-pathy	disease
				-sclerosis	hardening
				-stenosis	narrowing

© 2016 Cengage Learning®

EXERCISE 7

Write the word root, prefix, suffix, and their meanings on the space provided.

EXAMPLE: thrombosclerosis
ROOT: thromb/o   MEANING: clot
PREFIX: no prefix   MEANING: none
SUFFIX: -sclerosis   MEANING: hardening

1. sphygmomanometer

    ROOT: _____ MEANING: _____

    PREFIX: _____ MEANING: _____

    SUFFIX: _____ MEANING: _____

2. angiopathy

    ROOT: _____ MEANING: _____

    PREFIX: _____ MEANING: _____

    SUFFIX: _____ MEANING: _____

3. thrombosis

    ROOT: _____ MEANING: _____

    PREFIX: _____ MEANING: _____

    SUFFIX: _____ MEANING: _____

4. stethoscope

    ROOT: _____ MEANING: _____

    PREFIX: _____ MEANING: _____

    SUFFIX: _____ MEANING: _____

5. bradycardia

ROOT: _____   MEANING: _____

PREFIX: _____   MEANING: _____

SUFFIX: _____   MEANING: _____

6. tachycardia

ROOT: _____   MEANING: _____

PREFIX: _____   MEANING: _____

SUFFIX: _____   MEANING: _____

7. arteriosclerosis

ROOT: _____   MEANING: _____

PREFIX: _____   MEANING: _____

SUFFIX: _____   MEANING: _____

8. angiostenosis

ROOT: _____   MEANING: _____

PREFIX: _____   MEANING: _____

SUFFIX: _____   MEANING: _____

9. angiography

ROOT: _____   MEANING: _____

PREFIX: _____   MEANING: _____

SUFFIX: _____   MEANING: _____

10. cardiogram

ROOT: _____   MEANING: _____

PREFIX: _____   MEANING: _____

SUFFIX: _____   MEANING: _____

EXERCISE 8

Analyze each term by writing the prefix, root, combining vowel, and suffix separated by vertical slashes. Based on the meaning of the word parts, write a definition for each term.

EXAMPLE: thrombosclerosis

	thromb	*/ o*	*/ sclerosis*
prefix	*root*	*combining vowel*	*suffix*

DEFINITION: hardening of clots

1. angiopathy

prefix	*root*	*combining vowel*	*suffix*

DEFINITION: _____

2. thrombosis

prefix	root	combining vowel	suffix

DEFINITION: _____

3. stethoscope

prefix	root	combining vowel	suffix

DEFINITION: _____

4. bradycardia

prefix	root	combining vowel	suffix

DEFINITION: _____

5. tachycardia

prefix	root	combining vowel	suffix

DEFINITION: _____

6. arteriosclerosis

prefix	root	combining vowel	suffix

DEFINITION: _____

7. angiostenosis

prefix	root	combining vowel	suffix

DEFINITION: _____

8. angiography

prefix	root	combining vowel	suffix

DEFINITION: _____

9. cardiogram

prefix	root	combining vowel	suffix

DEFINITION: _____

Cardiovascular System General Medical Terms

Review the cardiovascular system general medical terms listed in Table 6-3. Complete the exercises for these terms.

TABLE 6-3 CARDIOVASCULAR SYSTEM GENERAL MEDICAL TERMS

Term with Pronunciation	Definition
blood pressure (BP)	the pressure exerted by circulating blood on the walls of the arteries

(continues)

TABLE 6-3 CARDIOVASCULAR SYSTEM GENERAL MEDICAL TERMS
(continued)

Term with Pronunciation	Definition
bruits (broo-**EEZ**)	abnormal blowing sounds or murmurs heard while listening to the blood flow through the arteries
cardiologist (**kar**-dee-**ALL**-oh-jist) cardi/o=heart -(o)logist=specialist	physician who specializes in diseases, disorders, and treatments related to the cardiovascular system
cardiology (**kar**-dee-**ALL**-oh-jee) cardi/o=heart -(o)logy=study of	study of the functions, structures, and disorders of the heart
diastole (digh-**ASS**-toh-lee)	period of time when the ventricles relax between contractions
occlusion (oh-**KLOO**-shun)	a blockage in a vessel, cavity, or passage of the body
sphygmomanometer (**sfig**-moh-man-**AH**-meh-ter) sphygm/o=pulse -meter=instrument to measure	instrument used to measure blood pressure
stethoscope (**STETH**-oh-skohp)	instrument used to listen to the sounds of the heart, chest, and lungs
systole (**SISS**-toh-lee)	period of time during ventricular contraction

© 2016 Cengage Learning®

EXERCISE 9

Write the medical term for each definition.

1. abnormal blowing sounds _____
2. blockage in a vessel or cavity _____
3. instrument used to listen to chest/heart sounds _____
4. instrument used to measure blood pressure _____
5. period of time during ventricular contraction _____
6. period of time of ventricular relaxation _____
7. physician heart specialist _____
8. pressure blood exerts on arterial walls _____
9. study of the heart _____

Cardiovascular System Disease and Disorder Terms

Cardiovascular system diseases and disorders include familiar problems such as hypertension and high blood pressure as well as more complex and less familiar diagnoses such as patent ductus arteriosis (i.e., an abnormal opening between the pulmonary artery and aorta). The medical terms are presented in alphabetical order. Review the pronunciation and definition for each term in Table 6-4 and complete the exercises.

TABLE 6-4 CARDIOVASCULAR SYSTEM DISEASE AND DISORDER TERMS

Term with Pronunciation	Definition
aneurysm (**AN**-yoo-rizm)	localized dilatation or ballooning of an artery at a weak point in the vessel wall
angina pectoris (**AN**-jin-ah, **or** an-**JIGH**-nah, **PECK**-tor-is)	severe pain and constriction around the heart; feeling of extreme pressure in the anterior chest
angiocarditis (an-jee-oh-kar-**DIGH**-tis) angi/o = vessels cardi/o = heart -itis = inflammation	Inflammation of the blood vessels of the heart
angiospasm (**AN**-jee-oh-spazm) angi/o = vessel -spasm = involuntary contraction	abnormal contraction of the blood vessels, primarily the arteries
aortic stenosis (ay-**OR**-tik sten-**OH**-sis) aort/o = aorta -ic = pertaining to sten/o = narrow, narrowing -osis = abnormal condition	abnormal narrowing of the aorta
arrhythmia (ah-**RITH**-mee-ah)	any irregular heartbeat
arteriosclerosis (ar-**tee**-ree-oh-skleh-**ROH**-sis) arteri/o = artery -sclerosis = hardening	hardening of the arteries
arteriosclerotic heart disease (ASHD) (ar-**tee**-ree-oh-skleh-**RAH**-tic) arteri/o = artery -sclerosis = hardening -ic = pertaining to	heart disease caused by hardening of the arteries
atherosclerosis (**ath**-eh-roh-skleh-**ROH**-sis) ather/o = fat -sclerosis = hardening	hardening and narrowing of the arteries due to deposits of fat and other debris along arterial walls (Figure 6-12)

(continues)

TABLE 6-4   CARDIOVASCULAR SYSTEM DISEASE AND DISORDER TERMS
(continued)

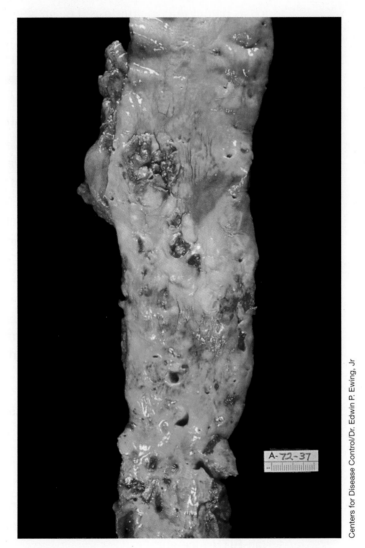

Centers for Disease Control/Dr. Edwin P. Ewing, Jr

Figure 6-12   Atherosclerosis; fatty plaque deposits along the interior wall of the aorta (Centers for Disease Control and Prevention/Dr. Edwin P. Ewing Jr.).

Term with Pronunciation	Definition
atrioventricular defect (**ay**-tree-oh-ven-**TRIK**-yoo-lar)	an abnormal opening between the atria and ventricles
bradycardia (**brad**-ih-**KAR**-dee-ah) brady = slow cardi/o = heart -ia = condition	slow heart rate; less than 60 beats per minute
bundle branch block (BBB)	interruption of the electrical impulse of the heart to the right or left bundle branch

(continues)

TABLE 6-4 CARDIOVASCULAR SYSTEM DISEASE AND DISORDER TERMS
(continued)

Term with Pronunciation	Definition
cardiac arrest	a sudden and immediate cessation of the heart's pumping action
cardiac tamponade (**KAR**-dee-ak tam-poh-**NAYD**)	compression of the heart due to the accumulation of blood in the pericardial sac
cardiomegaly (**kar**-dee-oh-**MEG**-ah-lee) cardi/o = heart -megaly = enlargement	enlargement of the heart; enlarged heart
cardiomyopathy (**kar**-dee-oh-my-**OP**-ah-thee) cardi/o = heart my/o = muscle -pathy = disease	any disease that affects the structure and function of the heart, and the heart muscle in particular

© 2016 Cengage Learning®

EXERCISE 10

Analyze each term. Write and define the root, prefix, and suffix, and their meanings. Using the word part definitions, write a definition for the term. Use a medical dictionary to check your definition.

EXAMPLE: cardiologist
ROOT: cardi/o   MEANING: heart
PREFIX: none   MEANING: none
SUFFIX: -logist   MEANING: specialist in the study of
DEFINITION: specialist in the study of the heart

1. angiocarditis

ROOT: _____ MEANING: _____

PREFIX: _____ MEANING: _____

SUFFIX: _____ MEANING: _____

DEFINITION: _____

2. arteriosclerosis

ROOT: _____ MEANING: _____

PREFIX: _____ MEANING: _____

SUFFIX: _____ MEANING: _____

DEFINITION: _____

3. atherosclerosis

ROOT: _____ MEANING: _____

PREFIX: _____ MEANING: _____

SUFFIX: _____   MEANING: _____

DEFINITION: _____

4. bradycardia

ROOT: _____   MEANING: _____

PREFIX: _____   MEANING: _____

SUFFIX: _____   MEANING: _____

DEFINITION: _____

5. cardiomegaly

ROOT: _____   MEANING: _____

PREFIX: _____   MEANING: _____

SUFFIX: _____   MEANING: _____

DEFINITION: _____

6. cardiomyopathy

ROOT: _____   MEANING: _____

PREFIX: _____   MEANING: _____

SUFFIX: _____   MEANING: _____

DEFINITION: _____

7. angiospasm

ROOT: _____   MEANING: _____

PREFIX: _____   MEANING: _____

SUFFIX: _____   MEANING: _____

DEFINITION: _____

EXERCISE 11

Replace the italicized phrase with the correct medical term.

1. The *ballooning artery* required immediate attention.

   _____

2. Nitroglycerin might relieve *severe pain and constriction around the heart*.

   _____

3. The child was born with an *abnormal narrowing of the aorta*.

   _____

4. Jules was concerned that his *irregular heartbeat* would prevent him from participating in the Boston Marathon.

   _____

5. Surgery to correct an *abnormal opening between the atria and ventricles* was scheduled for Rashel.

_____

6. Elsa's *heart compression* was caused by a stab wound to the chest.

_____

EXERCISE 12

Match the medical term in Column 1 with the correct definition in Column 2.

COLUMN 1

_____ 1. aneurysm

_____ 2. angina pectoris

_____ 3. aortic stenosis

_____ 4. arrhythmia

_____ 5. ASHD

_____ 6. atherosclerosis

_____ 7. BBB

_____ 8. bradycardia

_____ 9. cardiac arrest

_____ 10. cardiomegaly

_____ 11. cardiomyopathy

COLUMN 2

a. arteriosclerotic heart disease

b. bundle branch block

c. dilatation of an artery

d. disease of the heart and heart muscle

e. enlarged heart

f. feeling of extreme anterior chest pressure

g. hardening of arteries due to fatty deposits

h. irregular heartbeat

i. narrowing of the aorta

j. slow heart rate

k. sudden heart stoppage

Review the pronunciation and definition for each term in Table 6-5 and complete the exercises.

TABLE 6-5   CARDIOVASCULAR SYSTEM DISEASE AND DISORDER TERMS

Term with Pronunciation	Definition
coarctation of the aorta (koh-ark-**TAY**-shun of the ay-**OR**-tah)	congenital condition characterized by the narrowing of a segment of the aorta
congestive heart failure (CHF) (kon-**JESS**-tiv heart failure)	heart condition characterized by impaired cardiac pumping resulting in failure of the ventricles to eject blood
coronary artery disease (CAD) (**KOR**-oh-nair-ee **AR**-ter-ee **DIS**-eez)	any abnormal condition of the arteries of the heart
coronary occlusion (**KOR**-oh-nair-ee oh-**KLOO**-zhun)	an obstruction of any one of the coronary arteries

(continues)

TABLE 6-5   CARDIOVASCULAR SYSTEM DISEASE AND DISORDER TERMS
(continued)

Term with Pronunciation	Definition
coronary thrombosis (**KOR**-oh-nair-ee throm-**BOH**-sis) thromb/o = clot -osis = condition of	development of a blood clot in a coronary artery
deep vein thrombosis (DVT)	presence of a blood clot in a deep vein
endocarditis (**en**-doh-kar-**DIGH**-tis) end/o = within cardi/o = heart -itis = inflammation	inflammation of the endocardium or inner layer of the heart wall
fibrillation (fih-brih-**LAY**-shun)	rapid and incomplete contractions of the atria or ventricles
hypertension (high-per-**TEN**-shun)	elevated or high blood pressure
hypertensive heart disease (HHD) (high-per-**TEN**-siv)	heart disease caused by long-term elevated or high blood pressure
hypotension (high-poh-**TEN**-shun)	abnormally low blood pressure
ischemia (iss-**KEE**-mee-ah) isch/o = deficiency, blockage -emia = blood	deficient or decreased blood supply to a body part; might be caused by atherosclerosis
mitral valve prolapse (**MY**-tral valve **PROH**-laps)	protrusion of one or both of the flaps of the mitral valve into the left atrium
mitral valve stenosis (**MY**-tral valve sten-**OH**-sis)	narrowing of the mitral valve due to scarring
myocardial infarction (MI) (my-oh-**KAR**-dee-al in-**FARK**-shun) my/o = muscle cardi/o = heart -al = pertaining to	death of heart muscle due to a lack of oxygen caused by an insufficient blood supply from the coronary arteries; heart attack
myocarditis (**my**-oh-kar-**DIGH**-tis) my/o = muscle cardi/o = heart -itis = inflammation	inflammation of the myocardium, the muscle layer of the heart
palpitation (pal-pih-**TAY**-shun)	abnormally rapid throbbing or fluttering of the heart

EXERCISE 13

Write the medical term for each definition.

1. rapid, incomplete atrial or ventricular contractions _____
2. rapid fluttering of the heart _____
3. abnormally low blood pressure _____
4. elevated or high blood pressure _____
5. narrowing of a segment of an aorta _____
6. inflammation of the endocardium _____
7. inflammation of the myocardium _____

EXERCISE 14

Analyze each term by writing the prefix, root, combining vowel, and suffix separated by vertical slashes. Based on the meaning of the word parts, write a definition for each term. Check your definition in a medical dictionary.

1. ischemia

   _____
   prefix　　　　　*root*　　　　　*combining vowel*　　　　　*suffix*
   DEFINITION: _____

2. endocarditis

   _____
   prefix　　　　　*root*　　　　　*combining vowel*　　　　　*suffix*
   DEFINITION: _____

3. myocarditis

   _____
   prefix　　　　　*root*　　　　　*combining vowel*　　　　　*suffix*
   DEFINITION: _____

4. cardiomyopathy

   _____
   prefix　　　　　*root*　　　　　*combining vowel*　　　　　*suffix*
   DEFINITION: _____

5. atherosclerosis

   _____
   prefix　　　　　*root*　　　　　*combining vowel*　　　　　*suffix*
   DEFINITION: _____

EXERCISE 15

Write out each abbreviation.

1. CHF _____
2. HHD _____
3. MI _____

4. DVT   _____
5. CAD   _____

EXERCISE 16

Circle the medical term that best fits the definition.

DEFINITION	CIRCLE ONE TERM
1. obstruction of a coronary artery	*coronary thrombosis* OR *coronary occlusion*
2. deficient blood supply	*ischemia* OR *hypotension*
3. narrowing of the mitral valve	*mitral valve prolapse* OR *mitral valve stenosis*
4. blood clot in a coronary artery	*coronary thrombosis* OR *coronary occlusion*
5. protrusion of a mitral valve flap into the atrium	*mitral valve prolapse* OR *mitral valve stenosis*

Review the pronunciation and definition for each term in Table 6-6 and complete the exercises.

TABLE 6-6 CARDIOVASCULAR SYSTEM DISEASE AND DISORDER TERMS

Term with Pronunciation	Definition
paroxysmal atrial tachycardia (PAT) (pair-ok-**SIZ**-mal atrial tak-ih-**KAR**-dee-ah) tachy- = fast cardi/o = heart -a = noun ending	rapid atrial contractions that begin and end suddenly; usually from 150 to 240 beats per minute
patent ductus arteriosus (**PAY**-tent **DUK**-tus ar-tee-ree-**OH**-sis)	congenital opening between the main pulmonary artery and the aorta
pericarditis (**pair**-ih-kar-**DIGH**-tis)	inflammation of the pericardium
pitting edema	abnormal swelling of the skin of the extremities that, when pressed firmly, maintains the depression or dimpling created by the pressure
polyarteritis (**pall**-ee-ar-teh-**RIGH**-tis)	inflammation of medium and small arteries
premature atrial contraction (PAC) (**PRE**-mah-chur **AY**-tree-al kon-**TRACK**-shun)	irregular heart rhythm characterized by atrial contractions occurring before the expected time

(continues)

TABLE 6-6   CARDIOVASCULAR SYSTEM DISEASE AND DISORDER TERMS
(continued)

Term with Pronunciation	Definition
premature ventricular contraction (PVC) (**PRE**-mah-chur ven-**TRIK**-yoo-lar kon-**TRACK**-shun)	irregular heart rhythm characterized by ventricular contractions occurring before the expected time
rheumatic fever (roo-**MAT**-ik)	a systemic disease characterized by fever, joint pain, carditis, and other manifestations; usually follows a streptococcal infection or scarlet fever
rheumatic heart disease (RHD) (roo-**MAT**-ik)	a manifestation of rheumatic fever characterized by endocarditis that often results in damaged heart valves
tachycardia (tak-ih-**KAR**-dee-ah) cardi/o = heart tachy- = fast -a = noun ending	abnormally rapid heartbeat, usually defined as more than 100 beats per minute
thrombophlebitis (**throm**-boh-fleh-**BIGH**-tis) thromb/o = clot phleb/o = vein -itis = inflammation	inflammation of a vein in the presence of blood clot formation
varicose veins (**VAIR**-ih-kohs)	enlarged, twisted, and often dilated veins, most commonly found in the legs and esophagus
vasoconstriction (**vay**-zoh-con-**STRIK**-shun) vas/o = vessel -constriction = narrowing	constriction or narrowing of the diameter of a blood vessel
ventricular tachycardia (ven-**TRIK**-yoo-lar tak-ih-**KAR**-dee-ah) ventricul/o = ventricle -ar = pertaining to cardi/o = heart tachy- = fast -a = noun ending	abnormally rapid heartbeat of the ventricles, usually between 150 and 200 beats per minute

© 2016 Cengage Learning®

EXERCISE 17

Replace the italicized phrases with the correct medical term or phrase.

1. Carlos experienced *sudden rapid atrial contractions* that ended abruptly.

   _____

2. Certain medications will cause *constriction of the diameter of a blood vessel.*

   _____

3. Beth's *congenital opening between the pulmonary artery and aorta* was corrected during surgery.

   _____

4. Li was taking a common steroid medication for *inflammation of several medium and small arteries.*

   _____

5. *Inflammation of the pericardium* treatment includes complete bedrest and a light diet.

   _____

6. *Enlarged and twisted veins* might be painful to the touch.

   _____

7. Anticoagulants are often used to treat *inflammation of a vein with a blood clot.*

   _____

8. An *abnormally rapid heartbeat* might involve the atria or ventricles.

   _____

EXERCISE 18

Write out the following abbreviations.

1. PAT   _____
2. PAC   _____
3. PVC   _____
4. RHD   _____

Cardiovascular System Diagnostic, Surgical, and Treatment Terms

Review the pronunciation and definition of the diagnostic, surgical, and treatment terms in Table 6-7. Complete the exercises.

TABLE 6-7 CARDIOVASCULAR SYSTEM DIAGNOSTIC, SURGICAL, AND TREATMENT TERMS

Term with Pronunciation	Definition
anastomosis (ah-**nas**-toh-**MOH**-sis) ana- = without stom/o = mouth, opening -osis = condition	surgical connection of two vessels or other tubular structures
aneurysmectomy (**an**-yoo-rizm-**EK**-toh-mee)	surgical removal of an aneurysm
angiography (an-jee-**OG**-rah-fee) angi/o = vessel -graphy = process of recording	process of recording an x-ray picture of blood vessels
arteriogram (ar-**TEER**-ee-oh-gram) arteri/o = artery -gram = record; picture	x-ray record or picture of an artery
arteriography (ar-**teer**-ee-**OG**-rah-fee) arteri/o = artery -graphy = process of recording	process of recording an x-ray picture of arteries
cardiac catheterization (**KAR**-dee-ak **kath**-eh-ter-ih-**ZAY**-shun)	an x-ray procedure during which a catheter is guided into the heart through a blood vessel for the purpose of injecting a contrast medium to view and image the heart chambers and coronary arteries; also called left heart catheterization or coronary arteriography (Figure 6-13)
cardiopulmonary resuscitation (CPR) (kar-dee-oh-**PULL**-mon-air-ee ree-**suss**-ih-**TAY**-shun)	procedure for life support consisting of artificial respiration and manual external cardiac compression
coronary artery bypass graft (CABG) (**KOR**-oh-nair-ee **AR**-ter-ee)	surgical procedure that requires implanting a piece of vein onto the heart to bypass a blockage in a coronary artery and to improve blood flow to the heart; commonly called bypass surgery (Figure 6-14)
cardioversion (kar-dee-oh-**VER**-zhun)	restoration of a normal heart rhythm by delivering synchronized electric shocks through paddles placed on the chest

(continues)

TABLE 6-7   CARDIOVASCULAR SYSTEM DIAGNOSTIC, SURGICAL, AND TREATMENT TERMS (continued)

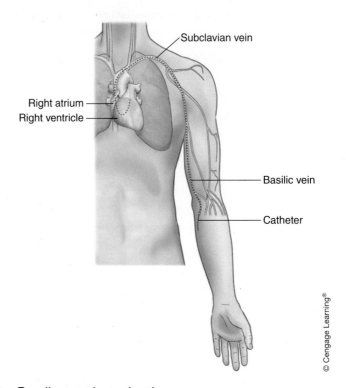

Figure 6-13   Cardiac catheterization.

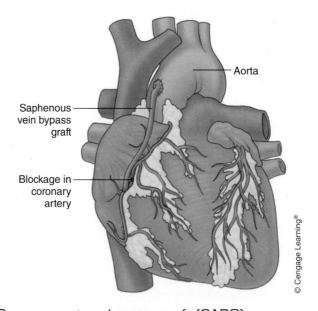

Figure 6-14   Coronary artery bypass graft (CABG).

(continues)

TABLE 6-7   CARDIOVASCULAR SYSTEM DIAGNOSTIC, SURGICAL, AND TREATMENT TERMS (continued)

Term with Pronunciation	Definition
defibrillation (dee-**fib**-rih-**LAY**-shun)	technique used to interrupt ventricular fibrillation and restore a normal heart rhythm by delivering electric shocks to specific areas around the heart
echocardiogram (**ek**-oh-**KAR**-dee-oh-gram) echo- = sound cardi/o = heart -gram = record; picture	graphic record of an ultrasound visualization of the heart
echocardiography (**ek**-oh-**kar**-dee-**OG**-rah-fee) echo- = sound cardi/o = heart -graphy = process of recording	ultrasound diagnostic procedure for the purpose of evaluating and recording the structures and motion of the heart
electrocardiogram (EKG, ECG) (ee-**lek**-troh-**KAR**-dee-oh-gram) electr/o = electricity cardi/o = heart -gram = record; picture	graphic record of the electrical activity of the heart (Figure 6-15)
electrocardiography (ee-**lek**-troh-**kar**-dee-**OG**-rah-fee) electr/o = electricity cardi/o = heart -graphy = process of recording	process of recording the electrical activity of the heart

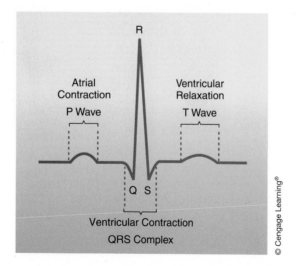

Figure 6-15   Electrocardiogram showing the contraction and relaxation of the heart.

(continues)

TABLE 6-7   CARDIOVASCULAR SYSTEM DIAGNOSTIC, SURGICAL, AND TREATMENT TERMS (continued)

Term with Pronunciation	Definition
endarterectomy (**end**-ar-ter-**EK**-toh-mee) end/o = within arter/i = artery -ectomy = surgical removal	surgical removal of the lining of an artery that is occluded due to fatty deposits
Holter monitoring	process of recording and monitoring heart rate and rhythms over a specific period, usually 24 hours
percutaneous transluminal coronary angioplasty (PTCA) (per-kyoo-**TAY**-nee-us trans-**LOO**-min-al **KOR**-oh-nair-ee **AN**-jee-oh-**plass**-tee)	surgical repair of a coronary artery by inserting a balloon on the end of a catheter into the artery, inflating the balloon, flattening the fatty deposits on the arterial wall, and stretching or increasing the diameter of the artery; a *stent* (wire-mesh tube) may be placed in the artery to provide support to the arterial wall (Figures 6-16A and 6-16B)
thallium stress test (**THAL**-ee-um)	assessment of cardiovascular health and function during and after the application of stress

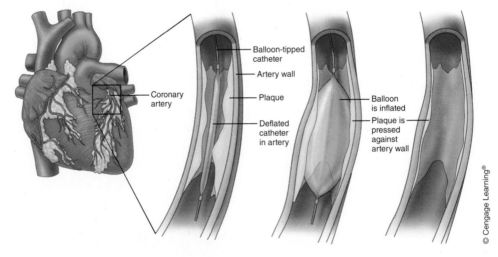

Coronary artery

Balloon-tipped catheter

Artery wall

Plaque

Deflated catheter in artery

Balloon is inflated

Plaque is pressed against artery wall

© Cengage Learning®

Figure 6-16A   Percutaneous transluminal coronary angioplasty (PTCA).

(continues)

TABLE 6-7   CARDIOVASCULAR SYSTEM DIAGNOSTIC, SURGICAL, AND TREATMENT TERMS (continued)

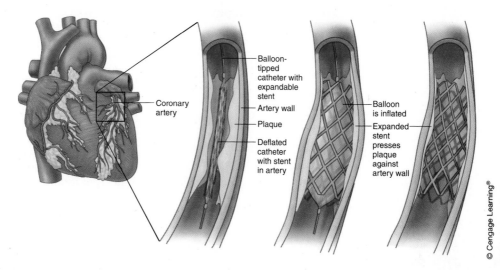

Figure 6-16B Percutaneous transluminal coronary angioplasty (PTCA) with stent placement.

Term with Pronunciation	Definition
transesophageal echocardiography (TEE) (**trans**-eh-soff-ah-**JEE**-al **ek**-oh-**kar**-dee-**OG**-rah-fee) trans- = through esophag/o = esophagus -al = pertaining to ech/o = sound cardi/o = heart -graphy = process of recording	process of viewing and recording the structures of the heart using ultrasound and placing the recording device into the esophagus
valvoplasty (**VAL**-voh-**plass**-tee) valv/o = valve -plasty = surgical repair	surgical repair of a heart valve

© 2016 Cengage Learning®

EXERCISE 19

Change the suffix -graphy to -gram. Rewrite the medical term. Based on the meaning of the new root, write a definition for the new term. Check the definition in a medical dictionary.

EXAMPLE: cardiography cardiogram x-ray film of the heart

1. angiography   NEW TERM: _____

   DEFINITION: _____

2. echocardiography NEW TERM: _____

DEFINITION: _____

3. electrocardiography NEW TERM: _____

DEFINITION: _____

4. arteriography NEW TERM: _____

DEFINITION: _____

EXERCISE 20

Analyze each term by writing the prefix, root, combining vowel, and suffix separated by vertical slashes. Based on the meaning of the word parts, write a definition for each term. Check your definition in a medical dictionary.

1. angiography

prefix	root	combining vowel	suffix

DEFINITION: _____

2. arteriogram

prefix	root	combining vowel	suffix

DEFINITION: _____

3. echocardiography

prefix	root	combining vowel	suffix

DEFINITION: _____

4. echocardiogram

prefix	root	combining vowel	suffix

DEFINITION: _____

5. electrocardiogram

prefix	root	combining vowel	suffix

DEFINITION: _____

6. electrocardiography

prefix	root	combining vowel	suffix

DEFINITION: _____

7. endarterectomy

prefix	root	combining vowel	suffix

DEFINITION: _____

8. valvoplasty

prefix	root	combining vowel	suffix

DEFINITION: _____

EXERCISE 21

Write out the following abbreviations.

1. CPR   _____

2. CABG   _____

3. EKG, ECG   _____

4. PTCA   _____

5. TEE   _____

Abbreviations

Review the cardiovascular system abbreviations in Table 6-8. Practice writing out the meaning of each abbreviation.

TABLE 6-8 ABBREVIATIONS

Abbreviation	Meaning
ASHD	arteriosclerotic heart disease
BBB	bundle branch block
BP	blood pressure
CABG	coronary artery bypass graft
CAD	coronary artery disease
CHF	congestive heart failure
CPR	cardiopulmonary resuscitation
DVT	deep vein thrombosis
HHD	hypertensive heart disease
MI	myocardial infarction
PAC	premature atrial contraction
PAT	paroxysmal atrial tachycardia
PTCA	percutaneous transluminal coronary angioplasty
PVC	premature ventricular contraction
RHD	rheumatic heart disease
TEE	transesophageal echocardiography

© 2016 Cengage Learning®

CHAPTER REVIEW

The Chapter Review can be used as a self-test. Go through each exercise and answer as many questions as you can without referring to previous exercises or earlier discussions within this chapter. Check your answers and fill in any blanks. Practice writing any terms you might have misspelled.

EXERCISE 22

Analyze each term. Write and define the root, prefix, and suffix. Using the word part definitions, write a definition for the term. Use a medical dictionary to check your definition.

1. cardiology

    ROOT: _____ MEANING: _____

    PREFIX: _____ MEANING: _____

    SUFFIX: _____ MEANING: _____

    DEFINITION: _____

2. cardiologist

    ROOT: _____ MEANING: _____

    PREFIX: _____ MEANING: _____

    SUFFIX: _____ MEANING: _____

    DEFINITION: _____

3. angiocarditis

    ROOT: _____ MEANING: _____

    PREFIX: _____ MEANING: _____

    SUFFIX: _____ MEANING: _____

    DEFINITION: _____

4. bradycardia

    ROOT: _____ MEANING: _____

    PREFIX: _____ MEANING: _____

    SUFFIX: _____ MEANING: _____

    DEFINITION: _____

5. cardiomegaly

    ROOT: _____ MEANING: _____

    PREFIX: _____ MEANING: _____

    SUFFIX: _____ MEANING: _____

    DEFINITION: _____

6. cardiomyopathy

    ROOT: _____ MEANING: _____

    PREFIX: _____ MEANING: _____

    SUFFIX: _____ MEANING: _____

    DEFINITION: _____

7. endocarditis

ROOT: _____ MEANING: _____

PREFIX: _____ MEANING: _____

SUFFIX: _____ MEANING: _____

DEFINITION: _____

8. polyarteritis

ROOT: _____ MEANING: _____

PREFIX: _____ MEANING: _____

SUFFIX: _____ MEANING: _____

DEFINITION: _____

9. tachycardia

ROOT: _____ MEANING: _____

PREFIX: _____ MEANING: _____

SUFFIX: _____ MEANING: _____

DEFINITION: _____

10. thrombophlebitis

ROOT: _____ MEANING: _____

PREFIX: _____ MEANING: _____

SUFFIX: _____ MEANING: _____

DEFINITION: _____

EXERCISE 23

Replace the italicized phrase with the correct medical term.

1. During Jackie's physical examination, the physician heard *an abnormal blowing sound.*

   _____

2. Bill was diagnosed with *hardening of the arteries.*

   _____

3. *A sudden and immediate stoppage of heart function* often results in death.

   _____

4. *Rapid and incomplete contractions of the heart* can be corrected with proper medication.

   _____

5. Bette's *abnormally low blood pressure* was due to loss of blood volume.

   _____

6. Jefferson's vascular problem was corrected by *the surgical removal of an aneurysm.*

   _____

7. Brad's echocardiogram revealed *an abnormal narrowing of the aorta.*

   _____

8. *Any irregular heartbeat* should be brought to the physician's attention.

   _____

9. *High blood pressure* can be a symptom of atherosclerosis.

   _____

10. A *heart attack* can occur at any age.

    _____

EXERCISE 24

Match the medical terms in Column 1 with the definitions in Column 2.

COLUMN 1

_____ 1. anastomosis

_____ 2. angina pectoris

_____ 3. angiospasm

_____ 4. arteriogram

_____ 5. blood pressure

_____ 6. cardiac tamponade

_____ 7. diastole

_____ 8. endarterectomy

_____ 9. ischemia

_____ 10. palpitation

_____ 11. sphygmomanometer

_____ 12. systole

_____ 13. valvoplasty

_____ 14. varicose veins

COLUMN 2

a. pressure exerted on arterial and venous walls

b. period of time when ventricles are relaxed

c. period of time when ventricles contract

d. instrument used to measure blood pressure

e. deficient blood supply to a body part

f. abnormal contraction of blood vessels

g. compression of the heart resulting from blood in the pericardial sac

h. severe chest pain

i. abnormal, rapid throbbing or fluttering of the heart

j. enlarged, twisted, and dilated veins

k. surgical connection of two vessels

l. x-ray record or picture of an artery

m. surgical removal of the lining of an artery

n. surgical repair of a heart valve

EXERCISE 25

Read the following discharge summary. Write the meaning of the italicized terms and phrases on the spaces provided.

DISCHARGE SUMMARY

BRIEF HISTORY: This 61-year-old woman was brought into the emergency room unconscious. (1) *Cardiopulmonary resuscitation* was begun immediately. During the ambulance transport, the portable (2) *electrocardiogram* demonstrated (3) *ventricular fibrillation*. The advanced (4) *cardiac* life support procedure was followed.

HOSPITAL COURSE: The patient was placed on the Coronary Care Unit. Family members confirmed a previous history of (5) *myocardial infarction* and a subsequent (6) *coronary artery bypass graft*. There was also a history of (7) *hypertension*. The patient's condition deteriorated, and she was in a coma during her entire hospitalization. The family was in close attendance and realized the severity of the situation. Consultation with the (8) *cardiologist* confirmed that there was extensive (9) *myocardial* tissue death due to (10) *ischemia*.

LABORATORY DATA: The chest x-ray showed (11) *cardiomegaly* and right upper lobe infiltrate. All laboratory tests were abnormal during the hospitalization. (12) *Arterial* blood gases indicated that mechanical ventilation was marginal at best.

DISPOSITION: The patient expired on November 12 with the family present.

1. _____

2. _____

3. _____

4. _____

5. _____

6. _____

7. _____

8. _____

9. _____

10. _____

11. _____

12. _____

EXERCISE 26

Circle the correct answer for each statement.

1. Which heart valve is also known as the bicuspid valve?
   a. aortic valve
   b. mitral valve
   c. pulmonary valve
   d. tricuspid valve

2. Which heart chamber pumps blood to the lungs?
   a. right atrium
   b. left atrium
   c. right ventricle
   d. left ventricle

3. Which heart chamber pumps blood to the aorta?
   a. right atrium
   b. left atrium
   c. right ventricle
   d. left ventricle

4. Select the term for hardening of the arteries.
   a. arteriosclerosis
   b. atherosclerosis
   c. angioconstriction
   d. angioplasty

5. Select the term that represents the largest artery in the body.
   a. pulmonary artery
   b. coronary artery
   c. vena cava
   d. aorta

6. Which heart valve is located between the right atrium and right ventricle?
   a. mitral valve
   b. tricuspid valve
   c. bicuspid valve
   d. pulmonary valve

7. Select the term for the smallest blood vessel.
   a. venule
   b. arteriole
   c. capillary
   d. vein

8. Select the term for the largest vein in the body.
   a. vena cava
   b. pulmonary vein
   c. aorta
   d. coronary vein

9. Select the phrase that means circulation of blood from the heart to the lungs.
   a. systemic circulation
   b. cardiac circulation
   c. oxygenation circulation
   d. pulmonary circulation

10. Select the phrase that means circulation of blood from the heart to the entire body.
    a. pulmonary circulation
    b. cardiac circulation
    c. systemic circulation
    d. oxygenation circulation

11. Restoration of a normal heart rhythm with electric shocks and paddles is called
    a. defibrillation
    b. cardioversion
    c. CPR
    d. cardiofibrillation

12. The technique used to interrupt extremely rapid ventricular contractions is called
    a. cardiofibrillation
    b. cardioversion
    c. defibrillation
    d. CPR

EXERCISE 27

Write out each abbreviation with a brief description.

EXAMPLE: ASHD = arteriosclerotic heart disease
DEFINITION: hardening of the arteries of the heart

1. AV node: _____
   DEFINITION: _____
2. BBB: _____
   DEFINITION: _____
3. BP: _____
   DEFINITION: _____

4. CABG: _____

DEFINITION: _____

5. CAD: _____

DEFINITION: _____

6. CHF: _____

DEFINITION: _____

7. EKG, ECG: _____

DEFINITION: _____

8. HHD: _____

DEFINITION: _____

9. MI: _____

DEFINITION: _____

10. PAC: _____

DEFINITION: _____

11. PAT: _____

DEFINITION: _____

12. PTCA: _____

DEFINITION: _____

13. PVC: _____

DEFINITION: _____

14. RHD: _____

DEFINITION: _____

15. SA node: _____

DEFINITION: _____

16. TEE: _____

DEFINITION: _____

CHALLENGE EXERCISE

Contact or visit your local hospital's patient education department. Request or obtain a pamphlet or pamphlets that describe the cardiac tests performed at the hospital. Read the pamphlet and write or explain the procedure, in your own words, to a family member or classmate.

Pronunciation Review

Review the terms in the chapter. Pronounce each term using the following phonetic pronunciations. Check off each term when you are comfortable saying it.

TERM	PRONUNCIATION
☐ anastomosis	ah-**nass**-toh-**MOH**-sis
☐ aneurysm	**AN**-yoo-rizm
☐ aneurysmectomy	**an**-yoo-rizm-**EK**-toh-mee
☐ angina pectoris	**AN**-jih-nah, *or* an-**JIGH**-nah, **PECK**-tor-is
☐ angiocarditis	**an**-jee-oh-kar-**DIGH**-tis
☐ angiograph	**AN**-jee-oh-graff
☐ angiography	an-jee-**OG**-rah-fee
☐ angiospasm	**AN**-jee-oh-spazm
☐ aorta	ay-**OR**-tah
☐ aortic stenosis	ay-**OR**-tik sten-**OH**-sis
☐ aortic valve	ay-**OR**-tik valve
☐ arrhythmia	ah-**RITH**-mee-ah
☐ arteriogram	ar-**TEER**-ee-oh-gram
☐ arteriole	are-**TEE**-ree-ohl
☐ arteriosclerosis	ar-**tee**-ree-oh-skleh-**ROH**-sis
☐ arteriosclerotic heart disease	ar-**tee**-reh-oh-skleh-**RAH**-tic disease
☐ artery	**AR**-teh-ree
☐ atherosclerosis	**ath**-eh-roh-skleh-**ROH**-sis
☐ atria	**AY**-tree-ah
☐ atrioventricular	**ay**-tree-oh-ven-**TRIK**-yoo-lar
☐ atrioventricular bundle	**ay**-tree-oh-ven-**TRIK**-yoo-lar bundle
☐ atrioventricular defect	**ay**-tree-oh-ven-**TRIK**-yoo-lar defect
☐ atrioventricular node	**ay**-tree-oh-ven-**TRIK**-yoo-lar node
☐ bicuspid valve	by-**KUSS**-pid valve
☐ bradycardia	brad-ih-**KAR**-dee-ah
☐ bruits	broo-**EEZ**
☐ bundle of His	bundle of **HISS**
☐ capillary	**KAP**-ih-lair-ee
☐ cardiac catheterization	**KAR**-dee-ak **kath**-eh-ter-ih-**ZAY**-shun
☐ cardiac tamponade	**KAR**-dee-ak tam-poh-**NAYD**
☐ cardiologist	kar-dee-**ALL**-oh-jist
☐ cardiology	kar-dee-**ALL**-oh-jee
☐ cardiomegaly	kar-dee-oh-**MEG**-ah-lee
☐ cardiomyopathy	kar-dee-oh-my-**OP**-ah-thee
☐ cardiopulmonary resuscitation	kar-dee-oh-**PULL**-mon-air-ee ree-**suss**-ih-**TAY**-shun
☐ coarctation of the aorta	koh-ark-**TAY**-shun of the ay-**OR**-tah
☐ congestive heart failure	kon-**JESS**-tiv heart failure
☐ coronary	**KOR**-oh-nair-ee
☐ coronary arteries	**KOR**-ah-nair-ee **AR**-ter-eez
☐ coronary artery bypass graft	**KOR**-oh-nair-ee **AR**-ter-ee bypass graft
☐ coronary artery disease	**KOR**-oh-nair-ee **AR**-ter-ee **DIS**-eez
☐ coronary occlusion	**KOR**-oh-nair-ee oh-**KLOO**-zhun
☐ coronary thrombosis	**KOR**-oh-nair-ee throm-**BOH**-sis

- ☐ coronary veins — **KOR**-oh-nair-ee vaynz
- ☐ deep vein thrombosis — deep vayn throm-**BOH**-sis
- ☐ defibrillation — dee-**fib**-rih-**LAY**-shun
- ☐ diastole — digh-**ASS**-toh-lee
- ☐ diastolic — **digh**-ah-**STALL**-ik
- ☐ echocardiogram — **ek**-oh-**KAR**-dee-oh-gram
- ☐ echocardiography — **ek**-oh-**kar**-dee-**OG**-rah-fee
- ☐ electrocardiogram — ee-**lek**-troh-**KAR**-dee-oh-gram
- ☐ electrocardiograph — ee-**lek**-troh-**KAR**-dee-oh-graff
- ☐ electrocardiography — ee-**lek**-troh-**kar**-dee-**OG**-rah-fee
- ☐ endarterectomy — **end**-ar-ter-**EK**-toh-mee
- ☐ endocarditis — **en**-doh-kar-**DIGH**-tis
- ☐ endocardium — en-doh-**KAR**-dee-um
- ☐ epicardium — **ep**-ih-**KAR**-dee-um
- ☐ fibrillation — fih-brih-**LAY**-shun
- ☐ Holter monitoring — Holter monitoring
- ☐ hypertension — high-per-**TEN**-shun
- ☐ hypertensive heart disease — high-per-**TEN**-siv heart disease
- ☐ hypotension — high-poh-**TEN**-shun
- ☐ inferior vena cava — in-**FEER**-ee-or **VEEN**-ah **KAY**-vah
- ☐ ischemia — iss-**KEE**-mee-ah
- ☐ mediastinum — **mee**-dee-ah-**STIGH**-num
- ☐ mitral valve — **MY**-tral valve
- ☐ mitral valve prolapse — **MY**-tral valve **PROH**-laps
- ☐ mitral valve stenosis — **MY**-tral valve sten-**OH**-sis
- ☐ myocardial infarction — my-oh-**KAR**-dee-al in-**FARK**-shun
- ☐ myocarditis — **my**-oh-kar-**DIGH**-tis
- ☐ myocardium — my-oh-**KAR**-dee-um
- ☐ occlusion — oh-**KLOO**-shun
- ☐ palpitation — pal-pih-**TAY**-shun
- ☐ paroxysmal atrial tachycardia — pair-ok-**SIZ**-mal **AY**-tree-al tak-ih-**KAR**-dee-ah
- ☐ patent ductus arteriosus — **PAY**-tent **DUK**-tus **ar**-tee-ree-**OH**-sis
- ☐ percutaneous transluminal coronary angioplasty — per-kyoo-**TAY**-nee-us trans-**LOO**-min-al **KOR**-oh-nair-ee **AN**-jee-oh-**plass**-tee
- ☐ pericardial fluid — pair-ih-**KAR**-dee-al fluid
- ☐ pericarditis — **pair**-ih-kar-**DIGH**-tis
- ☐ pericardium — pair-ih-**KAR**-dee-um
- ☐ polyarteritis — **pall**-ee-ar-teh-**RIGH**-tis
- ☐ premature atrial contraction — **PRE**-mah-chur **AY**-tree-al kon-**TRACK**-shun
- ☐ premature ventricular contraction — **PRE**-mah-chur ven-**TRIK**-yoo-lar kon-**TRACK**-shun
- ☐ pulmonary artery — **PULL**-moh-neh-ree artery
- ☐ pulmonary circulation — **PULL**-moh-neh-ree circulation
- ☐ pulmonary valve — **PULL**-moh-neh-ree valve
- ☐ pulmonary vein — **PULL**-moh-neh-ree vein

□ rheumatic fever — roo-**MAT**-ik fever

□ rheumatic heart disease — roo-**MAT**-ik heart disease

□ septum — **SEP**-tum

□ sinoatrial node — **sigh**-noh-**AY**-tree-al node

□ sphygmomanometer — **sfig**-moh-man-**AH**-meh-ter

□ stethoscope — **STETH**-oh-skohp

□ superior vena cava — superior **VEEN**-ah **KAY**-vah

□ systemic circulation — sis-**TEM**-ik circulation

□ systole — **SISS**-toh-lee

□ systolic — sis-**TALL**-ik

□ tachycardia — tak-ih-**KAR**-dee-ah

□ tetralogy of Fallot — teh-**TRALL**-oh-jee of fal-**LOH**

□ thallium stress test — **THAL**-ee-um stress test

□ thrombophlebitis — **throm**-boh-fleh-**BIGH**-tis

□ transesophageal echocardiography — **trans**-eh-soff-ah-**JEE**-al **ek**-oh- **kar**-dee-**OG**-rah-fee

□ tricuspid valve — try-**KUSS**-pid valve

□ valvoplasty — **VAL**-voh-**plass**-tee

□ varicose veins — **VAR**-ih-kohs veins

□ vasoconstriction — **vay**-zoh-con-**STRIK**-shun

□ vein — vayn

□ ventricles — **VEN**-trih-kuls

□ ventricular tachycardia — ven-**TRIK**-yoo-lar tak-ih-**KAR**-dee-ah

□ venule — **VEN**-yool

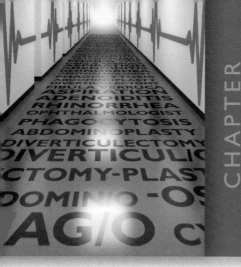

7 Blood and Lymphatic System

OBJECTIVES

At the completion of this chapter, the student should be able to:

1. Identify, define, and spell word roots associated with the blood and the lymphatic systems.
2. Label the basic structures of the blood and lymph systems.
3. Discuss the functions of the blood and the lymph systems.
4. Provide the correct spelling of blood and lymph terms, given the definition of the terms.
5. Analyze blood and lymph terms by defining the roots, prefixes, and suffixes of these terms.
6. Identify, define, and spell disease, disorder, and procedure terms related to the blood and lymph systems.

OVERVIEW

Blood is made up of **plasma**, the fluid portion of blood, and several types of blood cells. Blood delivers oxygen, nutrients, and essential chemicals to the cells and removes carbon dioxide and other waste products from the cells. Blood moves throughout the body by way of arteries and veins, which are discussed in Chapter 6.

The lymph system is made up of fluid, vessels, nodes, organs, and cells. The lymph system and its structures play an important role in the immune function of the body and also help maintain the fluid balance of body tissues. Blood and lymph structures are presented individually.

Blood and Lymph System Word Roots

To understand and use blood and lymph medical terms, it is necessary to acquire a thorough knowledge of the associated word roots. Review the word roots in Table 7-1 and complete the exercises that follow.

TABLE 7-1 BLOOD AND LYMPH WORD ROOTS

Word Root/Combining Form	Meaning
adenoid/o	adenoid
agglutin/o	to clump
angi/o	vessel
ather/o	fat; fatty plaque

(continues)

TABLE 7-1   BLOOD AND LYMPH WORD ROOTS (continued)

Word Root/Combining Form	Meaning
bas/o	base
blast/o	immature cell
coagul/o	clotting
cyt/o	cell
eosin/o	red; rosy
erythr/o	red
granul/o	granules
hem/o	blood
hemat/o	blood
immun/o	protection; immune; safe
is/o	equal
kary/o	nucleus
leuk/o	white
lymph/o	lymph; lymphatic tissue
lymphaden/o	lymph gland
lymphangi/o	lymph vessel
morph/o	form; shape
myel/o	bone marrow; spinal cord
nucle/o	nucleus
phag/o	to eat; swallow
poikil/o	varied; irregular
sarc/o	flesh; connective tissue
spher/o	sphere; round
splen/o	spleen
thromb/o	clot; thrombus
thym/o	thymus
tonsill/o	tonsils

EXERCISE 1

Write the meaning of the following word roots.

1. leuk/o   _____

2. erythr/o   _____

3. thromb/o   _____

4. nucle/o   _____

5. immun/o   _____

6. morph/o   _____

7. lymph/o   _____

8. hem/o; hemat/o _____

9. blast/o _____

10. agglutin/o _____

11. phag/o _____

12. thym/o _____

13. splen/o _____

14. lymphangi/o _____

EXERCISE 2

Write the word root and its meaning.

1. basophil

    ROOT: _____   MEANING: _____

2. leukocytopenia

    ROOT: _____   MEANING: _____

3. coagulation

    ROOT: _____   MEANING: _____

4. karyocyte

    ROOT: _____   MEANING: _____

5. eosinophil

    ROOT: _____   MEANING: _____

6. poikilocytosis

    ROOT: _____   MEANING: _____

7. sarcoma

    ROOT: _____   MEANING: _____

8. spherocytosis

    ROOT: _____   MEANING: _____

9. lymphadenopathy

    ROOT: _____   MEANING: _____

10. myelogram

    ROOT: _____   MEANING: _____

11. isometric

    ROOT: _____   MEANING: _____

12. granulocyte

    ROOT: _____   MEANING: _____

EXERCISE 3

Write the correct word root(s) for the following definitions.

1. lymph gland   _____

2. clotting   _____

3. cell   _____

4. red   _____

5. blood   _____

6. clot   _____

7. white   _____

8. lymph vessel   _____

9. protection   _____

10. form; shape   _____

Components of Blood

The major components of blood are plasma and cells. Plasma is the liquid portion of blood and makes up about 55% of the total blood volume. The plasma is about 90% water and contains dissolved substances such as electrolytes, glucose, gases, protein, and fats. Blood cells make up about 45% of the total blood volume. Blood cells are illustrated in Figure 7-1. Refer to this figure as you read about these cells.

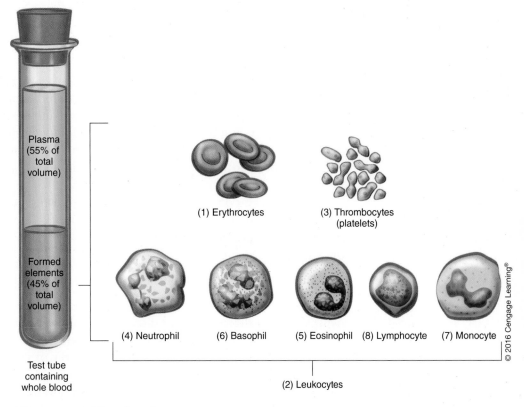

Figure 7-1 Blood cells.

© 2016 Cengage Learning®

The blood cells include (1) **erythrocytes** (eh-**RITH**-roh-sights), red blood cells; (2) **leukocytes** (**LOO**-koh-sights), white blood cells; and (3) **platelets** (**PLAYT**-lets) or **thrombocytes** (**THROM**-boh-sights). Leukocytes are further classified as (4) **neutrophils** (**NOO**-troh-fills); (5) **eosinophils** (ee-oh-**SIN**-oh-fills); (6) **basophils** (**BAY**-soh-fills); (7) **monocytes** (**MON**-oh-sights); and (8) **lymphocytes** (**LIM**-foh-sights). Blood cells are formed in the red bone marrow.

Erythrocytes

Erythrocytes, also called red blood cells (RBCs), are small, biconcave-shaped discs that are thinner in the center than around the edges. Erythrocytes are the most numerous of all blood cells. **Hemoglobin** (hee-moh-**GLOH**-bin), which is an iron-protein substance, is the main component of erythrocytes. The primary purpose of erythrocytes is to deliver oxygen to all cells.

Leukocytes

Leukocytes, also called white blood cells (WBCs), are larger than erythrocytes but fewer in number. Leukocytes function as part of our immune system and help fight disease. Refer to Figure 7-1 as you learn about the different types of leukocytes. There are five types of leukocytes, which are grouped into two categories: **granulocytes** (**GRAN**-yoo-loh-sights) and **agranulocytes** (ay-**GRAN**-yoo-loh-sights). Granulocytes have grains or granules in their cytoplasm. These granules absorb different types of stains (also called dyes) that make the cells more visible under a microscope. The three types of granulocytes include:

- (4) Neutrophils do not absorb any stain and appear neutral in color.
- (5) Eosinophils absorb stain and turn a rosy red color.
- (6) Basophils absorb stain and turn dark blue.

Neutrophils are **phagocytes** (**FAG**-oh-sights), which mean they fight disease by engulfing and digesting or destroying bacteria and damaged tissue. **Phagocytosis** (**fag**-oh-sigh-**TOH**-sis) is the process of engulfing and destroying a substance. Eosinophils increase in number and help defend the body during an allergic reaction. Basophils release **histamine** (**HISS**-tah-meen) and **heparin** (**HEP**-ah-rin), which help the body respond to an allergic reaction. Histamine increases blood flow, and heparin prevents the blood from clotting.

Agranulocytes do not have granules in their cytoplasm and do not absorb stains. Agranulocytes are categorized by the size of the cell and the shape of the nucleus. There are two types of agranulocytes:

- (7) Monocytes, the largest leukocytes with a kidney bean-shaped nucleus.
- (8) Lymphocytes, with a large spherical-shaped nucleus.

Monocytes and lymphocytes fight disease by phagocytosis. Some lymphocytes identify foreign substances and disease-causing organisms, such as bacteria and viruses. These lymphocytes then produce **antibodies** (**AN**-tih-**bod**-eez) that target and destroy or neutralize a specific substance, bacteria, or virus. The substance, bacteria, or virus that triggers the production of antibodies is called an **antigen** (**AN**-tih-jen). Antigen literally means against (*anti-*) growth or development (*-gen*). Figure 7-2 illustrates how the antibodies react to an antigen.

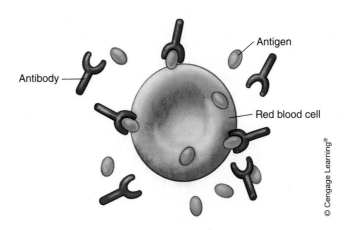

© Cengage Learning®

Figure 7-2 Illustrated antigen/antibody reaction.

Thrombocytes

Thrombocytes, or platelets, are small cells that are essential for normal blood **coagulation** (**koh**-ag-yoo-**LAY**-shun) or clotting.

Blood Groups

Human blood is grouped according to the presence or absence of specific antigens that are present on the surface of red blood cells. Three commonly referenced red blood cell antigens are the *A, B,* and *Rh* antigens. The ABO system is commonly used to group or type blood. Group A blood has A antigens, group B blood has B antigens, group AB blood has both A and B antigens, and group O blood has neither antigen.

The presence or absence of the Rh antigen further identifies an individual's blood type. Rh positive (Rh+) means that the red blood cells have the Rh antigen, and Rh negative (Rh–) means that the red blood cells do not contain the Rh antigen. For example, type A positive (A+) means both antigen A and the Rh antigen are present. Blood type A negative (A–) means antigen A is present and the Rh antigen is *not* present. In addition to the blood group antigens associated with red blood cells, blood group antibodies are present in the serum, or plasma, of human blood. Table 7-2 summarizes the ABO blood groups and identifies the antigens and antibodies associated with each group.

TABLE 7-2 ABO BLOOD TYPES WITH RH DESIGNATIONS

Blood Type	Antigen A/B	Rh Antigen	Antibodies
A+ (A positive)	A	Present	Antibody B
A– (A negative)	A	Not present	Antibody B
B+ (B positive)	B	Present	Antibody A
B– (B negative)	B	Not present	Antibody A
AB+ (AB positive)	A and B	Present	None
AB– (AB negative)	A and B	Not present	None
O+ (O positive)	None	Present	Antibody A and B
O– (O negative)	None	Not present	Antibody A and B

© 2016 Cengage Learning®

Identifying an individual's blood group is critical when the individual requires a blood transfusion. An individual should be transfused with blood of the same ABO group and the same Rh designation. If an individual with type A blood receives a transfusion of type B blood, an incompatibility reaction occurs. The B antibodies in the serum of the type A blood react with the B antigens on the red blood cells of the type B blood. There are two types of incompatibility reactions, **agglutination** and **hemolysis**. Agglutination (ah-**gloo**-tih-**NAY**-shun) means red blood cells clump together and inhibit blood flow. **Hemolysis** (hee-**MALL**-ih-sis) means red blood cells are destroyed.

The Rh antigen does not have naturally occurring antibodies. However, if an individual with Rh– blood is transfused with Rh+ blood, the Rh– individual might produce antibodies to the Rh antigen present in the transfused blood. Once an individual has Rh antibodies, subsequent transfusions with Rh+ blood results in the hemolysis (destruction) of the transfused Rh+ blood cells. Therefore, it is important that transfused blood is the same blood type and Rh designation as the blood of the individual receiving the transfusion.

The production of Rh antibodies might also occur during pregnancy. When an Rh– mother gives birth to an Rh+ infant, the infant's Rh+ blood comes in contact with the mother's Rh– blood. This contact stimulates the production of Rh antibodies in the mother's blood. In subsequent pregnancies, an Rh+ fetus is at risk for a condition called **hemolytic** (**hee**-moh-**LIT**-ik) **disease of the newborn**. In this situation, the Rh antibodies in the mother's blood might enter the fetal bloodstream and react with the fetal Rh+ blood cells. The reaction causes hemolysis of fetal red blood cells, which is a life-threatening condition.

Hemolytic disease of the newborn may be prevented by administering RhoGAM, a commercially prepared immune protein, shortly after the birth of an Rh+ infant by an Rh– mother. RhoGAM helps prevent the formation of Rh antibodies. RhoGAM may also be administered during subsequent pregnancies when an Rh incompatibility exists.

EXERCISE 4

Match the component of blood in Column 1 with the correct definition in Column 2.

COLUMN 1

_____ 1. agranulocytes

_____ 2. basophils

_____ 3. eosinophils

_____ 4. granulocytes

_____ 5. hemoglobin

_____ 6. lymphocytes

_____ 7. monocytes

_____ 8. neutrophils

_____ 9. phagocytes

_____ 10. platelets

COLUMN 2

a. absorb different types of stain

b. do not absorb stain

c. iron-protein substance

d. largest leukocyte

e. releases histamine and heparin

f. necessary for coagulation

g. engulf, digest, and/or destroy unwanted material

h. produce antibodies

i. increases in an allergic reaction

j. phagocytic white blood cell

EXERCISE 5

Label the blood cells illustrated in Figure 7-3. Write your answer on the spaces provided.

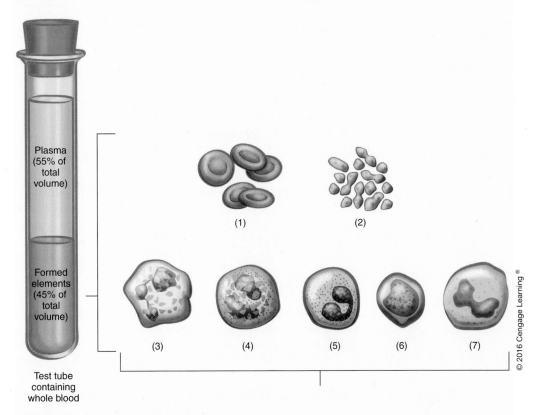

Plasma (55% of total volume)

Formed elements (45% of total volume)

Test tube containing whole blood

(1)   (2)   (3)   (4)   (5)   (6)   (7)

© 2016 Cengage Learning®

Figure 7-3 Blood cell labeling exercise.

1. _____

2. _____

3. _____

4. _____

5. _____

6. _____

7. _____

EXERCISE 6

Write the medical term that best fits each definition.

1. clumping together of red blood cells   _____

2. destruction of red blood cells   _____

3. determine(s) blood type A+   _____

4. determine(s) blood type O–   _____

5. determine(s) blood type B   _____

6. determine(s) blood type AB–   _____

7. plasma antibody(ies) in blood type A   _____

8. plasma antibody(ies) in blood type O   _____

9. plasma antibody(ies) in blood type B   _____

10. plasma antibody(ies) in blood type AB   _____

Lymphatic System

Lymphatic system components are illustrated in Figure 7-4. Refer to this figure as you read about the components.

The lymphatic system includes **lymph** (LIMF) **fluid**, (1) **lymph vessels**, (2) **lymph nodes**, **lymphocytes** (**LIM**-foh-sights), (3) **thymus** (**THIGH**-mus), (4) **spleen**, and (5) **tonsils**. As previously stated, the lymphatic system is an important part of the immune system and also helps maintain our internal fluid balance.

Lymph Fluid

Lymph fluid is clear, transparent, and colorless; it consists of proteins, electrolytes, fats, glucose, and lymphocytes. Lymph fluid is derived from the blood and the fluid that collects in body tissue.

Lymph Vessels

The smallest lymph vessels are called lymphatic capillaries. Lymph capillaries collect the fluid that filters out of the blood capillaries and into the interstitial (in-ter-**STIH**-shill) spaces. Interstitial spaces are located between the cells of body tissue. Figure 7-5 illustrates the relationship between lymph capillaries and blood capillaries. Once the fluid enters the lymph capillaries, it is called lymph fluid.

The lymph capillaries transport the lymph fluid to the larger lymphatic vessels. The lymphatic vessels allow water and dissolved substances to be returned to the blood. Lymph vessels continue to merge and eventually lead to the two **lymphatic ducts**: the right lymphatic duct and the thoracic duct.

Lymph Nodes

Lymph nodes are collections of lymphatic tissue located at intervals along the course of the lymph vessels. Lymph nodes contain specialized lymphocytes that are capable of destroying **pathogens** (**PATH**-oh-jenz). A pathogen is any substance that causes disease (*path/o* = disease; *-gen* = growth, development). These specialized cells, called **macrophages** (**MACK**-roh-fay-jezs) function as phagocytes and engulf and destroy certain pathogens.

As lymph fluid moves through the lymph nodes, macrophages destroy harmful substances such as bacteria and viruses. At the same time, other structures within the lymph node function as filters to remove other impurities. Eventually, lymph fluid is deposited into the venous circulation and is mixed with venous blood.

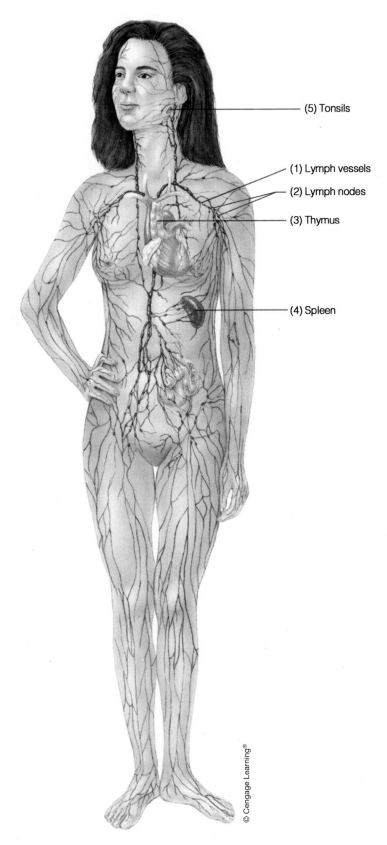

Figure 7-4 Components of the lymph system.

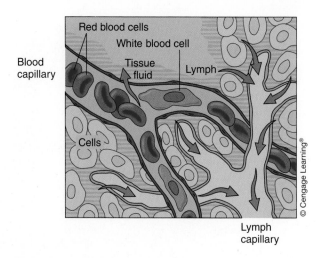

Figure 7-5 Relationship between blood capillaries and lymph capillaries.

Thymus

The **thymus** is a lymph and endocrine gland. It is located in the mediastinum near the middle of the chest. The thymus secretes a hormone called **thymosin** (thigh-**MOH**-sin), which stimulates the production of **T lymphocytes**, also called **T cells**. T cells are an important part of our immune system because they circulate throughout the body and attack foreign and/or abnormal cells. The thymus develops around the fifth week of gestation and continues to function through puberty. At this time, the thymus begins to diminish in function and size, and is usually dormant by age 40.

Spleen

The **spleen** is the largest lymph organ in the body. It is situated in the upper-left quadrant of the abdomen just below the diaphragm and behind the stomach. Figure 7-6 illustrates the spleen. The spleen filters blood in much the same way the lymph nodes filter lymph fluid. Macrophages in the spleen remove pathogens from the blood. The spleen also forms lymphocytes and monocytes; destroys worn-out erythrocytes; and stores surplus erythrocytes.

Tonsils

The **tonsils**, masses of lymphatic tissue, are located in the mouth at the back of the throat and are divided into three groups. The (1) **pharyngeal tonsils** (**fair**-in-**JEE**-al **TON**-sills), also called the **adenoids** (**ADD**-eh-noydz), are near the opening of the nasal cavity into the pharynx. The (2) **palatine** (**PAL**-ah-tine) **tonsils** are located on each side of the throat at the back of the oral cavity. The (3) **lingual** (**LING**-gwal) **tonsils** are near the base of the tongue. The tonsils are the first lines of defense against bacteria and other harmful substances that might enter the body through the nose and mouth. Figure 7-7 illustrates the location of the tonsils.

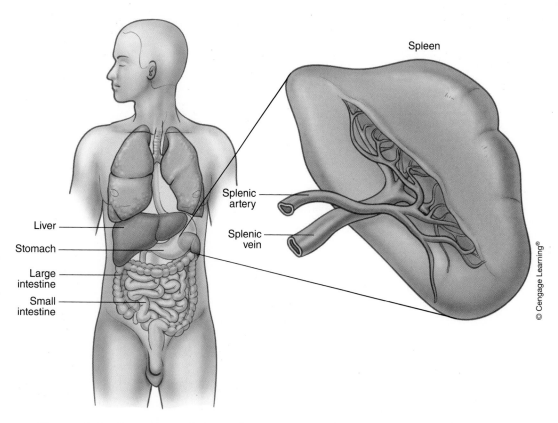

Figure 7-6 Location of the spleen.

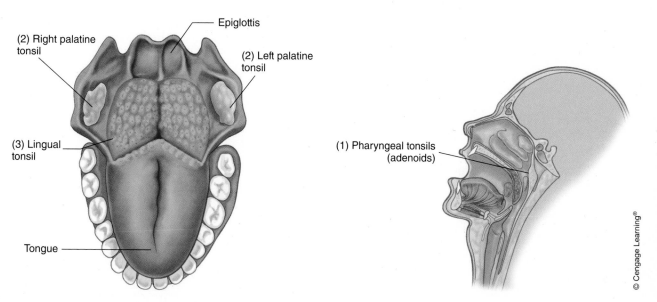

Figure 7-7 Location of the tonsils.

EXERCISE 7

Label the structures of the lymphatic system in Figure 7-8. Write your answers in the spaces provided.

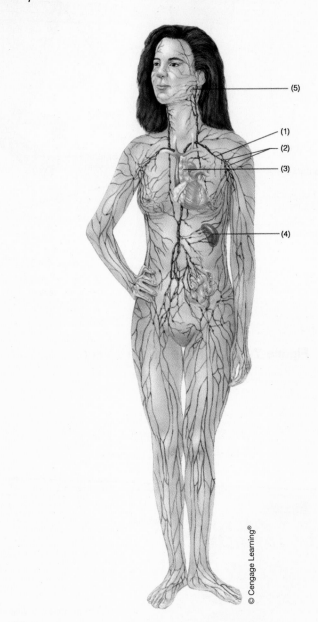

Figure 7-8 Lymphatic system labeling exercise.

1. _____

2. _____

3. _____

4. _____

5. _____

EXERCISE 8

Match the lymph terms in Column 1 with the definitions in Column 2.

COLUMN 1

_____ 1. interstitial space

_____ 2. lingual tonsils

_____ 3. lymph capillaries

_____ 4. lymph ducts

_____ 5. lymph fluid

_____ 6. macrophages

_____ 7. palatine tonsils

_____ 8. pharyngeal tonsils

_____ 9. spleen

_____ 10. T lymphocytes

COLUMN 2

a. adenoids

b. attack abnormal cells

c. between the cells of body tissue

d. composed of blood and body tissue fluid

e. collect interstitial fluid

f. merged lymph vessels

g. filters blood

h. engulf and destroy bacteria

i. near the base of the tongue

j. on each side of the throat

Blood and Lymphatic System Medical Terminology

Blood/lymph system medical terms are organized into three main categories: (1) general medical terms; (2) disease and condition terms; and (3) diagnostic procedure, surgery, and laboratory test terms. The prefixes and suffixes commonly used in blood/lymph terms are listed in Table 7-3. Review these word parts and complete the related exercises.

TABLE 7-3   PREFIXES AND SUFFIXES FOR THE BLOOD AND LYMPHATIC SYSTEM TERMS

Prefix	Meaning	Suffix	Meaning
inter-	between	-emia	blood condition
macro-	large	-globin	protein
mono-	one	-lysis, -lytic	destruction; related to destruction
pan-	all	-oid	like; resembling
		-oma	tumor
		-osis	condition
		-pathy	disease; illness
		-penia	deficiency; decreased number
		-philia	attraction to
		-poiesis	formation or production of
		-stasis	stopping or controlling

EXERCISE 9

Write the prefix, suffix, and their meanings for each medical term.

1. interstitial

   PREFIX: _____   MEANING: _____

   SUFFIX: _____   MEANING: _____

2. hemoglobin

   PREFIX: _____   MEANING: _____

   SUFFIX: _____   MEANING: _____

3. monocyte

   PREFIX: _____   MEANING: _____

   SUFFIX: _____   MEANING: _____

4. macrophage

   PREFIX: _____   MEANING: _____

   SUFFIX: _____   MEANING: _____

5. hemolysis

   PREFIX: _____   MEANING: _____

   SUFFIX: _____   MEANING: _____

6. leukopenia

   PREFIX: _____   MEANING: _____

   SUFFIX: _____   MEANING: _____

7. lymphadenopathy

   PREFIX: _____   MEANING: _____

   SUFFIX: _____   MEANING: _____

8. erythropoiesis

   PREFIX: _____   MEANING: _____

   SUFFIX: _____   MEANING: _____

9. hemophilia

   PREFIX: _____   MEANING: _____

   SUFFIX: _____   MEANING: _____

10. granulocytosis

   PREFIX: _____   MEANING: _____

   SUFFIX: _____   MEANING: _____

EXERCISE 10

Analyze each term. Write the root, prefix, suffix, and their meanings. Based on the meanings of the word parts, write a definition of each term. Check the definition in a medical dictionary.

EXAMPLE: adenoidectomy
ROOT: adenoid/o = adenoids
PREFIX: none
SUFFIX: -ectomy = surgical removal
DEFINITION: surgical removal of the adenoids

1. lymphadenopathy

   ROOT: _____ MEANING: _____

   PREFIX: _____ MEANING: _____

   SUFFIX: _____ MEANING: _____

   DEFINITION: _____

2. lymphoid

   ROOT: _____ MEANING: _____

   PREFIX: _____ MEANING: _____

   SUFFIX: _____ MEANING: _____

   DEFINITION: _____

3. leukocytopenia

   ROOT: _____ MEANING: _____

   PREFIX: _____ MEANING: _____

   SUFFIX: _____ MEANING: _____

   DEFINITION: _____

4. hemolysis

   ROOT: _____ MEANING: _____

   PREFIX: _____ MEANING: _____

   SUFFIX: _____ MEANING: _____

   DEFINITION: _____

5. macrophage

   ROOT: _____ MEANING: _____

   PREFIX: _____ MEANING: _____

   SUFFIX: _____ MEANING: _____

   DEFINITION: _____

6. hemoglobin

    ROOT: _____   MEANING: _____

    PREFIX: _____   MEANING: _____

    SUFFIX: _____   MEANING: _____

    DEFINITION: _____

7. hemostasis

    ROOT: _____   MEANING: _____

    PREFIX: _____   MEANING: _____

    SUFFIX: _____   MEANING: _____

    DEFINITION: _____

8. lymphoma

    ROOT: _____   MEANING: _____

    PREFIX: _____   MEANING: _____

    SUFFIX: _____   MEANING: _____

    DEFINITION: _____

9. leukemia

    ROOT: _____   MEANING: _____

    PREFIX: _____   MEANING: _____

    SUFFIX: _____   MEANING: _____

    DEFINITION: _____

Blood and Lymphatic System General Medical Terms

Review the pronunciation and meaning of each term in Table 7-4. Note that some terms are built from word parts and some are not. Complete the exercises for these terms.

TABLE 7-4 BLOOD AND LYMPHATIC SYSTEM GENERAL MEDICAL TERMS

Term with Pronunciation	Definition
agglutination (ah-**gloo**-tih-**NAY**-shun)	clumping together of cells
coagulation (koh-**ag**-yoo-**LAY**-shun)	process of blood clotting
corpuscle (**KOR**-pus-ehl)	any blood cell, red or white
hematologist (**hee**-mah-**TALL**-oh-jist) hemat/o = blood -(o)logist = specialist	physician specialist in the study of blood, blood-forming organs, and related disorders and diseases

(continues)

TABLE 7-4   BLOOD AND LYMPHATIC SYSTEM GENERAL MEDICAL TERMS (continued)

Term with Pronunciation	Definition
hematology (**hee**-mah-**TALL**-oh-jee) hemat/o = blood -(o)logy = study of blood and blood-forming organs	the study of blood and disorders of blood and blood-forming organs
hemostasis (**hee**-moh-**STAY**-sis) hem/o = blood -stasis = stopping or controlling	stopping or controlling the flow of blood
heparin (**HEP**-ah-rin)	anticoagulant substance in the blood
histamine (**HISS**-tah-meen)	a substance released from body cells in response to an allergic reaction
pathogen (**PATH**-oh-jen) path/o = disease -gen = producing; forming	any substance that causes disease
phagocyte (**FAG**-oh-sight) phag/o = to eat -cyte = cell	cell that engulfs and destroys or digests bacteria or other unwanted substances
phagocytosis (**fag**-oh-sigh-**TOH**-sis) phag/o = to eat cyt/o = cell -osis = condition	process of a cell engulfing and destroying bacteria or other unwanted substances

© 2016 Cengage Learning®

EXERCISE 11

Circle the term that best completes each statement.

1. *Agglutination* or *coagulation* describes blood clotting.

2. An anticoagulant substance is *histamine* or *heparin*.

3. Any blood cell may be called a *corpuscle* or *hemocyte*.

4. *Phagocytosis* or *phagocyte* describes a cell that destroys bacteria.

5. A *phagocyte* or *pathogen* causes disease.

6. *Hematologist* or *hematology* means the study of blood.

7. Stopping the flow of blood is called *hemostasis* or *hemorrhage*.

Blood and Lymphatic System Disease and Disorder Terms

Blood/lymph system diseases and disorders include familiar problems such as anemia as well as more complex and less familiar diagnoses such as polycythemia vera (**pol-ee-sigh-THEE**-mee-ah **VAIR**-ah). The medical terms are presented in alphabetical order in Table 7-5. Review the pronunciation and definition for each term and complete the exercises.

TABLE 7-5 BLOOD AND LYMPHATIC SYSTEM DISEASE AND DISORDER TERMS

Term with Pronunciation	Definition
acquired immune deficiency syndrome (AIDS)	a syndrome of infections that occur during the final stage of infection by the human immunodeficiency virus (HIV); characterized by the progressive loss of immune system function
adenoiditis (**add**-eh-noyd-**EYE**-tis) adenoid/o = adenoids -itis = inflammation	inflammation of the adenoids
anemia (ah-**NEE**-mee-ah) an- = without -emia = blood condition	deficiency in the quantity or quality of blood
aplastic anemia (ah-**PLAST**-ik ah-**NEE**-mee-ah) a- = without; lack of plast/o = development -ic = pertaining to an- = without -emia = blood condition	deficiency of red blood cell production due to a disorder of the bone marrow
dyscrasia (dis-**KRAY**-zee-ah)	any abnormal condition of blood
embolism (**EM**-boh-lizm)	obstruction of a blood vessel by a foreign substance or a blood clot; occurs when a foreign body or clot travels through the bloodstream and becomes lodged in the vessel
embolus (**EM**-boh-lus)	a blood clot, or other substance such as air, gas, or a fatty deposit that circulates in the blood
erythremia (ehr-ih-**THREE**-mee-ah) erythr/o = red -emia = blood condition	an abnormal increase in the number of red blood cells

(continues)

TABLE 7-5 BLOOD AND LYMPHATIC SYSTEM DISEASE AND DISORDER TERMS (continued)

Term with Pronunciation	Definition
erythrocytopenia (eh-**rith**-roh-**sigh**-toh-**PEE**-nee-ah) erythr/o = red cyt/o = cell -penia = deficiency; decreased number	decrease in the number of erythrocytes
granulocytosis (**gran**-yoo-loh-sigh-**TOH**-sis) granul/o = granules cyt/o = cell -osis = condition	an increase in the number of granulocytes
hemolysis (hee-**MALL**-ih-sis) hem/o = blood -lysis = destruction; break down	destruction or break down of red blood cells
hemolytic anemia (**hee**-moh-**LIT**-ik ah-**NEE**-mee-ah) hem/o = blood -lytic = pertaining to destruction an- = without -emia = blood	decrease in the quantity or quality of blood due to the premature destruction of red blood cells
hemolytic disease of newborns (**hee**-moh-**LIT**-ik) fetal Rh+ blood hem/o = blood -lytic = pertaining to destruction	destruction of newborn or fetal red blood cells caused by a reaction between Rh− blood and fetal Rh+ blood
hemophilia (**hee**-moh-**FILL**-ee-ah) hem/o = blood phil/o = attraction to -ia = condition	bleeding disorder caused by a deficiency of coagulation factors in the blood in which the blood does not clot
hemorrhage (**HEM**-eh-rij) hem/o = blood -(r)rhage = excessive flow; bursting forth	excessive loss of blood, internal or external
Hodgkin's disease (**HODJ**-kins)	malignant neoplasm of lymph tissue; also called Hodgkin's lymphoma

(continues)

TABLE 7-5 BLOOD AND LYMPHATIC SYSTEM DISEASE
AND DISORDER TERMS (continued)

Term with Pronunciation	Definition
iron deficiency anemia (ah-**NEE**-mee-ah) an- = without -emia = blood condition	anemia caused by an inadequate amount of iron for the production of hemoglobin
leukemia (loo-**KEE**-mee-ah) leuk/o = white -emia = blood condition	abnormal increase in the number of immature white blood cells caused by a malignancy of the blood-forming organs
leukopenia (**loo**-koh-**PEE**-nee-ah leuk/o = white -penia = deficiency; decreased number	decrease in the number of leukocytes
lymphadenitis (lim-fad-en-**EYE**-tis) lymphaden/o = lymph gland -itis = inflammation	inflammation of a lymph gland
lymphadenopathy (lim-**fad**-eh-**NOP**-ah-thee) lymphaden/o = lymph gland -pathy = disease	any disease of a lymph gland
lymphedema (**lim**-feh-**DEE**-mah) lymph/o = lymph -edema = swelling	swelling due to an abnormal accumulation of lymph fluid within the tissues
lymphoma (lim-**FOH**-mah) lymph/o = lymph -oma = tumor	a tumor arising from lymph tissue, usually malignant

© 2016 Cengage Learning®

EXERCISE 12

Analyze each term. Write the root, prefix, suffix, and their meanings. Based on the meanings of the word parts, write a definition of each term. Check the definition in a medical dictionary.

1. erythremia

ROOT: _____ MEANING: _____

PREFIX: _____ MEANING: _____

SUFFIX: _____ MEANING: _____

DEFINITION: _____

2. erythrocytopenia

ROOT: _____   MEANING: _____

PREFIX: _____   MEANING: _____

SUFFIX: _____   MEANING: _____

DEFINITION: _____

3. hemolysis

ROOT: _____   MEANING: _____

PREFIX: _____   MEANING: _____

SUFFIX: _____   MEANING: _____

DEFINITION: _____

4. hemorrhage

ROOT: _____   MEANING: _____

PREFIX: _____   MEANING: _____

SUFFIX: _____   MEANING: _____

DEFINITION: _____

5. leukemia

ROOT: _____   MEANING: _____

PREFIX: _____   MEANING: _____

SUFFIX: _____   MEANING: _____

DEFINITION: _____

6. leukocytopenia

ROOT: _____   MEANING: _____

PREFIX: _____   MEANING: _____

SUFFIX: _____   MEANING: _____

DEFINITION: _____

7. lymphadenopathy

ROOT: _____   MEANING: _____

PREFIX: _____   MEANING: _____

SUFFIX: _____   MEANING: _____

DEFINITION: _____

8. lymphadenitis

ROOT: _____   MEANING: _____

PREFIX: _____   MEANING: _____

SUFFIX: _____   MEANING: _____

DEFINITION: _____

9. lymphoma

ROOT: _____   MEANING: _____

PREFIX: _____   MEANING: _____

SUFFIX: _____   MEANING: _____

DEFINITION: _____

EXERCISE 13

Replace the italicized phrase with the correct medical term.

1. Rosita was given an antibiotic for *inflammation of the adenoids.*

   _____

2. A *circulating blood clot* might cause obstruction of a blood vessel.

   _____

3. Roger's diagnosis was *inflammation of the lymph glands.*

   _____

4. A *deficiency in the quantity or quality of blood* is characterized by fatigue.

   _____

5. Li's blood tests revealed *an increase in the number of granulocytes.*

   _____

6. The patient denied knowledge of *any abnormal condition of blood.*

   _____

7. After surgery, the patient experienced an *obstruction of a blood vessel by a blood clot.*

   _____

8. *The inability of the blood to clot* required Erik's parents to watch him closely for cuts and bruises.

   _____

9. *Anemia due to red blood cell destruction* might require blood transfusions as part of the treatment.

   _____

10. Arsenic poisoning might lead to *anemia due to bone marrow destruction.*

   _____

11. *Destruction of a newborn's red blood cells* is caused by a reaction between maternal and fetal blood.

   _____

12. The condition known as *a malignant neoplasm or tumor of lymph tissue* is named for the physician who first identified the disease.

   _____

Review the pronunciation and definition for each term in Table 7-6 and complete the exercises.

TABLE 7-6   BLOOD AND LYMPHATIC SYSTEM DISEASE
AND DISORDER TERMS

Term with Pronunciation	Definition
mononucleosis (**mon**-oh-noo-klee-**OH**-sis) mono- = one nucle/o = nucleus -osis = condition	an abnormal increase in the number of monocytes (i.e., white blood cells with one nucleus) accompanied by enlargement of the spleen and lymph nodes
multiple myeloma (**MULL**-tih-p'l my-eh-**LOH**-mah) myel/o = bone marrow -oma = tumor	a malignant neoplasm of the bone marrow
non-Hodgkin's lymphoma (NHL) (**HODJ**-kins lim-**FOH**-mah) lymph/o = lymph -oma = tumor	malignant neoplasm of lymph tissue that cannot be categorized as Hodgkin's disease
pancytopenia (**pan**-sigh-toh-**PEE**-nee-ah) pan- = all cyt/o = cell -penia = deficiency; decreased number	decrease in the number of all blood cells
pernicious anemia (per-**NISH**-us ah-**NEE**-mee-ah) an- = without -emia = blood condition	anemia resulting from a decrease in the formation of mature erythrocytes
polycythemia (**pol**-ee-sigh-**THEE**-mee-ah) poly- = many cyt/o = cells -emia = blood condition	an increase in the number of erythrocytes in the blood
polycythemia vera (**pol**-ee-sigh-**THEE**-mee-ah **VAIR**-ah) poly- = many cyt/o = cells -emia = blood condition	an abnormal increase in the number of erythrocytes, granulocytes, and thrombocytes

(continues)

TABLE 7-6   BLOOD AND LYMPHATIC SYSTEM DISEASE
AND DISORDER TERMS (continued)

Term with Pronunciation	Definition
purpura (**PURR**-pyoo-rah)	hemorrhages beneath the skin
rouleaux (roo-**LOH**)	abnormal stacking of erythrocytes (Figure 7-9)

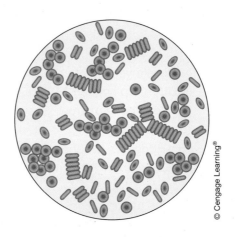

© Cengage Learning®

Figure 7-9   Rouleaux.

septicemia (**sep**-tih-**SEE**-mee-ah)	presence of disease-causing bacteria in the blood
sickle cell anemia (**SIK**-ul sell ah-**NEE**-mee-ah) an- = without -emia = blood condition	hereditary form of hemolytic anemia characterized by crescent-shaped erythrocytes (Figure 7–10)
spherocytosis (**sfee**-roh-sigh-**TOH**-sis) spher/o = round cyt/o = cell -osis = condition	abnormal condition of round or spherical-shaped erythrocytes
splenomegaly (splee-neh-**MEG**-ah-lee) splen/o = spleen -megaly = enlarged	enlargement of the spleen
thalassemia (thal-ah-**SEE**-mee-ah)	hereditary form of hemolytic anemia

(continues)

TABLE 7-6 BLOOD AND LYMPHATIC SYSTEM DISEASE
AND DISORDER TERMS (continued)

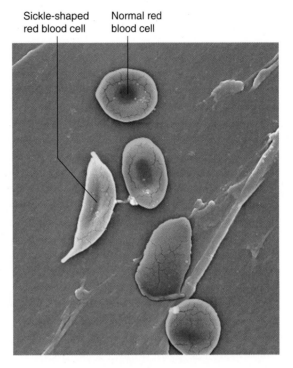

Sickle-shaped
red blood cell

Normal red
blood cell

Figure 7-10 Sickle cell anemia (Centers for Disease Control and Prevention/Sickle Cell Foundation of Georgia: Jackie George, Beverly Sinclair).

Term with Pronunciation	Definition
thrombocytopenia (**throm**-boh-**sigh**-toh-**PEE**-nee-ah) thromb/o = clot cyt/o = cell -penia = deficiency; decreased number	decrease in the number of thrombocytes
thrombosis (throm-**BOH**-sis) thromb/o = clot -osis = condition	presence of a blood clot within a blood vessel
thrombus (**THROM**-bus) thromb/o = clot	a blood clot; attaches to the wall of an artery or vein (Figure 7-11)
tonsillitis (ton-sih-**LIGH**-tis) tonsil/o = tonsils -itis = inflammation	inflammation of the tonsils

(continues)

TABLE 7-6 BLOOD AND LYMPHATIC SYSTEM DISEASE AND DISORDER TERMS (continued)

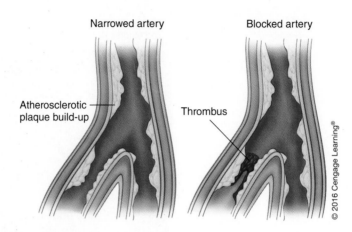

Narrowed artery   Blocked artery

Atherosclerotic plaque build-up

Thrombus

© 2016 Cengage Learning®

Figure 7-11 Thrombus.

© 2016 Cengage Learning®

EXERCISE 14

Analyze each term by writing the prefix, root, combining vowel, and suffix separated by vertical slashes. Based on the meaning of the word parts, write a definition for each term. Check your definition in a medical dictionary.

EXAMPLE: angiography

	/ angi	/ o	/ graphy
prefix	*root*	*combining vowel*	*suffix*

DEFINITION: process of recording an x-ray picture of a vessel

1. pancytopenia

prefix	*root*	*combining vowel*	*suffix*

DEFINITION: _____

2. polycythemia

prefix	*root*	*combining vowel*	*suffix*

DEFINITION: _____

3. spherocytosis

prefix	*root*	*combining vowel*	*suffix*

DEFINITION: _____

4. splenomegaly

prefix	*root*	*combining vowel*	*suffix*

DEFINITION: _____

5. thrombocytopenia

prefix	root	combining vowel	suffix

DEFINITION: _____

6. thrombosis

prefix	root	combining vowel	suffix

DEFINITION: _____

7. tonsillitis

prefix	root	combining vowel	suffix

DEFINITION:_____

8. mononucleosis

prefix	root	combining vowel	suffix

DEFINITION: _____

EXERCISE 15

Circle the medical term that best fits the definition.

DEFINITION	**CIRCLE ONE TERM**
1. anemia due to a decrease in the formation of mature erythrocyte	*thalassemia* OR *pernicious anemia*
2. anemia characterized by crescent-shaped erythrocytes	*sickle cell anemia* OR *spherocytosis*
3. hereditary form of hemolytic anemia	*pernicious anemia* OR *thalassemia*
4. hemorrhages beneath the skin	*rouleaux* OR *purpura*
5. malignant neoplasm of the bone marrow	*multiple myeloma* OR *polycythemia vera*
6. abnormal stacking of erythrocytes	*polycythemia vera* OR *rouleaux*
7. abnormal increase in all blood cells	*polycythemia vera* OR *pancytopenia*

Blood and Lymphatic System Diagnostic, Laboratory, and Treatment Terms

Review the pronunciation and definition of the laboratory, diagnostic, and treatment terms in Table 7-7. The terms are presented in alphabetic order, with the exception of the components of a complete blood count (CBC), listed in Table 7-8. Laboratory tests included in a CBC are presented as a set.

TABLE 7-7   BLOOD AND LYMPHATIC SYSTEM DIAGNOSTIC, LABORATORY, AND TREATMENT TERMS

Term with Pronunciation	Definition
bleeding time	a laboratory blood test that measures the time required for bleeding to stop
blood transfusion (trans-**FYOO**-zhun)	administration of blood or components of blood to replace the loss of blood
bone marrow biopsy (**BY**-op-see)	removal of a sample of the bone marrow for microscopic examination
complete blood count (CBC)	a blood test that analyzes the quantity and quality of the cellular components of blood
erythrocyte sedimentation rate (ESR) (eh-**RITH**-roh-sight **sed**-ih-men-**TAY**-shun)	a blood test that measures the rate at which red blood cells settle out of unclotted blood, also called sed rate
lymphangiogram (lim-**FAN**-jee-oh-gram) lymph/o = lymph angi/o = vessel -gram = record; picture	a record or picture of an x-ray examination of lymph vessels
prothrombin time (PT) (proh-**THROM**-bin)	a blood test that evaluates the ability of the blood to clot, also called protime

© 2016 Cengage Learning®

TABLE 7-8   COMPONENTS OF A COMPLETE BLOOD COUNT

Component with Pronunciation	Definition
red blood cell (RBC) count	identifies the number of red blood cells, erythrocytes, in a sample of blood
hemoglobin (Hgb) (**hee**-moh-**GLOH**-bin) hem(e) = blood -globin = protein	measures the number of grams of hemoglobin in a sample of blood
hematocrit (Hct) (hee-**MAT**-oh-krit) hemat/o = blood -crit = to separate	identifies the percentage of red blood cells in a specific volume of blood
red blood cell indices (**IN**-dih-seez) • MCV, mean corpuscular volume • MCH, mean corpuscular hemoglobin • MCHC, mean corpuscular hemoglobin concentration	mathematical calculations that identify erythrocyte size and erythrocyte hemoglobin concentration; MCV is the average size of an erythrocyte; MCH is the average amount of hemoglobin present in an average erythrocyte; and MCHC is the average percentage of hemoglobin in an average erythrocyte

(continues)

TABLE 7-8   COMPONENTS OF A COMPLETE BLOOD COUNT (continued)

Component with Pronunciation	Definition
white blood cell (WBC) count	identifies the number of white blood cells in a sample of blood
white blood cell differential (diff) (diff-er-**EN**-shal)	identifies the percentage of each type of white blood cell in a sample of blood
platelet count (**PLAYT**-let)	identifies the number of platelets in a sample of blood

© 2016 Cengage Learning®

A sample complete blood count report is illustrated in Figure 7-12.

BLUEBERRY COMMUNITY HOSPITAL BLUEBERRY, MAINE 55592			HEMATOLOGY PATIENT, NAME PATIENT NO. 121548	
TEST	**COLLECTED**	**TIME**	**RESULTS**	**RANGE**
CBC	02/04/20XX	10:00 A.M.		
WBC			5.75	4.80–10.00
Neutrophils			85% H*	55–70%
Monocytes			4%	2–8%
Lymphocytes			30%	20–40%
Eosinophils			2%	1–4%
Basophils			0.7%	0.5–1%
HGB			11.0 L*	12.0–16.0
HCT			32.6 L*	37.0–47.0
PLT			311.0	150.0–400.0
RBC			4.02 L*	4.20–5.40
MCV			81.1	80.6–96.0
MCH			27.3	27.0–33.0
MCHC			33.6	32.0–36.0
MPV			8.5	7.2–11.1
*Indicates abnormal results: H = higher than normal and L = lower than normal				

© Cengage Learning®

Figure 7-12   Complete blood count report.

EXERCISE 16

Match the term in Column 1 with the correct definition in Column 2.

COLUMN 1	COLUMN 2
_____ 1. administration of blood	a. percentage of red blood cells in blood
_____ 2. complete blood count	b. percentage of each type of leukocyte in blood
_____ 3. examination of bone marrow	c. number of erythrocytes in blood
_____ 4. hematocrit	d. number of leukocytes in blood
_____ 5. hemoglobin	e. number of thrombocytes in blood
_____ 6. platelet count	f. lymphangiogram
_____ 7. prothrombin time	g. grams of hemoglobin in blood
_____ 8. red blood cell count	h. erythrocyte size and hemoglobin content of blood
_____ 9. red blood cell indices	i. evaluates blood clotting ability
_____ 10. white blood cell count	j. cellular components in blood
_____ 11. white blood cell differential	k. bone marrow biopsy
_____ 12. x-ray of a lymph vessel	l. blood transfusion

EXERCISE 17

Write out and define the following abbreviations.

1. CBC: _____

   DEFINITION: _____

2. ESR: _____

   DEFINITION: _____

3. Hct: _____

   DEFINITION: _____

4. Hgb: _____

   DEFINITION: _____

5. RBC count: _____

   DEFINITION: _____

6. RBC indices: _____

   DEFINITION: _____

7. WBC count: _____

   DEFINITION: _____

Abbreviations

Review the blood and lymphatic system abbreviations in Table 7-9. Practice writing the meaning of each abbreviation.

TABLE 7-9 ABBREVIATIONS

Abbreviation	Meaning
AIDS	acquired immune deficiency syndrome
CBC	complete blood count
diff	white blood cell differential
ESR	erythrocyte sedimentation rate
Hct	hematocrit
Hgb	hemoglobin
HIV	human immunodeficiency virus
MCH	mean corpuscular hemoglobin
MCHC	mean corpuscular hemoglobin concentration
MCV	mean corpuscular volume
NHL	non-Hodgkin's lymphoma
PT	prothrombin time
RBC	red blood cell; red blood cell count
sed rate	erythrocyte sedimentation rate
WBC	white blood cell; white blood cell count

© 2016 Cengage Learning®

CHAPTER REVIEW

The Chapter Review can be used as a self-test. Go through each exercise and answer as many questions as you can without referring to previous exercises or earlier discussions within this chapter. Check your answers and fill in any blanks. Practice writing any terms you might have misspelled.

EXERCISE 18

Analyze each term by writing the prefix, root, combining vowel, and suffix separated by vertical slashes. Based on the meaning of the word parts, write a definition for each term. Check your definition in a medical dictionary.

1. agranulocyte

prefix	*root*	*combining vowel*	*suffix*

DEFINITION: _____

2. phagocyte

prefix	*root*	*combining vowel*	*suffix*

DEFINITION: _____

3. hematology

prefix	root	combining vowel	suffix

DEFINITION: _____

4. phagocytosis

prefix	root	combining vowel	suffix

DEFINITION: _____

5. erythrocytopenia

prefix	root	combining vowel	suffix

DEFINITION: _____

6. lymphadenopathy

prefix	root	combining vowel	suffix

DEFINITION: _____

7. mononucleosis

prefix	root	combining vowel	suffix

DEFINITION: _____

8. pancytopenia

prefix	root	combining vowel	suffix

DEFINITION: _____

9. splenomegaly

prefix	root	combining vowel	suffix

DEFINITION: _____

10. lymphangiogram

prefix	root	combining vowel	suffix

DEFINITION: _____

11. hemostasis

prefix	root	combining vowel	suffix

DEFINITION: _____

12. anemia

prefix	root	combining vowel	suffix

DEFINITION: _____

13. leukopenia

prefix	root	combining vowel	suffix

DEFINITION: _____

14. polycythemia

prefix	*root*	*combining vowel*	*suffix*

DEFINITION: _____

15. hematocrit

prefix	*root*	*combining vowel*	*suffix*

DEFINITION: _____

EXERCISE 19

Replace the italicized phrase with the correct medical term.

1. Jolinda decided to continue her residency in the *study of blood.*

   _____

2. *Inflammation of the adenoids* is often seen in "strep" throat.

   _____

3. Victoria's stroke was caused by a *circulating blood clot.*

   _____

4. *Destruction of red blood cells* might be part of an anemic condition.

   _____

5. *Excessive blood loss* is a clinical indication for a blood transfusion.

   _____

6. Mononucleosis is often characterized by *enlargement of the spleen.*

   _____

7. A *blood clot* might resolve without medical intervention.

   _____

8. Following surgery, Reetha was treated for *a disease-causing bacteria in the blood.*

   _____

9. A *decrease in the number of thrombocytes* might contribute to a bleeding disorder.

   _____

10. *Blood clotting* is dependent on the quality and quantity of available platelets.

   _____

EXERCISE 20

Read the following progress note and write a definition for the italicized terms or phrases on the spaces provided. Use a medical dictionary to check your definition.

PROGRESS NOTE
Rebecca is a 19-year-old college sophomore who was seen today for a low-grade fever, fatigue, and sore throat off and on for the past three weeks. She states she did not "have time" to come in earlier because she has been "cramming for exams." Examination reveals inflamed (1) *pharyngeal tonsils* and tenderness in the axilla and neck area consistent with (2) *lymphadenopathy*. Palpation of the abdomen is positive for marked (3) *splenomegaly*. Results of the (4) CBC and (5) white blood cell differential showed an atypical (6) *lymphocytosis*. Based on these findings, I ordered a serum analysis to confirm infectious (7) *mononucleosis*. Rebecca is advised to take it easy until we have the serum analysis results. I discussed the potential complications of infectious mononucleosis, which include (8) *granulocytopenia*, (9) *thrombocytopenia*, and (10) *hemolytic anemia*. Rebecca agreed to seek treatment at the local emergency room should her symptoms worsen.

1. _____
2. _____
3. _____
4. _____
5. _____
6. _____
7. _____
8. _____
9. _____
10. _____

EXERCISE 21

Select the best answer for each statement or question.

1. Which white blood cell does not absorb stains?
   a. basophil
   b. eosinophil
   c. granulocyte
   d. agranulocyte

2. Select the lymph structure(s) also known as the adenoids.
   a. thymus
   b. pharyngeal tonsils
   c. palatine tonsils
   d. lingual tonsils

3. Which white blood cell releases histamine and heparin?
   a. basophil
   b. eosinophil
   c. monocyte
   d. neutrophil

4. Select the white blood cell that stains rosy-red.
   a. basophil
   b. eosinophil
   c. monocyte
   d. neutrophil

5. Which substance is the main component of erythrocytes?
   a. hematocrit
   b. antibodies
   c. hemoglobin
   d. heparin

6. Select the medical term for abnormal stacking of erythrocytes.
   a. agglutination
   b. rouleaux
   c. coagulation
   d. hemolysis

7. Which type of anemia is characterized by erythrocyte destruction?
   a. aplastic anemia
   b. pernicious anemia
   c. sickle cell anemia
   d. hemolytic anemia

8. Select the blood/lymph vessel that collects interstitial fluid.
   a. lymph capillaries
   b. venule
   c. lymph ducts
   d. arterioles

9. Which blood/lymph organ filters blood?
   a. thymus
   b. spleen
   c. adenoids
   d. tonsils

10. Select the lymph cells that attack other abnormal cells.
    a. monocytes
    b. lymphocytes
    c. T lymphocytes
    d. macrophages

CHALLENGE EXERCISE

Search the Internet site WebMD for information about AIDS. Based on the informa-tion on that site, answer the following questions: What is the name of the pathogenic organism that causes AIDS? How is AIDS transmitted? What precautions should health care professionals take to minimize the risk of infection?

Pronunciation Review

Review the terms in the chapter. Pronounce each term using the following phonetic pronunciations. Check off each term when you are comfortable saying it.

TERM	PRONUNCIATION
☐ adenoid	**ADD**-eh-noyd
☐ adenoiditis	**add**-eh-noyd-**EYE**-tis
☐ agglutination	**ah**-gloo-tih-**NAY**-shun
☐ agranulocyte	ay-**GRAN**-yoo-loh-sight
☐ anemia	ah-**NEE**-mee-ah
☐ antibodies	**AN**-tih-bod-eez
☐ aplastic anemia	ah-**PLAS**-tik ah-**NEE**-mee-ah
☐ basophil	**BAY**-soh-fill
☐ blood transfusion	blood trans-**FYOO**-zhun
☐ bone marrow biopsy	bone marrow **BY**-op-see
☐ coagulation	**koh**-ag-yoo-**LAY**-shun
☐ corpuscle	**KOR**-pus-ehl
☐ dyscrasia	diss-**KRAY**-zee-ah
☐ embolism	**EM**-boh-lizm
☐ embolus	**EM**-boh-lus
☐ eosinophil	ee-oh-**SIN**-oh-fill
☐ erythremia	eh-rih-**THREE**-mee-ah
☐ erythrocyte	eh-**RITH**-roh-sight
☐ erythrocyte sedimentation rate	eh-**RITH**-roh-sight **sed**-ih-men-**TAY**-shun rate
☐ erythrocytopenia	eh-**rith**-roh-**sigh**-toh-**PEE**-nee-ah
☐ granulocyte	**GRAN**-yoo-loh-sight
☐ granulocytosis	**gran**-yoo-loh-sigh-**TOH**-sis
☐ hematocrit	hee-**MAT**-oh-krit
☐ hematologist	**hee**-mah-**TALL**-oh-jist
☐ hematology	**hee**-mah-**TALL**-oh-jee
☐ hemoglobin	**hee**-moh-**GLOH**-bin
☐ hemolysis	hee-**MALL**-ih-sis
☐ hemolytic anemia	hee-moh-LIT-ik ah-NEE-mee-ah
☐ hemophilia	**hee**-moh-**FILL**-ee-ah
☐ hemorrhage	**HEM**-eh-rij
☐ hemostasis	**hee**-moh-**STAY**-sis
☐ heparin	**HEP**-ah-rin
☐ histamine	**HISS**-tah-meen
☐ Hodgkin's disease	**HODJ**-kins disease
☐ interstitial	in-ter-**STIH**-shill

☐ iron deficiency anemia   iron deficiency ah-**NEE**-mee-ah
☐ leukemia   loo-**KEE**-mee-ah
☐ leukocyte   **LOO**-koh-sight
☐ leukopenia   **loo**-koh-**PEE**-nee-ah
☐ lingual tonsils   **LING**-gwal **TON**-sills
☐ lymph   LIMF
☐ lymph nodes   LIMF nodes
☐ lymph vessels   LIMF vessels
☐ lymphadenitis   lim-fad-en-**EYE**-tis
☐ lymphadenopathy   lim-fad-eh-**NOP**-ah-thee
☐ lymphangiogram   lim-**FAN**-jee-oh-gram
☐ lymphocyte   **LIM**-foh-sight
☐ lymphoma   lim-**FOH**-mah
☐ macrophage   **MAK**-roh-fayj
☐ monocyte   **MON**-oh-sight
☐ mononucleosis   **mon**-oh-noo-klee-**OH**-sis
☐ multiple myeloma   **MULL**-tih-p'l my-eh-**LOH**-mah
☐ neutrophil   **NOO**-troh-fill
☐ palatine tonsils   **PAL**-ah-tine **TON**-sills
☐ pancytopenia   **pan**-sigh-toh-**PEE**-nee-ah
☐ pathogen   **PATH**-oh-jen
☐ pernicious anemia   per-**NISH**-us ah-**NEE**-mee-ah
☐ phagocyte   **FAG**-oh-sight
☐ phagocytosis   fag-oh-sigh-**TOH**-sis
☐ pharyngeal tonsils   **fair**-in-**JEE**-al **TON**-sills
☐ plasma   **PLAZ**-mah
☐ platelet   **PLAYT**-let
☐ platelet count   **PLAYT**-let count
☐ polycythemia   **pol**-ee-sigh-**THEE**-mee-ah
☐ polycythemia vera   **pol**-ee-sigh-**THEE**-mee-ah **VAIR**-ah
☐ prothrombin   proh-**THROM**-bin
☐ prothrombin time   proh-**THROM**-bin time
☐ purpura   **PURR**-pyoo-rah
☐ rouleaux   roo-**LOH**
☐ septicemia   **sep**-tih-**SEE**-mee-ah
☐ sickle cell anemia   **SIK**-ul sell ah-**NEE**-mee-ah
☐ spherocytosis   **sfee**-roh-sigh-**TOH**-sis
☐ splenomegaly   splee-neh-**MEG**-ah-lee
☐ thalassemia   thal-ah-**SEE**-mee-ah
☐ thrombocyte   **THROM**-boh-sight
☐ thrombocytopenia   **throm**-boh-**sigh**-toh-**PEE**-nee-ah
☐ thrombosis   throm-**BOH**-sis
☐ thrombus   **THROM**-bus
☐ thymosin   thigh-**MOH**-sin
☐ thymus   **THIGH**-mus
☐ tonsillitis   **ton**-sih-**LIGH**-tis
☐ tonsils   **TON**-sills
☐ white blood cell differential   white blood cell diff-er-**EN**-shal

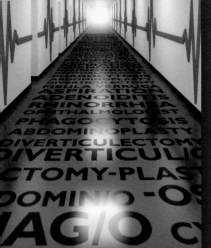

8 Respiratory System

OBJECTIVES

At the completion of this chapter, the student should be able to:

1. Identify, define, and spell word roots associated with the respiratory system.
2. Label the basic structures of the respiratory system.
3. Discuss the functions of the respiratory system.
4. Provide the correct spelling of respiratory terms, given the definition of the terms.
5. Analyze respiratory terms by defining the roots, prefixes, and suffixes of these terms.
6. Identify, define, and spell disease, disorder, and procedure terms related to the respiratory system.

OVERVIEW

The respiratory system is made up of the nose, pharynx, larynx, trachea, bronchi, and lungs. The structures of the respiratory system function together for the following purposes: to provide oxygen to all body cells, to remove the waste product carbon dioxide from all body cells, to assist the body's defense mechanisms against foreign material, and to produce sound necessary for speech. The respiratory system moves oxygen and carbon dioxide by external respiration and internal respiration.

External respiration is the exchange of air between the lungs and the external environment. When a person inhales, the oxygen in the air is drawn into the lungs. During exhalation, carbon dioxide is released into the environment.

Internal respiration is the exchange of oxygen and carbon dioxide between the cells and the blood. The blood delivers oxygen to every cell, via the cardiovascular system, and picks up carbon dioxide. The carbon dioxide is then returned to the lungs and, as previously noted, expelled from the body when you exhale.

Respiratory System Word Roots

To understand and use respiratory system medical terms, it is necessary to acquire a thorough knowledge of the associated word roots. Word roots associated with the respiratory system are listed with the combining vowel. Review the word roots in Table 8-1 and complete the exercises that follow.

TABLE 8-1 RESPIRATORY SYSTEM ROOT WORDS

Word Root/Combining Form	Meaning
alveol/o	alveolus
bronch/o; bronch/i	bronchus
bronchiol/o	bronchus
epiglott/o	epiglottis
laryng/o	larynx
nas/o	nose
orth/o	straight
pector/o	chest
pharyng/o	pharynx
phren/o	diaphragm
pleur/o	pleura
pneum/o; pneumon/o	lung; air
pulmon/o	lungs
rhin/o	nose
sinus/o	sinus
spir/o	breathe; breath
tonsill/o	tonsils
thorac/o	chest
trache/o	trachea

© 2016 Cengage Learning®

EXERCISE 1

Write the definitions of the following word roots.

1. alveol/o　　_____

2. bronch/o　　_____

3. bronchiol/o　_____

4. epiglott/o　 _____

5. laryng/o　　_____

6. nas/o　　　 _____

7. orth/o　　　_____

8. pector/o　　_____

9. pharyng/o　_____

10. phren/o　　_____

11. pleur/o　　 _____

12. pneum/o　　_____

13. pneumon/o　_____

14. pulmon/o　 _____

15. rhin/o   _____

16. sinus/o   _____

17. thorac/o   _____

18. trache/o   _____

EXERCISE 2

Write the word root and its meaning on the space provided.

1. alveolar

   ROOT: _____   MEANING: _____

2. sinusitis

   ROOT: _____   MEANING: _____

3. pleurisy

   ROOT: _____   MEANING: _____

4. rhinitis

   ROOT: _____   MEANING: _____

5. pneumothorax

   ROOT: _____   MEANING: _____

6. nasopharynx

   ROOT: _____   MEANING: _____

7. bronchopneumonia

   ROOT: _____   MEANING: _____

8. laryngitis

   ROOT: _____   MEANING: _____

9. thoracocentesis

   ROOT: _____   MEANING: _____

10. epiglottis

    ROOT: _____   MEANING: _____

11. tonsillitis

    ROOT: _____   MEANING: _____

12. phrenic

    ROOT: _____   MEANING: _____

EXERCISE 3

Write the correct word root(s) for the following definitions.

1. lungs   _____

2. nose   _____

3. diaphragm   _____

4. chest   _____

5. straight   _____

6. pleura   _____

7. alveolus   _____

8. trachea   _____

9. breathe; breath _____

10. tonsils   _____

Structures of the Respiratory System

The structures of the respiratory system include the (1) **nose**, (2) **nasal cavity**, (3) **pharynx** (**FAIR**-inks), (4) **larynx** (**LAIR**-inks), (5) **trachea** (**TRAY**-kee-ah), (6) **lungs**, (7) **bronchi** (**BRONG**-kigh), (8) **bronchiole** (**BRONG**-kee-ohl), (9) **alveoli** (al-**VEE**-oh-ligh), and (10) **diaphragm** (**DIGH**-ah-fram). Figure 8-1 illustrates these structures. Refer to this figure as you read about each structure.

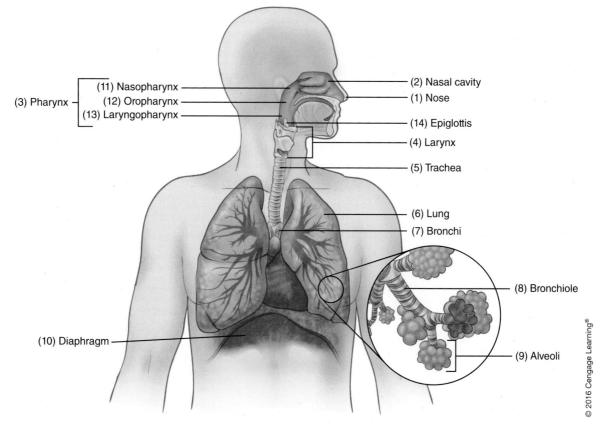

Figure 8-1 Structures of the respiratory system.

© 2016 Cengage Learning®

Nose

The (1) nose and mouth direct air into the body. The entrances to the nose are the **nares** (**NAIRZ**), also called *nostrils*. Air enters the nose through the right and left chambers of the (2) nasal cavity. A cartilage wall called the **septum** divides the chambers. Air also passes through the **paranasal sinuses**, which are cavities in the skull that open into the nasal cavity. The nose and sinuses are lined with mucous membranes and hairlike projections called **cilia**. The mucous membranes warm the air on its way into the lungs. The cilia sweep dirt and foreign particles toward the throat away from the lungs.

Pharynx and Larynx

The (3) pharynx, or throat, connects the nose and mouth to the (4) larynx, or voice box. The pharynx has three sections: the (11) **nasopharynx** (**nay**-zoh-**FAIR**-inks), the upper section; the (12) **oropharynx** (**or**-oh-**FAIR**-inks), the middle section; and the (13) **laryngopharynx** (lah-**ring**-oh-**FAIR**-inks), the lower portion. These sections are illustrated in Figure 8-1. The pharynx serves as the passageway for air, food, and liquids. As food and liquids pass through the pharynx, they must be prevented from entering the lungs. A small flap of cartilage, called the (14) **epiglottis** (ep-ih-**GLOT**-iss), closes over the trachea and prevents food and liquids from entering the larynx. The adenoids and tonsils are located in the pharynx.

The larynx, also called the voice box, contains **vocal cords** that make vocal sounds. As air passes through the spaces between the vocal cords, sound is produced. The spaces between the vocal cords are called the **glottis** (**GLOT**-iss). The larynx is made up of cartilage. The most prominent cartilage, usually seen on men, is actually the thyroid cartilage, often called the "Adam's apple." The larynx is connected to the trachea. Figure 8-2 illustrates the larynx and vocal cords.

Trachea, Bronchi, and Lungs

The trachea, bronchi, lungs, and related structures are illustrated in Figures 8-3, 8-4, and 8-5. Refer to these figures as you read about these structures.

The (1) **trachea** is commonly called the windpipe. It is the passageway for air and consists of muscular tissue that is kept open by a series of C-shaped cartilage rings. Before entering the lungs, the trachea branches into two tubes, called (2) **bronchi** (**BRONG**-kigh). One **bronchus** (**BRONG**-kus) enters the right lung,

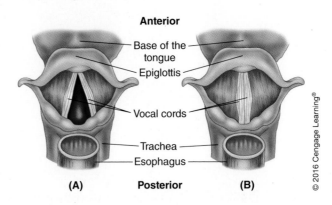

Figure 8-2 Superior view of the larynx and vocal cords. (A) Vocal cords open during breathing. (B) Vocal cords vibrate together during speech.

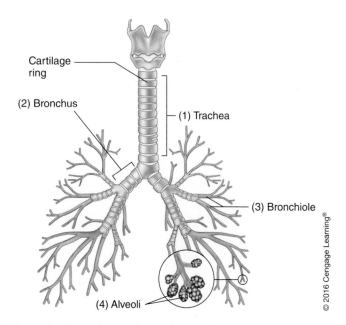

Figure 8-3   The trachea, bronchus, bronchiole, and alveoli.

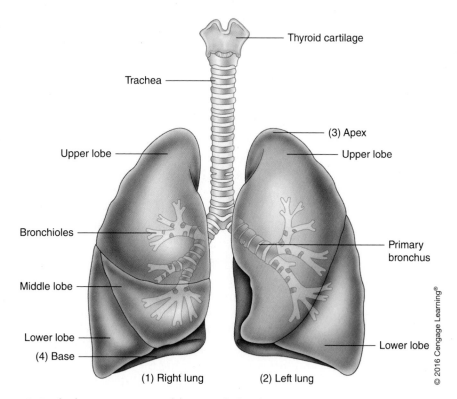

Figure 8-4   Lobes, apex, and base of the lungs.

and the other enters the left lung. Bronchi, as well as nerves and blood vessels, enter the lungs at a specific location called the **hilum** (**HIGH**-lum).

In the lungs, the bronchi divide into progressively smaller tubes called (3) **bronchioles** (**BRONG**-kee-ohlz). The bronchioles end in clusters of air sacs called

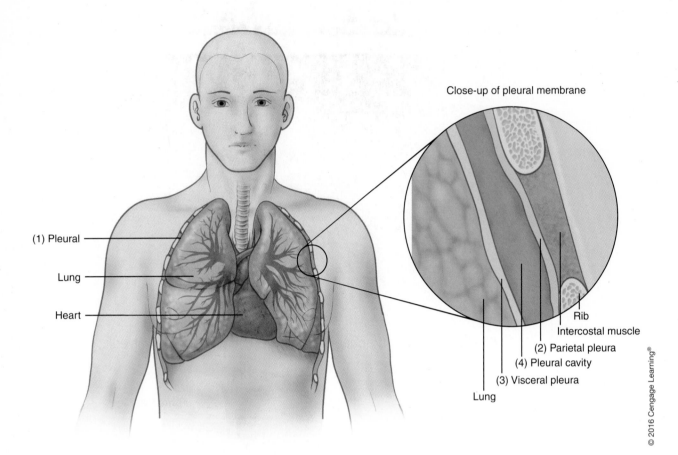

Close-up of pleural membrane

(1) Pleural

Lung

Heart

Rib
Intercostal muscle
(2) Parietal pleura
(4) Pleural cavity
(3) Visceral pleura
Lung

© 2016 Cengage Learning®

Figure 8-5   Parietal pleura, visceral pleura, and pleural cavity.

(4) **alveoli** (al-**VEE**-oh-ligh) (Figure 8-3). The alveoli are surrounded by capillaries. Oxygen and carbon dioxide pass between the alveoli and capillaries into the blood. The cardiovascular system delivers the oxygen-rich blood to the cells, and returns oxygen-poor blood to the lungs.

The lungs are cone-shaped, spongy organs that house the bronchi, bronchioles, alveoli, blood vessels, nerves, and elastic tissue. The lungs are divided into lobes: The (1) **right lung** has three lobes, and the (2) **left lung** has two lobes. The superior aspect of the lung is called the (3) **apex**, and the inferior aspect of the lung is called the (4) **base** (Figure 8-4).

A double-folded membrane called the (1) **pleural** (**PLOO**-ral) membrane or **pleura** (**PLOO**-rah) surrounds the lungs. The (2) **parietal** (pah-**RIGH**-eh-tal) **membrane** is the outer layer. It lines the wall of the thoracic cavity, covers the diaphragm, and forms a sac containing the lungs. The (3) **visceral** (**VISS**-eh-ral) **membrane** is the inner layer and is attached directly to the lungs. The small space between the layers is the (4) **pleural cavity** or space. The pleural cavity is filled with pleural fluid that prevents friction between the lungs and ribs during respiration.

The diaphragm is a muscular partition that separates the thoracic and abdominal cavities. During inhalation, the diaphragm drops to enlarge the thoracic cavity and draw air into the lungs. During exhalation, the diaphragm returns to its normal position and helps push air out of the lungs. Drawing air into the lungs is called **inhalation** or **inspiration**. Pushing air out of the lungs is called **exhalation** or **expiration**.

EXERCISE 4

Match the respiratory system structures in Column 1 with the correct definition in Column 2.

COLUMN 1

_____ 1. alveoli

_____ 2. bronchi

_____ 3. bronchioles

_____ 4. capillaries

_____ 5. diaphragm

_____ 6. hilum

_____ 7. larynx

_____ 8. lungs

_____ 9. Nares

_____ 10. pharynx

_____ 11. pleura

_____ 12. trachea

COLUMN 2

a. muscular partition between the thoracic and abdominal cavities

b. entrances to the nose

c. entrance into the lungs for bronchi, nerves, and blood vessels

d. very small blood vessel in the lungs

e. membranes surrounding the lungs

f. voice box

g. throat

h. tubes leading to the lungs

i. airway; windpipe

j. air sacs

k. cone-shaped, spongy organs

l. "little" bronchi

EXERCISE 5

Label the structures of the respiratory system identified in Figure 8-6. Write your answer on the spaces provided.

1. _____

2. _____

3. _____

4. _____

5. _____

6. _____

7. _____

8. _____

9. _____

10. _____

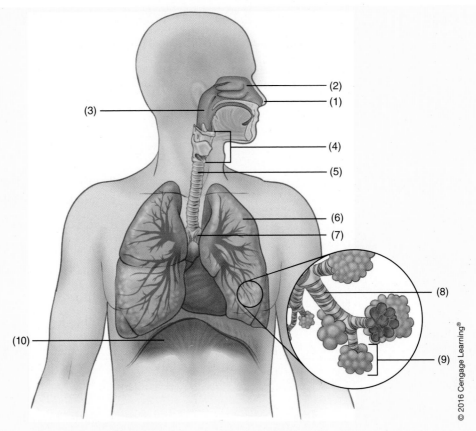

Figure 8-6 Respiratory system labeling exercise.

Respiratory System Medical Terminology

Respiratory system medical terms are organized into three main categories: (1) general medical terms; (2) disease and condition terms; and (3) diagnostic procedure, surgery, and laboratory test terms. Word roots, prefixes, and suffixes that are often a part of respiratory medical terms are listed in Table 8-2. Review these word parts and complete the related exercises.

TABLE 8-2 ROOTS, PREFIXES, AND SUFFIXES FOR THE RESPIRATORY SYSTEM TERMS

Root	Meaning	Prefix	Meaning	Suffix	Meaning
anthrac/o	coal	eu-	normal	-capnia	carbon dioxide
atel/o	incomplete			-ectasis	stretching; dilatation
coni/o	dust			-meter	instrument to measure
hem/o	blood			-metry	measuring
hemat/o	blood			-phonia	sound; voice
muc/o	mucus			-pnea	breathing
ox/i	oxygen			-ptysis	coughing; spitting up
py/o	pus			-(r)rhagia	hemorrhage
				-(r)rhea	copious discharge
				-thorax	chest

EXERCISE 6

Write the root, prefix, or suffix for each meaning.

1. breathing   _____
2. coal   _____
3. carbon dioxide   _____
4. coughing; spitting up   _____
5. copious discharge   _____
6. dust   _____
7. hemorrhage   _____
8. mucus   _____
9. oxygen   _____
10. stretching out; dilatation   _____

EXERCISE 7

Write the root, prefix, suffix, and their meanings for each term. Based on the meanings, write a definition of the term. Use a medical dictionary to check the definition.

EXAMPLE: tonsillitis
ROOT: tonsill/o   MEANING: tonsils
PREFIX: no prefix
SUFFIX: -itis   MEANING: inflammation
DEFINITION: inflammation of the tonsils

1. anoxia

   ROOT: _____ MEANING: _____

   PREFIX: _____ MEANING: _____

   SUFFIX: _____ MEANING: _____

   DEFINITION: _____

2. eupnea

   ROOT: _____ MEANING: _____

   PREFIX: _____ MEANING: _____

   SUFFIX: _____ MEANING: _____

   DEFINITION: _____

3. atelectasis

   ROOT: _____ MEANING: _____

   PREFIX: _____ MEANING: _____

   SUFFIX: _____ MEANING: _____

   DEFINITION: _____

4. pyothorax

ROOT: _____ MEANING: _____

PREFIX: _____ MEANING: _____

SUFFIX: _____ MEANING: _____

DEFINITION: _____

5. orthopnea

ROOT: _____ MEANING: _____

PREFIX: _____ MEANING: _____

SUFFIX: _____ MEANING: _____

DEFINITION: _____

6. hemothorax

ROOT: _____ MEANING: _____

PREFIX: _____ MEANING: _____

SUFFIX: _____ MEANING: _____

DEFINITION: _____

7. hemoptysis

ROOT: _____ MEANING: _____

PREFIX: _____ MEANING: _____

SUFFIX: _____ MEANING: _____

DEFINITION: _____

8. pyorrhea

ROOT: _____ MEANING: _____

PREFIX: _____ MEANING: _____

SUFFIX: _____ MEANING: _____

DEFINITION: _____

9. oximetry

ROOT: _____ MEANING: _____

PREFIX: _____ MEANING: _____

SUFFIX: _____ MEANING: _____

DEFINITION: _____

Respiratory System General Medical Terms

Review the pronunciation and meaning of each term in Table 8-3. Note that some terms are built from word parts and some are not. Complete the exercises for these terms.

TABLE 8-3   RESPIRATORY SYSTEM GENERAL MEDICAL TERMS

Term with Pronunciation	Definition
aspirate (**ASS**-pih-rayt)	to withdraw or suction fluid; to draw foreign material into the lungs
nebulizer (**NEB**-yoo-ligh-zer)	mechanic device for delivering a fine spray or mist into the respiratory tract
oximeter (ock-**SIM**-eh-ter) ox/o = oxygen -meter = instrument to measure	instrument for measuring oxygen saturation in the blood
patent (**PAY**-tent)	open
pulmonologist (**pull**-mon-**ALL**-oh-jist) pulmon/o = lungs -(o)logist = specialist	physician who specializes in respiratory diseases
respiratory therapist (RT)	allied health professional who administers respiratory therapy treatments
spirometer (spigh-**ROM**-eh-ter) spir/o = breathing -meter = instrument to measure	instrument used to measure breathing
ventilator (**VENT**-ih-lay-tor)	mechanical device used to assist with or substitute for patient's breathing

© 2016 Cengage Learning®

EXERCISE 8

Replace the italicized phrase with the correct respiratory term.

1. The respiratory therapist instructed Beth on the use of the *piece of equipment that creates a fine spray or mist.*

   _____

2. Brian set a goal to become a *physician who specializes in respiratory diseases.*

   _____

3. The *instrument that measures oxygen saturation* was placed on the patient's finger.

   _____

4. The hospital board of directors decided it was time to purchase a new *instrument that measures breathing.*

   _____

5. As part of Juan's treatment, the physician decided to *withdraw or suction* the fluid from his bronchi.

———————————————

6. An *open* trachea is necessary for a successful surgical intervention.

———————————————

7. The *machine to assist breathing* is a piece of medical equipment that sustains life.

———————————————

Respiratory System Disease and Disorder Terms

Respiratory system diseases and disorders include familiar problems such as influenza as well as more complex and less familiar diagnoses such as *Pneumocystis carinii* pneumonia. The medical terms are presented in alphabetical order in Table 8-4. Review the pronunciation and definition for each term and complete the exercises.

TABLE 8-4   RESPIRATORY SYSTEM DISEASE AND DISORDER TERMS

Term with Pronunciation	Definition
acapnia (ay-**KAP**-nee-ah) a- = without -capnia = carbon dioxide	absence of carbon dioxide in the blood; less than normal blood levels of carbon dioxide
adenoiditis (**ad**-eh-noyd-**EYE**-tis) adenoid/o = adenoids -itis = inflammation	inflammation of the adenoids
adult respiratory distress syndrome (ARDS)	respiratory failure associated with a variety of acute conditions that directly or indirectly injure the lung, for example, primary bacterial or viral pneumonias, aspiration of gastric contents, and trauma
anoxia (an-**OCKS**-ee-ah) an- = absence; lack of ox/i = oxygen -a = noun ending	absence or lack of the normal level of oxygen in the blood
anthracosis (an-thrah-**KOH**-sis) anthrac/o = coal -osis = condition	accumulation of carbon deposits in the lungs; black lung disease; coal worker's pneumoconiosis

(continues)

TABLE 8-4   RESPIRATORY SYSTEM DISEASE AND DISORDER TERMS
(continued)

Term with Pronunciation	Definition
aphonia (ay-**FOH**-nee-ah) a- = absence; lack of -phonia = sound or voice	inability to produce sound or speech
apnea (ap-**NEE**-ah) a- = absence; lack of -pnea = breathing	absence or lack of breathing; temporary cessation of breathing
asbestosis (as-bess-**TOH**-sis)	accumulation of asbestos particles in the lungs
asphyxia (as-**FICKS**-ee-ah)	oxygen deprivation; suffocation
asthma (**AZ**-mah)	spasm or swelling of the mucous membranes of the bronchial tubes resulting in wheezing and difficulty in breathing
atelectasis (at-eh-**LEK**-tah-sis) atel/o = incomplete -ectasis = expansion; dilatation	incomplete expansion, usually of the lung
bronchiectasis (**brong**-kee-**EK**-tah-sis) bronch/o = bronchus; bronchi -ectasis = expansion; dilatation	abnormal dilatation or expansion of the bronchi
bronchitis (brong-**KIGH**-tis bronch/o = bronchus, bronchi -itis = inflammation	inflammation of the bronchi
bronchogenic carcinoma (**brong**-koh-**JEN**-ic kar-sin-OH-mah) bronch/o = bronchus -genic = pertaining to development carcin- = cancer; malignant -oma = tumor	a malignant lung tumor originating in the bronchi; lung cancer
bronchopneumonia (**brong**-koh-noo-**MOH**-nee-ah) bronch/o = bronchus pneumon/o = lungs; air -ia = noun ending	inflammation of the bronchi and lungs caused primarily by bacteria

(continues)

TABLE 8-4 RESPIRATORY SYSTEM DISEASE AND DISORDER TERMS
(continued)

Term with Pronunciation	Definition
bronchospasm (**BRONG**-koh-spasm) bronch/o = bronchus -spasm = involuntary contraction	involuntary contraction of the smooth muscle of the walls of the bronchi

© 2016 Cengage Learning®

EXERCISE 9

Analyze each term by writing the prefix, root, combining vowel, and suffix separated by vertical slashes. Based on the meaning of the word parts, write a definition for each term.

EXAMPLE: angiography

	/ angi	/ o	/ graphy
prefix	*root*	*combining vowel*	*suffix*

DEFINITION: process of recording an x-ray picture of a vessel

1. apnea

prefix	*root*	*combining vowel*	*suffix*

DEFINITION: _____

2. atelectasis

prefix	*root*	*combining vowel*	*suffix*

DEFINITION: _____

3. bronchiectasis

prefix	*root*	*combining vowel*	*suffix*

DEFINITION: _____

4. bronchitis

prefix	*root*	*combining vowel*	*suffix*

DEFINITION: _____

5. bronchospasm

prefix	*root*	*combining vowel*	*suffix*

DEFINITION: _____

6. anoxia

prefix	*root*	*combining vowel*	*suffix*

DEFINITION: _____

7. acapnia

_____
prefix   _root_   _combining vowel_   _suffix_

DEFINITION: _____

8. anthracosis

_____
prefix   _root_   _combining vowel_   _suffix_

DEFINITION: _____

EXERCISE 10

Write a definition for each medical term.

1. After years of working in construction, Ben developed _asbestosis._

2. The patient was devastated by the diagnosis of _bronchogenic carcinoma._

3. A common cause of _bronchopneumonia_ is streptococcal bacteria.

4. _Aphonia_ was a temporary outcome of the patient's larynx surgery.

5. Because he has _asthma,_ Joel brings his inhaler to school.

EXERCISE 11

Write the medical term for the italicized phrases.

1. Arthur had recurrent episodes of _inflamed adenoids._

   _____

2. _Oxygen deprivation_ was listed as the immediate cause of death.

   _____

3. According to the respiratory therapist's progress note, the patient exhibited a _lack of oxygen._

   _____

4. The 80-year-old woman was hospitalized for _respiratory failure._

   _____

5. _Absence or lack of breathing_ while asleep may cause symptoms of sleep deprivation.

   _____

6. Coal miners are especially susceptible to _black lung disease._

   _____

7. Because of an *abnormal dilatation of the bronchi,* Tanner had trouble breathing.

   _____

8. Ruby's postoperative complications included an *incomplete expansion* of the right lung.

   _____

Review the pronunciation and definition for each term in Table 8-5 and complete the exercises.

TABLE 8-5 RESPIRATORY SYSTEM DISEASE AND DISORDER TERMS

Term with Pronunciation	Definition
chronic obstructive pulmonary disease (COPD)	a progressive and irreversible condition characterized by obstruction of bronchial airflow and diminished lung capacity
coryza; rhinitis (koh-**RIGH**-zuh) (righ-**NIGH**-tis) rhin/o = nose -itis = inflammation	inflammation of the mucous membranes of the nose; a common cold
croup (KROOP)	a childhood disease characterized by a barking cough, dyspnea, and laryngeal spasms
cystic fibrosis (CF) (**SIS**-tik figh-**BROH**-sis)	a hereditary disorder characterized by excess mucus production in the respiratory tract
deviated septum (**DEE**-vee-ay-ted)	misalignment of the nasal septum due to malformation or injury
dysphonia (diss-**FOH**-nee-ah) dys- = difficult -phonia = voice; sound	difficulty producing speech or vocal sounds
dyspnea (disp-**NEE**-ah) dys- = difficult -pnea = breathing	difficulty breathing
emphysema (em-fih-**SEE**-mah)	distention and destruction of alveolar walls causing decreased elasticity of the lungs (Figure 8-7)
epistaxis, rhinorrhagia (ep-ih-**STAK**-sis) (**righ**-noh-**RAY**-jee-ah) rhin/o = nose -(r)rhagia = hemorrhage	discharge of blood from the nose; nosebleed

(continues)

TABLE 8-5 RESPIRATORY SYSTEM DISEASE AND DISORDER TERMS
(continued)

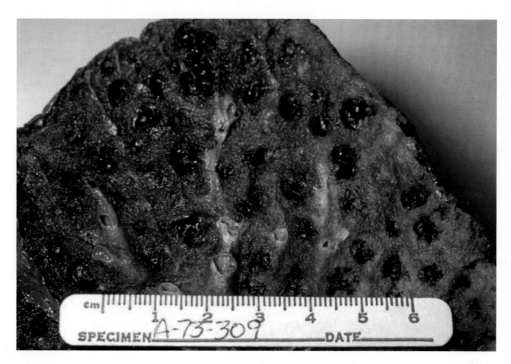

Figure 8-7 Lung tissue with emphysema lesions (Centers for Disease Control and Prevention/Edwin P. Ewing Jr.).

Term with Pronunciation	Definition
hemoptysis (hee-**MOP**-tih-sis) hem/o = blood -ptysis = spitting up	coughing up blood-tinged sputum; spitting up blood
hemothorax (**hee**-moh-**THOR**-aks) hem/o = blood -thorax = chest; chest cavity	blood in the chest cavity or pleural space
hypercapnia (**high**-per-**KAP**-nee-ah) hyper- = excessive; increase -capnia = carbon dioxide	increased or excessive carbon dioxide in the blood
hyperpnea (**high**-perp-**NEE**-ah) hyper- = excessive; increase -pnea = breathing	excessive or increased breathing

EXERCISE 12

Analyze each term by writing the prefix, root, combining vowel, and suffix separated by vertical slashes. Based on the meaning of the word parts, write a definition for each term. Use a medical dictionary to check the definition.

1. rhinitis

prefix	root	combining vowel	suffix

   DEFINITION: _____

2. dysphonia

prefix	root	combining vowel	suffix

   DEFINITION: _____

3. dyspnea

prefix	root	combining vowel	suffix

   DEFINITION: _____

4. rhinorrhagia

prefix	root	combining vowel	suffix

   DEFINITION: _____

5. eupnea

prefix	root	combining vowel	suffix

   DEFINITION: _____

6. hemoptysis

prefix	root	combining vowel	suffix

   DEFINITION: _____

7. hemothorax

prefix	root	combining vowel	suffix

   DEFINITION: _____

8. hypercapnia

prefix	root	combining vowel	suffix

   DEFINITION: _____

9. hyperpnea

prefix	root	combining vowel	suffix

   DEFINITION: _____

EXERCISE 13

Match the condition in Column 1 with the correct definition in Column 2.

COLUMN 1	COLUMN 2
_____ 1. COPD	a. barking cough, dyspnea, and laryngeal spasms
_____ 2. coryza	b. coughing up blood-tinged sputum
_____ 3. croup	c. common cold
_____ 4. cystic fibrosis	d. distention and destruction of alveolar walls
_____ 5. deviated septum	e. excessive carbon dioxide in the blood
_____ 6. emphysema	f. excessive breathing
_____ 7. epistaxis	g. hereditary disorder with excess mucus production
_____ 8. hypercapnia	h. misalignment of the nasal septum
_____ 9. hyperpnea	i. nosebleed
_____ 10. hemoptysis	j. progressive, irreversible, diminished lung capacity

Review the pronunciation and definition for each term in Table 8-6 and complete the exercises.

TABLE 8-6 RESPIRATORY SYSTEM DISEASE AND DISORDER TERMS

Term with Pronunciation	Definition
hypocapnia (**high**-poh-**KAP**-nee-ah) hypo- = decreased; deficient -capnia = carbon dioxide	deficient carbon dioxide levels in the blood
hypopnea (**high**-pop-**NEE**-ah) hypo- = decreased; deficient -pnea = breathing	decreased or deficient breathing
hypoxemia (**high**-pocks-**EE**-mee-ah) hypo- = decreased; deficient ox/i = oxygen- emia = blood	deficient or decreased oxygen in the blood
hypoxia (high-**POCKS**-ee-ah) hypo- = decreased; deficient ox/i = oxygen -a = noun ending	deficient or decreased oxygen supply to body tissue
influenza (flu) (in-floo-**EN**-zah)	highly contagious infection of the respiratory tract caused by a virus

(continues)

TABLE 8-6   RESPIRATORY SYSTEM DISEASE AND DISORDER TERMS
(continued)

Term with Pronunciation	Definition
laryngitis (lair-in-**JIGH**-tis) laryng/o = larynx -itis = inflammation	inflammation of the larynx
laryngospasm (lah-**RING**-oh-spasm) laryng/o = larynx -spasm = involuntary contraction	involuntary or spasmodic contractions of the larynx
Legionnaire's disease (**lee**-jeh-**NAIRZ**)	a lobar pneumonia caused by the *Legionella pneumophila* bacteria
lobar pneumonia (**LOH**-bar noo-**MOH**-nee-ah)	a severe infection of one or more of the five lobes of the lung
mucopurulent (**myoo**-koh-**PYOOR**-yoo-lent)	containing both mucus and pus
mucous (adjective) (**MYOO**-kus) muc/o = mucus -ous = pertaining to	pertaining to mucus or mucus-secreting tissue
mucus (noun) (**MYOO**-kus)	a slimy, viscous secretion of mucous membranes and glands
nasopharyngitis (**nay**-zoh-**fair**-in-**JIGH**-tis) nas/o = nose pharyng/o = pharynx -itis = inflammation	inflammation of the nose and pharynx (i.e., throat)
obstructive sleep apnea	temporary absence of breathing during sleep due to repetitive pharyngeal collapse
orthopnea (or-**THOP**-nee-ah) orth/o = straight -pnea = breathing	ability to breathe only when upright or in the upright position
pansinusitis (**pan**-sigh-nus-**EYE**-tis) pan- = all sinus/o = nasal sinus -itis = inflammation	inflammation of all nasal sinuses
pertussis (per-**TUSS**-is)	a highly contagious respiratory disease characterized by coughing and a loud whooping on inspiration; commonly called whooping cough

(continues)

TABLE 8-6 RESPIRATORY SYSTEM DISEASE AND DISORDER TERMS
(continued)

Term with Pronunciation	Definition
pleural effusion (**PLOO**-ral eh-**FYOO**-zhun)	escape of fluid into the pleural space
pleuritis, pleurisy (ploo-**RIGH**-tis, **PLOOR**-ih-see) pleur/o = pleura -itis = inflammation	inflammation of the pleural membrane

© 2016 Cengage Learning®

EXERCISE 14

Analyze each term by writing the prefix, root, combining vowel, and suffix separated by vertical slashes. Based on the meaning of the word parts, write a definition for each term. Use a medical dictionary to check the definition.

1. hypocapnia

prefix	root	combining vowel	suffix

   DEFINITION: _____

2. hypopnea

prefix	root	combining vowel	suffix

   DEFINITION: _____

3. laryngitis

prefix	root	combining vowel	suffix

   DEFINITION: _____

4. laryngospasm

prefix	root	combining vowel	suffix

   DEFINITION: _____

5. nasopharyngitis

prefix	root	combining vowel	suffix

   DEFINITION: _____

6. mucous

prefix	root	combining vowel	suffix

   DEFINITION: _____

7. orthopnea

prefix	*root*	*combining vowel*	*suffix*

DEFINITION: _____

8. pansinusitis

prefix	*root*	*combining vowel*	*suffix*

DEFINITION: _____

9. pleuritis

prefix	*root*	*combining vowel*	*suffix*

DEFINITION: _____

EXERCISE 15

Replace the italicized phrase with the correct medical term.

1. A premature infant might exhibit *a deficiency of oxygen in the blood.*

   _____

2. Cystic fibrosis is often characterized by copious amounts of *a slimy, viscous secretion.*

   _____

3. The symptoms of *whooping cough* are often frightening to the parents.

   _____

4. *The flu* is a highly contagious infection of the respiratory tract.

   _____

5. Albert's sputum sample was *characterized by mucus and pus.*

   _____

6. *Escape of fluid into the pleural space* can be a postoperative complication.

   _____

7. *A temporary absence of breathing during sleep* is more common in men than in women.

   _____

8. Erythromycin is the preferred treatment for *pneumonia caused by the Legionella pneumophila bacteria.*

   _____

Review the pronunciation and definition for each term in Table 8-7 and complete the exercises.

TABLE 8-7   RESPIRATORY SYSTEM DISEASE AND DISORDER TERMS

Term with Pronunciation	Definition
Pneumocystis carinii pneumonia (**noo**-moh-**SISS**-tis kah-**RIN**-ee-eye noo-**MOH**-nee-ah)	a type of pneumonia caused by a parasite
pneumonia (noo-**MOH**-nee-ah)	an acute inflammation of the lungs
pneumoconiosis (noo-moh-**koh**-nee-**OH**-sis) pneum/o = lungs con/i = dust -osis = condition	any disease of the lung by chronic inhalation of dust, usually mineral dusts of occupational or environmental origin
pulmonary edema (**PULL**-mon-air-ee eh-**DEE**-mah) pulmon/o = lungs -ary = pertaining to	swelling of the lungs caused by an abnormal accumulation of fluid in the lungs
pulmonary embolism (**PULL**-mon-air-ee **EM**-boh-lizm) pulmon/o = lungs -ary = pertaining to	obstruction of one or more of the pulmonary arteries by a thrombus (clot)
pulmonary heart disease (cor pulmonale) (**PULL**-mon-air-ee) (cor pull-mon-**ALL**-ee)	heart failure caused by pulmonary disease
pyothorax, empyema (pigh-oh-**THOH**-raks, em-pigh-**EE**-mah) py/o = pus -thorax = chest	presence of pus in the chest or pleural space
rales (**RALZ**)	abnormal chest sound caused by congested or spasmodic bronchi
respiratory distress syndrome (RDS) of newborns	disorder associated with premature birth and characterized by diffuse atelectasis and immature development of alveolar membranes; also called hyaline membrane disease
rhinorrhea (**righ**-noh-**REE**-ah) rhin/o = nose -(r)rhea = copious discharge; drainage	thin, watery discharge from the nose; runny nose

(continues)

TABLE 8-7 RESPIRATORY SYSTEM DISEASE AND DISORDER TERMS (continued)

Term with Pronunciation	Definition
rhonchi (**RONG**-kigh)	rales or rattling in the throat, resembles snoring
sputum (**SPYOO**-tum)	material coughed up from the lungs
stridor (**STRIGH**-dor)	harsh, high-pitched sound during respiration
tonsillitis (**ton**-sih-**LIGH**-tis) tonsill/o = tonsils -itis = inflammation	inflammation of the palatine tonsils
tracheostenosis (tray-kee-oh-sten-**OH**-sis) trache/o = trachea -stenosis = narrowing	narrowing of the trachea
tuberculosis (TB) (**too**-ber-kyoo-**LOH**- sis)	an infectious disease of the lungs caused by a specific type of bacillus
upper respiratory infection (URI)	infection of the pharynx, larynx, trachea, and bronchi

© 2016 Cengage Learning®

EXERCISE 16

Write the root, suffix, and their meanings for each term. Using the word part meanings, write a definition for the term. Check the definition in a medical dictionary.

1. pneumonoconiosis

   ROOT: _____ MEANING: _____

   SUFFIX: _____ MEANING: _____

   DEFINITION: _____

2. pulmonary edema

   ROOT: _____ MEANING: _____

   SUFFIX: _____ MEANING: _____

   DEFINITION: _____

3. pyothorax

   ROOT: _____ MEANING: _____

   SUFFIX: _____ MEANING: _____

   DEFINITION: _____

4. rhinorrhea

ROOT: _____   MEANING: _____

SUFFIX: _____   MEANING: _____

DEFINITION: _____

5. tonsillitis

ROOT: _____   MEANING: _____

SUFFIX: _____   MEANING: _____

DEFINITION: _____

6. tracheostenosis

ROOT: _____   MEANING: _____

SUFFIX: _____   MEANING: _____

DEFINITION: _____

EXERCISE 17

Match the medical term in Column 1 with the correct definition in Column 2.

COLUMN 1

_____ 1. pneumonia

_____ 2. pneumonoconiosis

_____ 3. pulmonary heart disease

_____ 4. rales

_____ 5. rhonchi

_____ 6. sputum

_____ 7. stridor

_____ 8. tuberculosis

_____ 9. URI

COLUMN 2

a. abnormal chest sound due to congested bronchi

b. acute inflammation of the lungs

c. harsh, high-pitched sound

d. heart failure caused by lung disease

e. infectious lung disease caused by a type of bacillus

f. infection of the pharynx, larynx, trachea, and bronchi

g. lung disease caused by inhaling dust

h. material coughed up from the lungs

i. rattling in the throat

Respiratory System Diagnostic and Treatment Terms

Review the pronunciation and definition of the surgery and diagnostic procedure terms in Table 8-8. Complete the exercises for each set of terms.

TABLE 8-8   RESPIRATORY SYSTEM DIAGNOSTIC AND TREATMENT TERMS

Term with Pronunciation	Definition
adenoidectomy (**add**-eh-noyd-**EK**-toh-mee) adenoid/o = adenoid gland -ectomy = surgical removal or excision	surgical removal of the adenoid glands
bronchoplasty (**BRONG**-koh-**plass**-tee) bronch/o = bronchi -plasty = surgical repair of	surgical repair of the bronchi
bronchoscope (**BRONG**-koh-skohp) bronch/o = bronchi -scope = instrument for viewing	instrument for viewing the bronchi
bronchoscopy (brong-**KOSS**-koh-pee) bronch/o = bronchi -scopy = process of viewing	visualization of the bronchi with a scope (Figure 8-8)

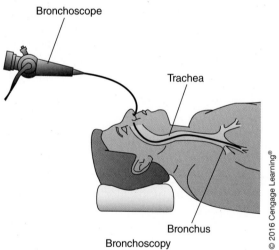

Bronchoscope

Trachea

Bronchus

Bronchoscopy

© 2016 Cengage Learning®

Figure 8-8   Bronchoscopy.

chest x-ray	process of recording an image of the lungs and mediastinum; a radiograph of the chest
esophagram (eh-**SOFF**-ah-gram) esophag/o = esophagus -gram = record	an x-ray record (picture) of the esophagus obtained by using barium as a contrast medium to visualize and identify abnormalities; also known as a barium swallow

(continues)

TABLE 8-8   RESPIRATORY SYSTEM DIAGNOSTIC AND TREATMENT TERMS
(continued)

Term with Pronunciation	Definition
laryngectomy (lair-in-**JEK**-toh-mee) laryng/o = larynx -ectomy = surgical removal or excision	surgical removal of the larynx
laryngocentesis (lah-**ring**-oh-sen-**TEE**-sis) laryng/o = larynx -centesis = surgical puncture to withdraw fluid	surgical puncture into the larynx to withdraw fluid
laryngoplasty (lah-**RING**-oh-**plass**-tee) laryng/o = larynx -plasty = surgical repair	surgical repair of the larynx
laryngoscope (lah-**RING**-oh-skohp) laryng/o = larynx -scope = instrument for viewing	instrument for viewing the larynx
laryngoscopy (lair-in-**GOSS**-koh-pee) laryng/o = larynx -scopy = process of visualization or viewing with a scope	visualization of the larynx with a scope
laryngostomy (lair-in-**GOSS**-toh-mee) laryng/o = larynx -(o)stomy = creation of a new or artificial opening	creation of an artificial opening into the larynx
laryngotracheotomy (lah-**ring**-oh-**tray**-kee-**OT**-oh-mee) laryng/o = larynx trache/o = trachea -(o)tomy = incision into	incision into the larynx and trachea
lobectomy (loh-**BEK**-toh-mee) lob/o = lobe of the lung -ectomy = surgical removal or excision	surgical removal of a lobe of the lung

EXERCISE 18

Analyze each term by writing the root(s), combining vowel, and suffix separated by vertical slashes. Based on the meaning of the word parts, write a definition for each term. Use a medical dictionary to check the definition.

1. adenoidectomy

   _____
   root   *combining vowel*   *suffix*
   DEFINITION: _____

2. bronchoplasty

   _____
   root   *combining vowel*   *suffix*
   DEFINITION: _____

3. bronchoscopy

   _____
   root   *combining vowel*   *suffix*
   DEFINITION: _____

4. laryngectomy

   _____
   root   *combining vowel*   *suffix*
   DEFINITION: _____

5. laryngoscopy

   _____
   root   *combining vowel*   *suffix*
   DEFINITION: _____

6. laryngoplasty

   _____
   root   *combining vowel*   *suffix*
   DEFINITION: _____

7. laryngostomy

   _____
   root   *combining vowel*   *suffix*
   DEFINITION: _____

8. laryngotracheotomy

   _____
   root   *combining vowel*   *suffix*
   DEFINITION: _____

9. lobectomy

   _____
   root   *combining vowel*   *suffix*
   DEFINITION: _____

EXERCISE 19

Write a medical term for each definition.

1. surgical puncture of the larynx to withdraw fluid   _____
2. incision into the larynx and trachea   _____
3. instrument for viewing the bronchi   _____
4. x-ray film of the lungs and mediastinum   _____
5. instrument for viewing the larynx   _____
6. creation of an artificial opening into the larynx   _____
7. surgical removal of a lobe of the lung   _____

Review the pronunciation and definition for each term in Table 8-9 and complete the exercises.

TABLE 8-9   RESPIRATORY SYSTEM DIAGNOSTIC AND TREATMENT TERMS

Term with Pronunciation	Definition
pleurocentesis (**ploo**-roh-sen-**TEE**-sis) pleur/o = pleura; pleural space -centesis = surgical puncture to withdraw fluid	surgical puncture into the pleural space to withdraw fluid
pneumonectomy (**noo**-mon-**EK**-toh-mee) pneumon/o = lung; air -ectomy = surgical removal or excision	surgical removal of a lung
rhinoplasty (**RIGH**-noh-**plass**-tee) rhin/o = nose -plasty = surgical repair of	surgical repair of the nose
septoplasty (**SEP**-toh-plass-tee) sept/o = septum; nasal septum -plasty = surgical repair of	surgical repair of the nasal septum
sinusotomy (sigh-nus-**OT**-oh-mee) sinus/o = sinus; nasal sinus -(o)tomy = incision into	incision into the nasal sinuses
thoracentesis (**thor**-ah-sen-**TEE**-sis) thorac/o = thorax; chest -centesis = surgical puncture to withdraw fluid	surgical puncture into the chest or thorax to withdraw fluid

(continues)

TABLE 8-9   RESPIRATORY SYSTEM DIAGNOSTIC AND TREATMENT TERMS
(continued)

Term with Pronunciation	Definition
thoracoscopy (**thor**-ah-**KOSS**-koh-pee) thorac/o = thorax; chest -scopy = process of viewing or visualization	visual examination of the thorax with a scope
thoracotomy (**thor**-ah-**KOT**-ah-mee) thorac/o = thorax; chest -(o)tomy = incision into	incision into the thorax or chest wall
tonsillectomy (ton-sill-**EK**-toh-mee) tonsil/o = tonsils -ectomy = surgical removal or excision	surgical removal of the tonsils
tracheostomy (**tray**-kee-**OSS**-toh-mee) trache/o = trachea -(o)stomy = creation of a new or artificial opening	creation of a new or artificial opening into the trachea
tracheotomy (tray-kee-**OT**-oh-mee) trache/o = trachea -(o)tomy = incision into	incision into the trachea

© 2016 Cengage Learning®

EXERCISE 20

Analyze each term by writing the root, combining vowel, and suffix separated by vertical slashes. Based on the meaning of the word parts, write a definition for each term. Use a medical dictionary to check the definition.

1. pleurocentesis

   _____ _____ _____
   root   *combining vowel*   *suffix*

   DEFINITION: _____

2. pneumonectomy

   _____ _____ _____
   root   *combining vowel*   *suffix*

   DEFINITION: _____

3. rhinoplasty

   _____ _____ _____
   root   *combining vowel*   *suffix*

   DEFINITION: _____

4. septoplasty

root	combining vowel	suffix

DEFINITION: _____

5. sinusotomy

root	combining vowel	suffix

DEFINITION: _____

6. thoracentesis

root	combining vowel	suffix

DEFINITION: _____

7. thoracotomy

root	combining vowel	suffix

DEFINITION: _____

8. tonsillectomy

root	combining vowel	suffix

DEFINITION: _____

9. tracheostomy

root	combining vowel	suffix

DEFINITION: _____

10. tracheotomy

root	combining vowel	suffix

DEFINITION: _____

11. thoracoscopy

root	combining vowel	suffix

DEFINITION: _____

EXERCISE 21

Replace the italicized phrase with the correct medical term.

1. *Lung removal* may be the only treatment for lung cancer.

   _____

2. As a result of a sports injury, Jacque was scheduled for *a repair of his nasal septum.*

   _____

3. Katie was hopeful that the *incision into her nasal sinuses* would relieve her pain.

   _____

4. To relieve pressure on the heart, the surgeon performed a *surgical puncture into the pleural space to withdraw fluid*.

   _____

5. After Rosita's motor vehicle accident, she underwent a *surgical repair of the nose*.

   _____

6. *Surgical removal of the tonsils* may be recommended following repeated "strep" infections.

   _____

7. The emergency room physician performed an *incision into the trachea* to restore breathing.

   _____

Review the pronunciation and definition for each pulmonary function test in Table 8-10 and complete the exercises.

TABLE 8-10   RESPIRATORY SYSTEM DIAGNOSTIC AND TREATMENT TERMS

Pulmonary Function Test	Definition
arterial blood gases (ABG) (ar-**TEE**-ree-al)	examination of arterial blood to determine blood levels of oxygen, carbon dioxide, and other gases
lung scan	a nuclear medicine study used to detect abnormalities related to air or blood flow to the lungs
oximeter (ock-**SIM**-eh-ter) ox/i = oxygen -meter = measurement; instrument for measuring	instrument for measuring the oxygen saturation of blood
oximetry (ock-**SIM**-eh-tree) ox/i = oxygen -metry = to measure	measuring the oxygen saturation of blood
perfusion (lung) scan (per-**FYOO**-shun)	a nuclear medicine study used to detect areas of inadequate blood flow to the lungs
pulmonary function tests (PFTs) (**PULL**-mon-air-ee) pulmon/o = lungs -ary = pertaining to	a group of tests designed to measure respiratory function and identify abnormalities

(continues)

TABLE 8-10   RESPIRATORY SYSTEM DIAGNOSTIC AND TREATMENT TERMS
(continued)

Pulmonary Function Test	Definition
spirometer (spigh-**ROM**-eh-ter) spir/o = breathing -meter = instrument for measuring	instrument used to measure breathing activity or lung volumes
spirometry (spigh-**ROM**-eh-tree) spir/o = breathing -metry = to measure	the process of measuring breathing or lung volumes
ventilation (lung) scan (vent-ih-**LAY**-shun)	a nuclear medicine study used to detect areas of inadequate air flow to the lungs
ventilation/perfusion (lung) scan (V/Q scan)	a nuclear medicine study used to detect abnormalities of air and blood flow to the lungs

© 2016 Cengage Learning®

EXERCISE 22

Write the correct term for each definition.

1. an instrument for measuring the oxygen saturation of blood

   _____

2. a group of tests designed to measure respiratory function

   _____

3. a nuclear medicine study of the lungs

   _____

4. the process of measuring breathing or lung volumes

   _____

5. the process of measuring the oxygen saturation of blood

   _____

6. an instrument used to measure breathing or lung volumes

   _____

7. method to determine the levels of oxygen and carbon dioxide in arterial blood

   _____

Abbreviation   Review the respiratory system abbreviations in Table 8-11. Practice writing the meaning of each abbreviation.

TABLE 8-11   ABBREVIATIONS

Abbreviation	Meaning
ABG	arterial blood gases
ARD	acute respiratory distress
ARDS	adult respiratory distress syndrome
ARF	acute respiratory failure
CF	cystic fibrosis
CO_2	carbon dioxide
COPD	chronic obstructive pulmonary disease
PCP	*Pneumocystis carinii* pneumonia
PFTs	pulmonary function tests
RDS	respiratory distress syndrome
SOB	shortness of breath
TB	tuberculosis
URI	upper respiratory (tract) infection
V/Q scan	ventilation/perfusion scan

© 2016 Cengage Learning®

CHAPTER REVIEW

The Chapter Review can be used as a self-test. Go through each exercise and answer as many questions as you can without referring to previous exercises or earlier discussions within this chapter. Check your answers and fill in any blanks. Practice writing any terms you might have misspelled.

EXERCISE 23

Using your knowledge of roots, prefixes, and suffixes write the medical term for each definition.

1. lack of oxygen in the blood _____

2. lack or temporary cessation of breathing _____

3. inflammation of the bronchi _____

4. normal breathing _____

5. blood in the thorax or chest cavity _____

6. narrowing of the trachea _____

7. incision into the larynx and trachea _____

8. surgical repair of the nose _____

9. coughing up blood or blood-tinged sputum _____

10. difficulty breathing _____

11. inflammation of the larynx _____

12. pus in the pleural space _____

13. rapid flow of blood from the nose _____

14. surgical removal of the adenoids _____

15. surgical removal of a lung _____

16. incision into the trachea _____

17. surgical puncture into the thorax to withdraw fluid _____

18. excessive or increased breathing _____

19. ability to breathe only when in an upright position _____

20. inflammation of the nose and throat _____

EXERCISE 24

Match the term in Column 1 with the definition in Column 2.

COLUMN 1

_____ 1. anthracosis

_____ 2. asphyxia

_____ 3. atelectasis

_____ 4. bronchiectasis

_____ 5. bronchogenic carcinoma

_____ 6. coryza

_____ 7. emphysema

_____ 8. mucopurulent

_____ 9. pertussis

_____ 10. pleural effusion

_____ 11. pneumonia

_____ 12. pulmonary edema

_____ 13. rhinorrhea

_____ 14. sputum

COLUMN 2

a. oxygen deprivation

b. common cold

c. lung cancer

d. runny nose

e. containing both mucus and pus

f. distention and destruction of the alveolar wall

g. acute lung inflammation

h. black lung disease

i. swelling of the lungs

j. dilatation of the bronchi

k. incomplete expansion of lungs

l. material coughed up from the lungs

m. whooping cough

n. escape of fluid into the pleural space

EXERCISE 25

Read the following discharge note. Write out all abbreviations and a definition for the italicized terms.

DISCHARGE NOTE

This 65-year-old man was admitted for (1) *ARD* that was brought on by an (2) *asthma* attack. The chest examination revealed (3) *stridor* and (4) *rhonchi* associated with (5) *bronchospasm*. The chest x-ray revealed moderate (6) *pulmonary edema* with minimal (7) *pleural effusion* and right lobar (8) *pneumonia*. During the hospitalization, the patient's (9) *ABGs* were normal. He was treated with low-dose prednisone. At discharge, the patient was stable. Final diagnoses: ARD, lobar pneumonia, and (10) *COPD*.

1. _____
2. _____
3. _____
4. _____
5. _____
6. _____
7. _____
8. _____
9. _____
10. _____

EXERCISE 26

Explain the difference between these related terms.

1. hypoxia, hypoxemia

_____

_____

2. mucous, mucus

_____

_____

3. anoxia, asphyxia

_____

_____

4. hemothorax, pneumothorax

_____

_____

5. rhinorrhagia, rhinorrhea

_____

_____

6. pneumonoconiosis, pneumonia

_____

_____

7. rhonchi, rales

_____

_____

EXERCISE 27

Select the best answer for each statement or question.

1. Select the structure that prevents food from entering the larynx.
   a. trachea
   b. epiglottis
   c. pharynx
   d. bronchi

2. Which structure is also called the windpipe?
   a. glottis
   b. pharynx
   c. larynx
   d. trachea

3. Select the medical term for "air sacs."
   a. lungs
   b. diaphragm
   c. alveoli
   d. bronchioles

4. Which term identifies the area at which the bronchi enter the lungs?
   a. hilum
   b. apex
   c. base
   d. diaphragm

5. Select the structure that is sometimes called the "muscle of respiration."
   a. nose
   b. mouth
   c. lungs
   d. diaphragm

6. Which structure is commonly called the "voice box"?
   a. trachea
   b. larynx
   c. pharynx
   d. glottis

7. Which term means the exchange of air between the lungs and the environment?
   a. internal respiration
   b. inspiration
   c. expiration
   d. external respiration

8. Select the medical term for a slimy, viscous discharge of the respiratory system.
   a. mucous
   b. mucus
   c. sputum
   d. pleural effusion

9. Which medical term means decreased oxygen levels in the blood?
   a. hypoxia
   b. anoxia
   c. hypoxemia
   d. hypocapnia

10. Select the medical term for a runny nose.
   a. rhinorrhea
   b. rhinorrhagia
   c. rhinitis
   d. epistaxis

CHALLENGE EXERCISE

Asthma is a difficult disease at any age, and particularly so for children. Visit your local public health department or local chapter of the American Lung Association and ask for information about asthma that is written specifically for children. What types of material are available? If these organizations are not available in your area, search the Internet for the American Lung Association. Are materials available from this site? If so, is there a charge?

Pronunciation Review

Using the CD, listen to each term, pronounce it, and check off the term once you are comfortable saying it.

TERM	PRONUNCIATION
☐ acapnia	ay-**KAP**-nee-ah
☐ adenoidectomy	**add**-eh-noyd-**EK**-toh-mee
☐ adenoiditis	**add**-eh-noyd-**EYE**-tis
☐ alveoli	al-**VEE**-oh-ligh
☐ anoxia	an-**OKS**-ee-ah
☐ anthracosis	an-thrah-**KOH**-sis
☐ aphonia	ay-**FOH**-nee-ah
☐ apnea	ap-**NEE**-ah
☐ arterial blood gases	ar-**TEE**-ree-al blood gases
☐ asbestosis	as-bess-**TOH**-sis
☐ asphyxia	as-**FIKS**-ee-ah
☐ aspirate	**ASS**-pih-rayt
☐ asthma	**AZ**-mah
☐ atelectasis	at-eh-**LEK**-tah-sis
☐ bronchi	**BRONG**-kigh
☐ bronchiectasis	**brong**-kee-**EK**-tah-sis
☐ bronchiole	**BRONG**-kee-ohl
☐ bronchitis	brong-**KIGH**-tis

☐ bronchogenic carcinoma   **brong**-koh-**JEN**-ic **kar**-sin-**OH**-mah
☐ bronchoplasty   **BRONG**-koh-**plass**-tee
☐ bronchoscope   **BRONG**-koh-skohp
☐ bronchoscopy   brong-**KOSS**-koh-pee
☐ bronchus   **BRONG**-kus
☐ cor pulmonale   cor pull-mon-**ALL**-ee
☐ coryza   koh-**RIGH**-zuh
☐ croup   KROOP
☐ cystic fibrosis   **SIS**-tik figh-**BROH**-sis
☐ deviated septum   **DEE**-vee-ay-ted septum
☐ diaphragm   **DIGH**-ah-fram
☐ dysphonia   diss-**FOH**-nee-ah
☐ dyspnea   disp-**NEE**-ah
☐ emphysema   em-fih-**SEE**-mah
☐ empyema   em-pigh-**EE**-mah
☐ epiglottis   **ep**-ih-**GLOT**-iss
☐ epistaxis   **ep**-ih-**STAK**-sis
☐ eupnea   yoop-**NEE**-ah
☐ glottis   **GLOT**-iss
☐ hemoptysis   hee-**MOP**-tih-sis
☐ hemothorax   **hee**-moh-**THOR**-aks
☐ hilum   **HIGH**-lum
☐ hypercapnia   **high**-per-**KAP**-nee-ah
☐ hyperpnea   **high**-perp-**NEE**-ah
☐ hypocapnia   **high**-poh-**KAP**-nee-ah
☐ hypopnea   **high**-pop-**NEE**-ah
☐ hypoxemia   **high**-pocks-**EE**-mee-ah
☐ hypoxia   high-**POCKS**-ee-ah
☐ influenza   in-floo-**EN**-zah
☐ laryngectomy   lair-in-**JEK**-toh-mee
☐ laryngitis   lair-in-**JIGH**-tis
☐ laryngocentesis   lah-**ring**-oh-sen-**TEE**-sis
☐ laryngopharynx   lah-**ring**-oh-**FAIR**-inks
☐ laryngoplasty   lah-**RING**-oh-**plass**-tee
☐ laryngoscope   lah-**RING**-oh-skohp
☐ laryngoscopy   lair-in-**GOSS**-koh-pee
☐ laryngospasm   lah-**RING**-oh-spasm
☐ laryngostomy   lair-in-**GOSS**-toh-mee
☐ laryngotracheotomy   lah-**ring**-oh-**tray**-kee-**OT**-oh-mee
☐ larynx   **LAIR**-inks
☐ Legionnaire's disease   **lee**-jeh-**NAIRZ** disease
☐ lobar pneumonia   **LOH**-bar noo-**MOH**-nee-ah
☐ lobectomy   loh-**BEK**-toh-mee
☐ mediastinum   **mee**-dee-ah-**STIGH**-num
☐ mucopurulent   **myoo**-koh-**PYOOR**-yoo-lent
☐ mucous   **MYOO**-kus
☐ mucus   **MYOO**-kus
☐ nares   **NAIRZ**
☐ nasal cavity   **NAY**-zal cavity
☐ nasopharyngitis   **nay**-zoh-**fair**-in-**JIGH**-tis
☐ nasopharynx   **nay**-zoh-**FAIR**-inks

☐ nebulizer	**NEB**-yoo-ligh-zer
☐ oropharynx	**or**-oh-**FAIR**-inks
☐ orthopnea	or-**THOP**-nee-ah
☐ oximeter	ock-**SIM**-eh-ter
☐ oximetry	ock-**SIM**-eh-tree
☐ pansinusitis	**pan**-sigh-nus-**EYE**-tis
☐ paranasal sinuses	**pair**-ah-**NAY**-sal sinuses
☐ patent	**PAY**-tent
☐ pertussis	per-**TUSS**-iss
☐ pharynx	**FAIR**-inks
☐ pleura	**PLOO**-rah
☐ pleural effusion	**PLOO**-ral eh-**FYOO**-zhun
☐ pleurisy	**PLOOR**-ih-see
☐ pleuritis	ploo-**RIGH**-tis
☐ pleurocentesis	**ploo**-roh-sen-**TEE**-sis
☐ *Pneumocystis carinii* pneumonia	**noo**-moh-**SISS**-tis kah-**RIN**-ee-eye noo-**MOH**-nee-ah
☐ pneumonectomy	**noo**-mon-**EK**-toh-mee
☐ pneumonia	noo-**MOH**-nee-ah
☐ pneumoconiosis	noo-moh-**koh**-nee-**OH**-sis
☐ pulmonary edema	**PULL**-mon-air-ee eh-**DEE**-mah
☐ pulmonary embolism	**PULL**-mon-air-ee **EM**-boh-lizm
☐ pulmonary heart disease	**PULL**-mon-air-ee heart disease
☐ pulmonologist	**pull**-mon-**ALL**-oh-jist
☐ pyothorax	pigh-oh-**THOH**-raks
☐ rales	**RALZ**
☐ rhinitis	righ-**NIGH**-tis
☐ rhinoplasty	**RIGH**-noh-**plass**-tee
☐ rhinorrhagia	**righ**-noh-**RAY**-jee-ah
☐ rhinorrhea	**righ**-noh-**REE**-ah
☐ rhonchi	**RONG**-kigh
☐ septoplasty	**SEP**-toh-plass-tee
☐ septum	**SEP**-tum
☐ sinusotomy	sigh-nus-**OT**-oh-mee
☐ spirometer	spigh-**ROM**-eh-ter
☐ spirometry	spigh-**ROM**-eh-tree
☐ sputum	**SPYOO**-tum
☐ stridor	**STRIGH**-dor
☐ thoracentesis	**thor**-ah-sen-**TEE**-sis
☐ thoracoscope	thoh-**RAK**-oh-skohp
☐ thoracoscopy	**thor**-ah-**KOSS**-koh-pee
☐ thoracotomy	**thor**-ah-**KOT**-ah-mee
☐ tonsillectomy	ton-sill-**EK**-toh-mee
☐ trachea	**TRAY**-kee-ah
☐ tracheostomy	tray-kee-**OSS**-toh-mee
☐ tracheotomy	tray-kee-**OT**-oh-mee
☐ tuberculosis	**too**-ber-kyoo-**LOH**- sis
☐ ventilation/perfusion scan	vent-ih-**LAY**-shun per-**FYOO**-zhun scan
☐ ventilator	**VENT**-ih-lay-tor
☐ wheeze	**WEEZ**

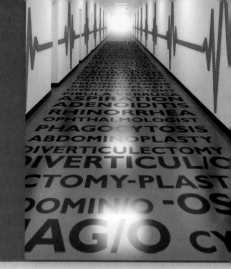

9 Digestive System

OBJECTIVES

At the completion of this chapter, the student should be able to:

1. Identify, define, and spell word roots associated with the digestive system.
2. Label the basic structures of the digestive system.
3. Discuss the functions of the digestive system.
4. Provide the correct spelling of digestive system terms, given the definition of the terms.
5. Analyze digestive system terms by defining the roots, prefixes, and suffixes of these terms.
6. Identify, define, and spell disease, disorder, and procedure terms related to the digestive system.

OVERVIEW

The digestive system, also called the gastrointestinal (GI) tract, alimentary canal, or the digestive tract, is made up of the mouth, pharynx, esophagus, stomach, small intestine, large intestine, and accessory organs, including the salivary glands, liver, gallbladder, and pancreas. The structures of the digestive system function together for the following purposes: (1) to digest food; (2) to absorb nutrients into the bloodstream; and (3) to eliminate solid waste products.

Digestive System Word Roots

To understand and use the digestive system medical terms, it is necessary to acquire a thorough knowledge of the associated word roots. The word roots are listed with the combining vowel in Table 9-1. Review these roots and complete the exercises that follow.

TABLE 9-1 DIGESTIVE SYSTEM ROOT WORDS

Word Root/Combining Form	Meaning
abdomin/o; celi/o	abdomen
an/o	anus
append/o; appendic/o	appendix
bil/i	bile
bucc/o	cheek
cec/o	cecum

(continues)

TABLE 9-1 DIGESTIVE SYSTEM ROOT WORDS (continued)

Word Root/Combining Form	Meaning
cheil/o	lips
chol/e	bile; gall
cholangi/o	bile duct
cholecyst/o	gallbladder
choledoch/o	common bile duct
col/o; colon/o	colon; large intestines
duoden/o	duodenum
enter/o	intestines; small intestines
esophag/o	esophagus
gastr/o	stomach
gingiv/o	gums
gloss/o; lingu/o	tongue
hepat/o	liver
ile/o	ileum
jejun/o	jejunum
lapar/o	abdominal wall
lip/o	fat
lith/o	stone
or/o; stomat/o	mouth
pancreat/o	pancreas
peritone/o	peritoneum
pharyng/o	pharynx
proct/o; rect/o	rectum
sial/o	salivary gland; saliva
sigmoid/o	sigmoid colon

© 2016 Cengage Learning®

EXERCISE 1

Write the meaning for each of the following word roots.

1. cholecyst/o _____

2. duoden/o _____

3. enter/o _____

4. proct/o _____

5. sigmoid/o _____

6. lapar/o _____

7. lith/o _____

8. gastr/o _____

9. chol/e _____

10. hepat/o   _____

11. esophag/o   _____

12. sial/o   _____

13. cholangi/o   _____

14. abdomin/o   _____

15. an/o   _____

EXERCISE 2

Write the word root and meaning in each term.

1. colonoscopy

   ROOT:_____   MEANING:_____

2. appendectomy

   ROOT:_____   MEANING: _____

3. colorectal

   ROOT:_____   MEANING:_____

4. pancreatitis

   ROOT: _____   MEANING:_____

5. rectocele

   ROOT:_____   MEANING:_____

6. laparoscopy

   ROOT:_____   MEANING:_____

7. oral

   ROOT: _____   MEANING:_____

8. ileocecal

   ROOT:_____   MEANING:_____

9. cholelithiasis

   ROOT:_____   MEANING:_____

10. gastrostomy

   ROOT: _____   MEANING: _____

11. gingivitis

   ROOT: _____   MEANING: _____

12. sigmoidoscopy

   ROOT: _____   MEANING: _____

EXERCISE 3

Write the correct combining form(s) for each meaning.

1. abdomen   _____
2. abdominal wall   _____
3. appendix   _____
4. bile   _____
5. cecum   _____
6. cheek   _____
7. common bile duct   _____
8. fat   _____
9. jejunum   _____
10. lips   _____
11. mouth   _____
12. pharynx   _____
13. rectum   _____
14. salivary gland   _____
15. tongue   _____

Structures of the Digestive System

Structures of the digestive system include the (1) **mouth**, also called the oral cavity, and all that is in it; (2) **salivary glands**; (3) **pharynx** (**FAIR**-inks), commonly called the throat; (4) **esophagus** (eh-**SOFF**-ah-gus), a 10-inch tube that extends from the pharynx to the stomach; (5) **stomach**; (6) **small intestine**; (7) **large intestine**; (8) **rectum** and **anus**; (9) **liver**; (10) **gallbladder**; and (11) **pancreas** (**PAN**-kree-ass). Figure 9-1 illustrates these structures.

Mouth/Oral Cavity, Pharynx, Esophagus and Salivary Glands

The mouth, also called the oral cavity, includes the (1) **lips**, (2) **gingiva** (**JIN**-jih-vah), (3) **teeth**, (4) **tongue**, (5) **hard** and (6) **soft palate** (**PAL**-at), and (7) **uvula** (**YOO**-vyoo-lah). Figure 9-2 illustrates the parts of the oral cavity. Refer to this figure as you learn about the mouth.

The lips form the opening to the oral cavity, and the teeth are used to mechanically break down food. The tongue moves the food around the mouth, provides us with our sense of taste, and helps push the food into the throat. The hard palate forms the roof of the mouth, and the soft palate prevents food from entering the nasal cavity. The uvula can trigger our gag reflex and also helps produce sounds and speech.

The **salivary glands** produce **saliva**, a watery substance that contains digestive enzymes. Figure 9-3 illustrates the location of the salivary glands. There are three pairs of salivary glands: (1) **parotid** (pah-**ROT**-id) **glands**, located in front of and slightly below the ear; (2) **sublingual** (sub-**LING**-gwall) **glands**, located underneath

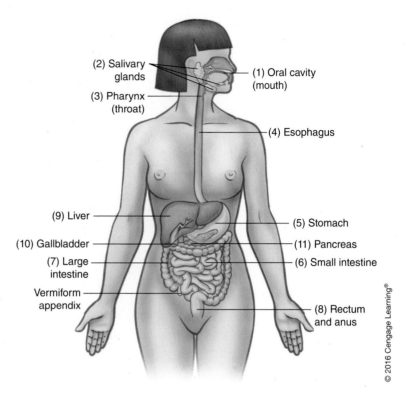

Figure 9-1 Major structures and accessory organs of the digestive system.

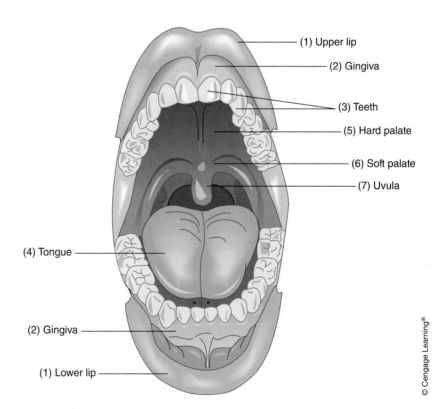

Figure 9-2 Oral cavity.

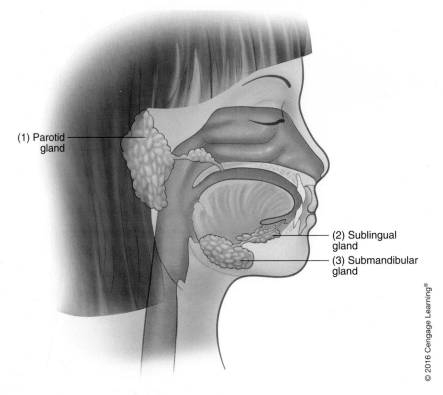

(1) Parotid gland

(2) Sublingual gland

(3) Submandibular gland

© 2016 Cengage Learning®

Figure 9-3 The salivary glands.

the tongue; and (3) **submandibular** (**sub**-man-**DIB**-yoo-lar) **glands**, located on the posterior floor of the mouth.

The **bolus** (**BOH**-lus), which is foodstuffs mixed with salivary secretions, passes through the pharynx into the esophagus, which is a muscular tube. At this point, the bolus is pushed to the stomach by wavelike muscular contractions called **peristalsis** (pair-ih-**STALL**-sis).

Stomach and Small Intestine

The stomach and small intestines are the major organs of digestion. Both the stomach and small intestine function in the digestive process. The small intestine absorbs nutrients into the bloodstream. Figure 9-4 illustrates the stomach and the first segment of the small intestines. Refer to the figure as you learn about the organs.

The bolus of food enters the (1) **stomach** through the (2) **lower esophageal** (eh-**soff**-ah-**JEE**-al) **sphincter** (**SFINGK**-ter), also called the **cardiac sphincter.** This muscular ring at the upper end of the stomach prevents food from moving back into the esophagus. In the stomach, the bolus mixes with digestive juices and hydrochloric acid. The areas of the stomach have specific names. The (3) **fundus** (**FUN**-dus) is the superior area; the (4) **body** is the middle area; the (5) **antrum** (**AN**-trum) is the inferior area. The (6) **pylorus** (pigh-**LOR**-us) is a narrow passage at the end of the antrum that connects the stomach with the small intestines. The (7) **pyloric sphincter** (pigh-**LOR**-ik **SFINGK**-ter), is a muscular ring that allows partially digested food to move into the small intestine.

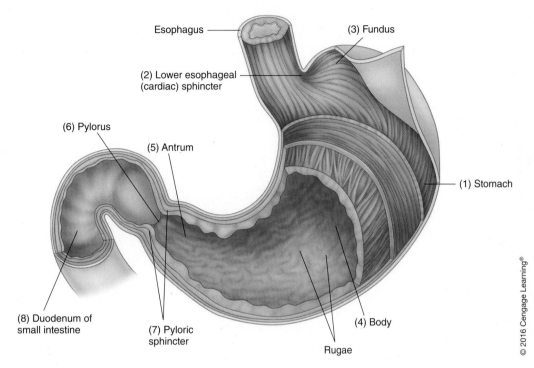

Esophagus

(3) Fundus

(2) Lower esophageal
(cardiac) sphincter

(6) Pylorus

(5) Antrum

(1) Stomach

(8) Duodenum of
small intestine

(7) Pyloric
sphincter

(4) Body

Rugae

Figure 9-4 Stomach and duodenum of the small intestine.

The first 10 to 12 inches of the small intestine is the (8) **duodenum** (doo-oh-**DEE**-num, doo-**ODD**-eh-num); it is here that most digestion occurs. The small intestine is approximately 20 feet in length and extends from the pyloric sphincter to the large intestine. The **jejunum** (jeh-**JOO**-num), the second segment of the small intestine, is approximately 8 feet long; and the **ileum** (**ILL**-ee-um), the third segment of the small intestine, is approximately 11 feet long. As the digested food passes through the small intestines, nutrients are passed into the bloodstream. The remaining waste is liquid and is passed into the large intestine.

Large Intestine

The large intestine is approximately 5 to 6 feet long and extends from the cecum to the anus. Figure 9-5 illustrates the large intestines. Refer to this figure as you learn about the large intestine.

The large intestine is connected to the small intestine by the (1) **ileocecal** (**ill**-ee-oh-**SEE**-kull) **sphincter**. The large intestine has distinct segments and two curves called **flexures** (**FLECK**-shurs). The segments and flexures include: the (2) **cecum** (**SEE**-kum), (3) **ascending colon**, (4) **hepatic** (heh-**PAT**- ic) **flexure**, (5) **transverse colon**, (6) **splenic** (**SPLEN**- ic) **flexure**, (7) **descending colon**, (8) **sigmoid colon**, and the (9) **rectum**. The (10) **anus** is the opening at the end of the rectum.

As liquid waste product moves through the large intestine, water and minerals are absorbed into the bloodstream. The solid to semisolid waste is stored in the rectum. The (11) internal and (12) external **anal sphincter** muscles control the flow of waste out of the body. Note the **vermiform appendix**, often called the appendix, at the lower end of the cecum.

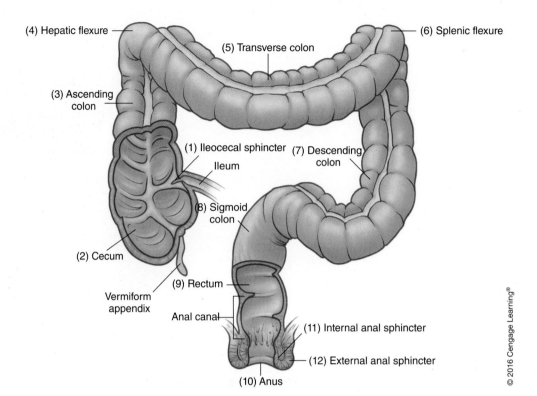

Figure 9-5   Large intestine.

Liver, Gallbladder, and Pancreas

The (1) **liver**, (2) **gallbladder**, and (3) **pancreas** are commonly called the accessory organs of the digestive system. Figure 9-6 illustrates these organs. Refer to this figure as you learn about these organs. The liver is the largest organ in the body and has a right and left lobe. The gallbladder is a pear-shaped organ located under the liver, and the pancreas is located behind the stomach.

The liver produces bile, which is necessary for the digestion of fats. Bile is stored in the gallbladder, a small saclike structure. The pancreas, which functions as a digestive organ and an endocrine gland, produces additional digestive juices that help digest all types of foods.

Bile and pancreatic digestive juices empty into the duodenum by a series of ducts. Note in Figure 9-6 that the (4) **right** and (5) **left hepatic ducts** come together to form the (6) **common hepatic duct**. The common hepatic duct joins with the (7) **cystic duct** to form the (8) **common bile duct**. The common bile duct joins with the (9) **pancreatic ducts** and enters the duodenum.

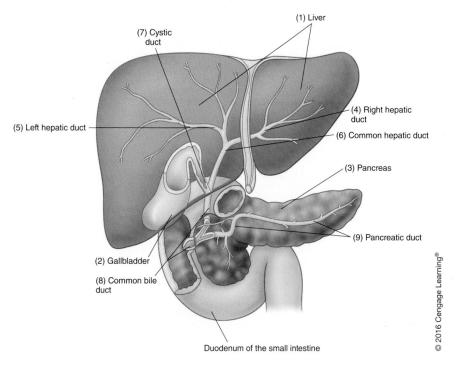

Figure 9-6   Liver, gallbladder, and pancreas.

EXERCISE 4

Write the names of the digestive system structures shown in Figure 9-7. Write your answers on the spaces provided.

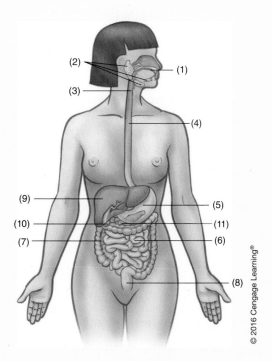

Figure 9-7   Label the structures of the digestive system.

1. _____
2. _____
3. _____
4. _____
5. _____
6. _____
7. _____
8. _____
9. _____
10. _____
11. _____

EXERCISE 5

Write the name of the digestive system organ or structure that fits each description.

1. adds digestive juices to the duodenum   _____
2. adds hydrochloric acid to foodstuffs   _____
3. nutrients absorbed into the bloodstream   _____
4. pouch for storing solid waste   _____
5. produces bile   _____
6. produce saliva   _____
7. stores bile   _____
8. water absorbed into the bloodstream   _____

EXERCISE 6

Match the sections and structures associated with the small and large intestine in Column 1 with the correct definition in Column 2.

COLUMN 1

_____ 1. anus
_____ 2. ascending colon
_____ 3. cecum
_____ 4. descending colon
_____ 5. duodenum
_____ 6. hepatic flexure
_____ 7. ileocecal valve

COLUMN 2

a. first segment, small intestine
b. beginning section, large intestine
c. second segment, small intestine
d. stores solid waste
e. last segment, large intestine
f. third segment, small intestine
g. connects small and large intestine

COLUMN 1	COLUMN 2
_____ 8. ileum	h. located above the cecum
_____ 9. jejunum	i. located across the abdomen
_____ 10. rectum	j. sphincter muscle, holds waste
_____ 11. sigmoid colon	k. located on the left side
_____ 12. splenic flexure	l. curve between the ascending and transverse colon
_____ 13. transverse colon	m. curve between the transverse and descending colon

Digestive System Medical Terminology

Digestive system medical terms are organized into three main categories: (1) general medical terms; (2) disease and condition terms; and (3) diagnostic procedure, surgery, and laboratory test terms. The roots, prefixes, and suffixes associated with digestive system terms are listed in Table 9-2. Review these word parts and complete the exercises.

TABLE 9-2   COMBINING FORMS, PREFIXES, AND SUFFIXES FOR DIGESTIVE SYSTEM TERMS

Root	Meaning	Prefix	Meaning	Suffix	Meaning
leuk/o	white	endo-	within	-centesis	surgical puncture
polyp/o	polyp	retro-	backward; located behind	-gram	record of
				-graphy	process of recording
				-iasis	abnormal condition
				-lithiasis	presence of stones
				-(o)stomy	creating a new or artificial opening
				-pepsia	digestion
				-phagia	eating, swallowing
				-plasty	surgical repair
				-(r)rhaphy	to suture
				-scope	instrument for viewing
				-scopy	process of viewing
				-tripsy	crushing

EXERCISE 7

Write the root, prefix, suffix, and their meanings for each medical term.

1. duodenoplasty

   ROOT: _____ MEANING: _____

   PREFIX: _____ MEANING: _____

   SUFFIX: _____ MEANING: _____

2. endoscope

   ROOT: _____ MEANING: _____

   PREFIX: _____ MEANING: _____

   SUFFIX: _____ MEANING: _____

3. endoscopy

   ROOT: _____ MEANING: _____

   PREFIX: _____ MEANING: _____

   SUFFIX: _____ MEANING: _____

4. gastroplasty

   ROOT: _____ MEANING: _____

   PREFIX: _____ MEANING: _____

   SUFFIX: _____ MEANING: _____

5. glossorrhaphy

   ROOT: _____ MEANING: _____

   PREFIX: _____ MEANING: _____

   SUFFIX: _____ MEANING: _____

6. ileostomy

   ROOT: _____ MEANING: _____

   PREFIX: _____ MEANING: _____

   SUFFIX: _____ MEANING: _____

7. lithotripsy

   ROOT: _____ MEANING: _____

   PREFIX: _____ MEANING: _____

   SUFFIX: _____ MEANING: _____

8. pancreatography

   ROOT: _____ MEANING: _____

   PREFIX: _____ MEANING: _____

   SUFFIX: _____ MEANING: _____

9. polypectomy

ROOT: _____ MEANING: _____

PREFIX: _____ MEANING: _____

SUFFIX: _____ MEANING: _____

10. retrograde

ROOT: _____ MEANING: _____

PREFIX: _____ MEANING: _____

SUFFIX: _____ MEANING: _____

EXERCISE 8

Based on your knowledge of the meanings of roots, prefixes, and suffixes, write a brief definition for each term. Use a medical dictionary to check your definition.

1. gastrocentesis _____

2. colonoscopy _____

3. endoscope _____

4. choledochogram _____

5. colostomy _____

6. gingivoplasty _____

7. glossorrhaphy _____

8. cholecystography _____

9. retroversion _____

10. polypectomy _____

Digestive System General Medical Terms

Review the pronunciation and meaning of each term in Table 9-3. Note that some terms are built from word parts and some are not. Complete the exercises for these terms.

TABLE 9-3   DIGESTIVE SYSTEM GENERAL MEDICAL TERMS

Term with Pronunciation	Definition
abdominal (ab-**DOM**-ih-nal) abdomin/o = abdomen -al = pertaining to	pertaining to the abdomen

(continues)

TABLE 9-3 DIGESTIVE SYSTEM GENERAL MEDICAL TERMS (continued)

Term with Pronunciation	Definition
anal (**AY**-nal) an/o = anus -al = pertaining to	pertaining to the anus
buccal (**BUCK**-al) bucc/o = cheek -al = pertaining to	pertaining to the cheek or mouth
fecal (**FEE**-kal) fec/o = feces -al = pertaining to	pertaining to feces
feces (**FEE**-seez)	stool; excrement; body waste from the large intestine
gastric (**GASS**-trik) gastr/o = stomach -ic = pertaining to	pertaining to the stomach
gastroenterologist (**gass**-troh-**en**-ter-**ALL**-oh-jist) gastr/o = stomach enter/o = intestines -(o)logist = specialist in the study of	physician who specializes in diseases and treatments of the digestive system
gastroenterology (**gass**-troh-**en**-ter-**ALL**-oh-jee) gastr/o = stomach enter/o = intestines -(o)logy = study of	study of the diseases and treatments related to the digestive system
ileocecal (**ill**-ee-oh-**SEE**-kal) ile/o = ileum cec/o = cecum -al = pertaining to	pertaining to the ileum and the cecum
nasogastric (nay-zoh-**GASS**-trik) nas/o = nose gastr/o = stomach -ic = pertaining to	pertaining to the nose and stomach
oral (**OR**-al) or/o = mouth -al = pertaining to	pertaining to the mouth

(continues)

TABLE 9-3   DIGESTIVE SYSTEM GENERAL MEDICAL TERMS (continued)

Term with Pronunciation	Definition
pancreatic (pan-kree-**AT**-ik) pancreat/o = pancreas -ic = pertaining to	pertaining to the pancreas
peritoneal (**pair**-ih-toh-**NEE**-al) peritone/o = peritoneum -al = pertaining to	pertaining to the peritoneum or the peritoneal membrane
proctologist (prok-**TALL**-oh-jist) proct/o = rectum; anus -(o)logist = specialist in the study of	physician who specializes in diseases and treatments of the anus and rectum
proctology (prok-**TALL**-oh-jee) proct/o = rectum, anus -(o)logy = study of	study of the diseases and treatments of the anus and rectum
sublingual (sub-**LING**-gwall) sub- = beneath; under ling/o = tongue -al = pertaining to	under the tongue; pertaining to under the tongue

© 2016 Cengage Learning®

EXERCISE 9

Analyze each term by writing the root, suffix, and their meanings. Based on the meaning of the word parts, write a definition of each term. Check the definition in a medical dictionary.

EXAMPLE: abdominal
ROOT: abdomin/o   MEANING: abdomen
SUFFIX:-al   MEANING: pertaining to
DEFINITION: pertaining to the abdomen

1. anal

ROOT: _____ MEANING: _____

SUFFIX: _____ MEANING: _____

DEFINITION: _____

2. buccal

ROOT: _____ MEANING: _____

SUFFIX: _____ MEANING: _____

DEFINITION: _____

3. fecal

ROOT: _____ MEANING: _____

SUFFIX: _____ MEANING: _____

DEFINITION: _____

4. gastric

ROOT: _____ MEANING: _____

SUFFIX: _____ MEANING: _____

DEFINITION: _____

5. ileocecal

ROOT: _____ MEANING: _____

SUFFIX: _____ MEANING: _____

DEFINITION: _____

6. oral

ROOT: _____ MEANING: _____

SUFFIX: _____ MEANING: _____

DEFINITION: _____

7. pancreatic

ROOT: _____ MEANING: _____

SUFFIX: _____ MEANING: _____

DEFINITION: _____

8. sublingual

ROOT: _____ MEANING: _____

SUFFIX: _____ MEANING: _____

DEFINITION: _____

EXERCISE 10

Write the medical term for each definition.

1. stool, excrement _____

2. physician specialist, digestive diseases _____

3. study of diseases, treatments, digestive system _____

4. pertaining to the peritoneum _____

5. pertaining to the nose and stomach _____

6. physician specialist, anus and rectum _____

7. study of diseases, treatments, anus and rectum _____

8. pertaining to the ileum and cecum _____

Digestive System Disease and Disorder Terms

Digestive system diseases and disorders include familiar problems such as diarrhea as well as more complex and less familiar diagnoses such as volvulus. The medical terms are presented in alphabetical order in Table 9-4. Review the pronunciation and definition for each term and complete the exercises.

TABLE 9-4 DIGESTIVE SYSTEM DISEASE AND DISORDER TERMS

Term with Pronunciation	Definition
achalasia (ak-ah-**LAY**-zee-ah)	decreased mobility of the lower two-thirds of the esophagus with lower esophageal sphincter constriction
anorexia nervosa (an-oh-**REK**-see-ah ner-**VOH**-sah)	loss of appetite and emaciation accompanied by an extreme and unfounded fear of obesity
aphagia (ah-**FAY**-jee-ah) a- = lack of; without -phagia = to swallow	loss of the ability to swallow
aphthous stomatitis (**AFF**-thuss stoh-mah-**TIGH**-tis) stomat/o = mouth -itis = inflammation	inflammatory, noninfectious ulcerated lesion of the lips, tongue, and mouth; canker sore
appendicitis (ah-**pen**-dih-**SIGH**-tis) appendic/o = appendix -itis = inflammation	inflammation of the vermiform appendix
ascites (ah-**SIGH**-teez)	abnormal accumulation of fluid in the peritoneal cavity
bulimia (buh-**LIM**-ee-ah)	condition characterized by alternately overeating and inducing vomiting
cholecystitis (**koh**-lee-sist-**EYE**-tis) cholecyst/o = gallbladder -itis = inflammation	inflammation of the gallbladder
choledocholithiasis (koh-lee-**doh**-koh-lih-**THIGH**-ah-sis) choledoch/o = bile duct lith/o = stones; calculi -iasis = abnormal condition	presence of calculi (stones) in the common bile duct (Figure 9-8)

(continues)

TABLE 9-4 DIGESTIVE SYSTEM DISEASE AND DISORDER TERMS (continued)

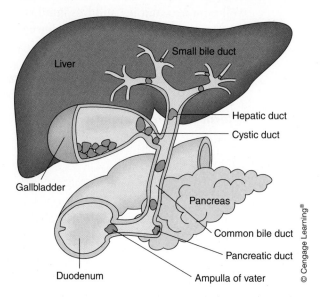

Figure 9-8 Simplified illustration of choledocholithiasis and cholelithiasis.

Term with Pronunciation	Definition
cholelithiasis (**koh**-lee-lih-**THIGH**-ah-sis) chole/o = bile lith/o = stones -iasis = abnormal condition	formation or presence of bile stones in the gallbladder; gallstones (Figure 9-8)
cirrhosis (sih-**ROH**-sis)	chronic disease of the liver characterized by the destruction of liver cells
colorectal carcinoma (cancer) (koh-loh-**REK**-tal kar-sin-**OH**-mah) col/o = colon rect/o = rectum -al = pertaining to carcin- = cancer; malignant -oma = tumor	malignant neoplasm of the colon and rectum
Crohn's disease (KROHNZ)	chronic inflammation of the ileum characterized by ulcerations along the intestinal wall and the formation of scar tissue; also called regional ileitis or regional enteritis
diarrhea (digh-ah-**REE**-ah)	frequent passage of loose, watery stools

(continues)

TABLE 9-4   DIGESTIVE SYSTEM DISEASE AND DISORDER TERMS (continued)

Term with Pronunciation	Definition
diverticulitis (**digh**-ver-**tik**-yoo-**LIGH**-tis) diverticul/o = diverticulum -itis = inflammation	inflammation of a diverticulum or several diverticula
diverticulosis (**digh**-ver-**tik**-yoo-**LOH**-sis) diverticul/o = diverticulum -osis = condition	presence of diverticula in the colon
diverticulum (**digh**-ver-**TIK**-yoo-lum)	a sac or pouch in the walls of an organ; often exhibited in the large intestine

© 2016 Cengage Learning®

EXERCISE 11

Write the root, prefix, suffix, and their meanings for each term. Based on the meanings of the word parts, write a definition for the term. Check the definitions using a medical dictionary.

1. aphagia

   ROOT: _____ MEANING: _____

   PREFIX: _____ MEANING: _____

   SUFFIX: _____ MEANING: _____

   DEFINITION: _____

2. appendicitis

   ROOT: _____ MEANING: _____

   PREFIX: _____ MEANING: _____

   SUFFIX: _____ MEANING: _____

   DEFINITION: _____

3. cholecystitis

   ROOT: _____ MEANING: _____

   PREFIX: _____ MEANING: _____

   SUFFIX: _____ MEANING: _____

   DEFINITION: _____

4. choledocholithiasis

   ROOT: _____ MEANING: _____

   PREFIX: _____ MEANING: _____

   SUFFIX: _____ MEANING: _____

   DEFINITION: _____

5. cholelithiasis

ROOT: _____ MEANING: _____

PREFIX: _____ MEANING: _____

SUFFIX: _____ MEANING: _____

DEFINITION: _____

6. diverticulitis

ROOT: _____ MEANING: _____

PREFIX: _____ MEANING: _____

SUFFIX: _____ MEANING: _____

DEFINITION: _____

7. diverticulosis

ROOT: _____ MEANING: _____

PREFIX: _____ MEANING: _____

SUFFIX: _____ MEANING: _____

DEFINITION: _____

EXERCISE 12

Replace the italicized phrase with the correct medical term.

1. Carlos' lower GI series identified the presence of *sacs or pouches in his large intestine.*

   _____

2. As a result of Marjorie's *overeating and induced vomiting,* Marjorie's parents requested a mental health consultation.

   _____

3. *Canker sores* may be caused by poor dietary habits.

   _____

4. Because of a family history of *malignancy of the colon and rectum,* Jerald made an appointment with his family physician.

   _____

5. Regina's *regional ileitis* was treated with prednisone.

   _____

6. *Decreased esophageal mobility and sphincter constriction* made it difficult for Luke to swallow.

   _____

7. Chronic alcoholism often leads to *abnormal accumulation of fluid in the perito-neal cavity.*

   _____

8. Repeated episodes of *loose, watery stools* caused baby Rosita's dehydration.

   _____

9. *Inflammation of the appendix* usually requires surgical intervention.

   _____

10. *Loss of appetite, emaciation, and an extreme fear of obesity* are more common in young women than in young men.

   _____

Review the pronunciation and definition for each term in Table 9-5 and complete the exercises.

TABLE 9-5 DIGESTIVE SYSTEM DISEASE AND DISORDER TERMS

Term with Pronunciation	Definition
duodenal ulcer (doo-oh-**DEE**-nal, doo-**OD**-eh-nal **ULL**-sir) duoden/o = duodenum -al = pertaining to	ulceration of the mucous membrane of the duodenum; peptic ulcer; caused by a bacterium or certain types of medications
dysentery	infection of the intestinal tract that results in an inflammation of the intestinal mucosa characterized by loose, bloody, mucuslike stools; infection may be caused by bacteria, viruses, or microbes
dyspepsia (diss-**PEP**-see-ah) dys- = abnormal; painful; difficult -pepsia = digestion	painful or abnormal digestion; indigestion
dysphagia (diss-**FAY**-jee-ah) dys- = abnormal; painful; difficult -phagia = swallowing	difficulty in swallowing
emaciation (ee-**may**-she-**AY**-shun)	state of being abnormally and extremely lean
eructation (eh-ruk-**TAY**-shun)	producing gas from the stomach and expelling it through the mouth; belch, burp
flatus (**FLAY**-tus)	gas in the digestive tract; expelling gas from the anus

(continues)

TABLE 9-5   DIGESTIVE SYSTEM DISEASE AND DISORDER TERMS (continued)

Term with Pronunciation	Definition
gastric ulcer (**GASS**-trik **ULL**-sir)	ulcer of the mucosa of the stomach; peptic ulcer; caused by a bacterium or certain medications
gastrodynia, gastralgia (gass-troh-**DIN**-ee-ah, gass-**TRAL**-jee-ah) gastr/o = stomach -dynia,-algia = pain	pain in the stomach; stomachache
gastroenteritis (**gass**-troh-**en**-ter-**EYE**-tis) gastr/o = stomach enter/o = intestines -itis = inflammation	inflammation of the stomach and intestinal tract
gastroesophageal reflux disease (GERD) (**gass**-troh-eh-**soff**-oh-**JEE**-al **REE**-flux) gastr/o = stomach esophag/o = esophagus -eal = pertaining to	reflux or moving backward of gastric contents into the esophagus
gingivitis (jin-jih-**VIGH**-tis) gingiv/o = gingiva; gums -itis = inflammation	inflammation of the gums or gingiva
hematemesis (hem-at-**EM**-eh-sis) hemat/o = blood -emesis = vomiting	vomiting blood
hepatitis (hep-ah-**TIGH**-tis) hepat/o = liver -itis = inflammation	inflammation of the liver
hernia (**HER**-nee-ah)	protrusion of an organ or part of an organ through the wall of a cavity; usually refers to some part of the intestinal tract protruding through the abdominal wall
herpetic stomatitis (her-**PEH**-tik **stoh**-mah-**TIGH**-tis) stomat/o = mouth -itis = inflammation	inflammatory infectious lesions of the oral cavity caused by the herpes simplex virus; cold sores, fever blisters
hiatal hernia (high-**AY**-tal **HER**-nee-ah)	herniation of a portion of the stomach through the esophageal opening in the diaphragm (Figure 9-9)

(continues)

TABLE 9-5   DIGESTIVE SYSTEM DISEASE AND DISORDER TERMS (continued)

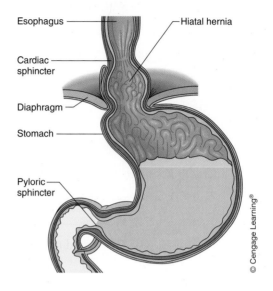

Figure 9-9   Hiatal hernia.

© 2016 Cengage Learning®

EXERCISE 13

Analyze each term by writing the prefix, root, combining vowel, and suffix separated by vertical slashes. Based on the meaning of the word parts, write a definition for each term. Check your definition in a medical dictionary.

EXAMPLE: abdominoplasty

	/ abdomin	/ o	/ plasty
prefix	*root*	*combining vowel*	*suffix*

DEFINITION: surgical repair of the abdomen

1. dyspepsia

prefix	*root*	*combining vowel*	*suffix*

DEFINITION: _____

2. gastrodynia

prefix	*root*	*combining vowel*	*suffix*

DEFINITION: _____

3. gastroenteritis

prefix	*root*	*combining vowel*	*suffix*

DEFINITION: _____

4. gingivitis

prefix	*root*	*combining vowel*	*suffix*

DEFINITION: _____

5. hepatitis

prefix	root	combining vowel	suffix

DEFINITION: _____

6. hematemesis

prefix	root	combining vowel	suffix

DEFINITION: _____

EXERCISE 14

Replace the italicized phrase with the correct medical term.

1. Marilyn developed a *peptic ulcer* for no apparent reason.

   _____

2. Surgery was scheduled to repair the *protrusion of the small intestine through the abdominal wall.*

   _____

3. After visiting a remote tropical village, Ling-Ling had *loose, bloody, mucuslike stools.*

   _____

4. *The state of being abnormally and extremely lean* is often associated with anorexia nervosa.

   _____

5. Gastric hypersecretion was the cause of Rodney's *belching.*

   _____

6. Many hospitals required immunization for *inflammation of the liver* for all employees.

   _____

7. *Fever blisters* often occur around the lips.

   _____

8. "Heartburn" might be caused by a *herniation of the stomach into the esophagus.*

   _____

9. *Vomiting blood* is a good indication of a gastrointestinal problem.

   _____

10. *GERD* causes a burning sensation in the upper gastrointestinal tract.

   _____

EXERCISE 15

Circle the medical term that best fits the definition.

DEFINITION	**CIRCLE ONE TERM**
1. indigestion	*flatus* OR *dyspepsia*
2. extremely, abnormally lean	*emaciation* OR *anorexia nervosa*
3. herniation through the diaphragm	*gastroesophageal reflux disease* OR *hiatal hernia*
4. belch, burp	*flatus* OR *eructation*
5. cold sore	*herpetic stomatitis* OR *gingivitis*
6. stomachache	*gastric ulcer* OR *gastrodynia*
7. expelling gas from the anus	*eructation* OR *flatus*
8. peptic ulcer	*gastroenteritis* OR *gastric ulcer*
9. flow of gastric contents into the esophagus	*GERD* OR *hiatal hernia*
10. inflammation of the liver	*hepatitis* OR *gingivitis*

Review the pronunciation and definition for each term in Table 9-6 and complete the exercises.

TABLE 9-6   DIGESTIVE SYSTEM DISEASE AND DISORDER TERMS

Term with Pronunciation	Definition
ileus (**ILL**-ee-us)	obstruction of the intestine
intestinal obstruction (in-**TESS**-tin-al ob-**STRUK**-shun)	complete or partial interruption of the movement of the contents of the small or large intestine
intussusceptions (in-**tuh**-suh-**SEP**-shun)	telescoping of one portion of the large intestine into another portion of the large intestine
irritable bowel syndrome (IBS)	increased motility of the small or large intestines resulting in abdominal pain, flatulence, nausea, anorexia, and trapped gas throughout the intestines; spastic colon
melena (**MELL**-eh-nah)	abnormal, black, tarry stool containing digested blood
nausea (**NAW**-zee-ah)	unpleasant sensation usually preceding vomiting
oral leukoplakia (**OR**-al **loo**-koh-**PLAY**-kee-ah)	presence of white spots or patches on the mucous membrane of the tongue or cheek; lesions may become malignant

(continues)

TABLE 9-6   DIGESTIVE SYSTEM DISEASE AND DISORDER TERMS (continued)

Term with Pronunciation	Definition
pancreatitis (**pan**-kree-ah-**TIGH**-tis) pancreat/o = pancreas -itis = inflammation	inflammation of the pancreas
peritonitis (**pair**-ih-toh-**NIGH**-tis) peritone/o = peritoneum -itis = inflammation	inflammation of the peritoneum
polyp (**PALL**-ip)	a small growth projecting from the mucous membrane of organs such as the colon, nose, or uterus
polyposis, chronic (pall-ee-**POH**-sis) polyp/o = polyp -osis = condition	presence of a large number of polyps in the large intestine
pruritus ani (proo-**RIGH**-tus **AN**-eye)	severe itching around the anus
sialolithiasis (**sigh**-ah-loh-lih-**THIGH**-ah-sis) sial/o = saliva; salivary glands lith/o = stones; calculi -iasis = abnormal condition	presence of salivary stones or calculi in the salivary gland or duct
thrush	a fungal infection of the mouth and throat that produces creamy white patches on the tongue and other oral surfaces (Figure 9-10)

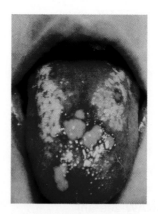

Figure 9-10   Thrush (Centers for Disease Control and Prevention).

(continues)

TABLE 9-6 DIGESTIVE SYSTEM DISEASE AND DISORDER TERMS (continued)

Term with Pronunciation	Definition
ulcerative colitis (**ULL**-ser-ah-tiv koh-**LIGH**-tis) col/o = colon; large intestine -itis = inflammation	a chronic inflammatory condition characterized by the formation of ulcerated lesions in the mucous membrane lining of the colon; inflammatory bowel disease (IBD)
volvulus (**VOL**-vyoo-lus)	twisting of loops of the bowel or colon that results in an intestinal obstruction (Figure 9-11)

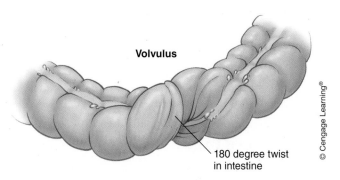

Volvulus

180 degree twist in intestine

© Cengage Learning®

Figure 9-11 Volvulus.

© 2016 Cengage Learning®

EXERCISE 16

Replace the italicized phrase with the correct medical term.

1. Jackson's postoperative course was complicated by an *intestinal obstruction.*

   _____

2. Gita was scheduled for surgery to correct *telescoping of the large intestine.*

   _____

3. Choton eliminated dairy products from his diet to relieve *spastic colon.*

   _____

4. A *twisting of loops of the bowel* might cause an intestinal obstruction.

   _____

5. Marie received high-dose, oral prednisone for her *chronic inflammatory condition of the colon.*

   _____

6. *Black, tarry stools* might be symptomatic of a bleeding ulcer.

   _____

7. Ella received a topical medication for *the creamy, white patches on her tongue.*

   _____

8. The oral surgeon informed Wade that he had *salivary calculi*.

_____

9. *Severe itching around the anus* might be caused by pinworms.

_____

10. *Inflammation of the pancreas* complicated Isun's postoperative treatment.

_____

11. A ruptured appendix might lead to *inflammation of the peritoneum*.

_____

12. After eating poorly cooked chicken, Bill experienced *a sensation that vomiting might occur*.

_____

EXERCISE 17

Match the conditions in Column 1 with the correct descriptions in Column 2.

COLUMN 1

_____ 1. IBD

_____ 2. IBS

_____ 3. ileus

_____ 4. intussusception

_____ 5. melena

_____ 6. oral leukoplakia

_____ 7. polyp

_____ 8. sialolithiasis

_____ 9. thrush

_____ 10. volvulus

COLUMN 2

a. black, tarry stools

b. chronic inflammatory condition of the lining of the colon

c. fungal infection of the oral cavity; creamy, white patches

d. growth projecting from the mucous membrane of the colon

e. obstruction of the intestine

f. salivary stones or calculi

g. spastic colon

h. telescoping of the large intestine into itself

i. twisted loops of the bowel or colon

j. white patches of the oral mucous membrane

Digestive System Diagnostic Medical Terms

Review the pronunciation and definition of the diagnostic terms in Table 9-7. Complete the exercises for each set of terms. Diagnostic procedures such as colonoscopy also function as a surgical or treatment approach. For example, during a diagnostic colonoscopy, the gastroenterologist discovers several suspicious-looking polyps. With the patient's consent, she removes the polyps. In this example, the diagnostic colonoscopy has become the surgical approach for a polypectomy.

TABLE 9-7   DIGESTIVE SYSTEM DIAGNOSTIC MEDICAL TERMS

Term with Pronunciation	Definition
abdominocentesis (ab-**dom**-ih-noh-sen-**TEE**-sis) abdomin/o = abdomen -centesis = surgical puncture to remove fluid	surgical puncture into the abdominal/peritoneal cavity to remove excess fluid; also known as paracentesis
cholangiogram (kohl-**AN**-jee-oh-gram) cholangi/o = bile ducts -gram = record; picture	record or picture of the bile ducts
cholangiography (**kohl**-an-jee-**OG**-rah-fee) cholangi/o = bile ducts -graphy = process of recording	recording a picture or record of the bile ducts
cholecystogram (**koh**-lee-**SISS**-toh-gram) cholecyst/o = gallbladder -gram = record; picture	record or picture of the gallbladder
cholecystography (**koh**-lee-sist-**OG**-rah-fee) cholecyst/o = gallbladder -graphy = process of recording	recording a picture or record of the gallbladder
colonoscopy (koh-lon-**OSS**-koh-pee) colon/o = colon; large intestine -scopy = process of visualization with a scope	endoscopic visualization and examination of the large intestine from the anus to the ileocecal junction
endoscopic retrograde cholangiopancreatogram (ERCP) (en-doh-**SKOP**-ic **REH**-troh-grayd kohl-**an**-jee-oh-**PAN**-kree-ah- toh-gram) endo- = within -scopic = pertaining to visualization with a scope cholangi/o = bile duct pancreat/o = pancreas -gram = record; picture	image or picture of the pancreatic and bile ducts; visualization is accomplished with a scope and injection of a contrast medium

(continues)

TABLE 9-7 DIGESTIVE SYSTEM DIAGNOSTIC MEDICAL TERMS (continued)

Term with Pronunciation	Definition
endoscopic retrograde cholangiopancreatography (ERCP) (en-doh-**SKOP**-ic **REH**-troh-grayd kohl-**an**-jee-oh-**pan**-kree-ah-**TOG**-rah-fee) cholangi/o = bile duct pancreat/o = pancreas -graphy = process of recording	process of recording an image of the pancreatic and bile ducts by inserting a scope into the throat, through the stomach, and injecting a contrast medium into the pancreatic and bile ducts
esophagogastroduodenoscopy (EGD) (eh-**soff**-ah-goh-**gass**-troh-doo-**wah**-den-**OSS**-koh-pee) esophag/o = esophagus gastr/o = stomach duoden/o = duodenum -scopy = process of visualization with a scope	endoscopic visualization and examination of the esophagus, stomach, and duodenum
esophagoscopy (eh-**soff**-ah-**GOSS**-koh-pee) esophag/o = esophagus -scopy = process of visualization with a scope	endoscopic visualization and examination of the esophagus
gastroscopy (gass-**TROSS**-koh-pee) gastr/o = stomach -scopy = process of visualization with a scope	endoscopic visualization and examination of the stomach
Helicobacter pylori (H. pylori) (hee-lih-koh-**BAK**-ter pigh-**LOR**-eye)	a blood test to determine the presence of *H. pylori* antibodies, which indicate infection with the bacteria; *H. pylori* is also found in the lining of the stomach and causes duodenal ulcers
laparoscopy (lap-ah-**ROSS**-koh-pee) lapar/o = abdominal wall -scopy = process of visualization with a scope	endoscopic visualization and examination of the abdominal and pelvic cavities
lower gastrointestinal series (**gass**-troh-in-**TESS**-tin-al) gastr/o = stomach intestin/o = intestines -al = pertaining to	x-ray examination of the rectum and large intestine aided by a contrast medium, usually barium; also called a barium enema

(continues)

TABLE 9-7   DIGESTIVE SYSTEM DIAGNOSTIC MEDICAL TERMS (continued)

Term with Pronunciation	Definition
occult blood test (uh-**KULT**)	microscopic examination of feces to detect the presence of blood that is not otherwise visible; screening test for colorectal cancer
proctoscopy (prok-**TOSS**-koh-pee) proct/o = rectum, anus -scopy = process of visualization with a scope	endoscopic visualization and examination of the anus and rectum
sigmoidoscopy (sig-moyd-**OSS**-koh-pee) sigmoid/o = sigmoid colon -scopy = process of visualization with a scope	endoscopic visualization and examination of the sigmoid colon
small bowel follow-through (SBF)	x-ray examination of the small intestine aided by a contrast medium; often done in conjunction with an upper gastrointestinal series
upper gastrointestinal series (**gass**-troh-in-**TESS**-tin-al) gastr/o = stomach intestin/o = intestines -al = pertaining to	x-ray examination of the esophagus, stomach, and a portion of the duodenum aided by a contrast medium, usually barium; also called a barium swallow

© 2016 Cengage Learning®

EXERCISE 18

Analyze each term by writing the root, combining vowel, and suffix separated by vertical slashes. Based on the meaning of the word parts, write a definition for each term. Check your definition in a medical dictionary.

1. abdominocentesis

root	*combining vowel*	*suffix*

    DEFINITION: _____

2. cholecystogram

root	*combining vowel*	*suffix*

    DEFINITION: _____

3. cholecystography

root	*combining vowel*	*suffix*

    DEFINITION: _____

4. cholangiography

_____
root   combining vowel   suffix

DEFINITION: _____

5. colonoscopy

_____
root   combining vowel   suffix

DEFINITION: _____

6. esophagoscopy

_____
root   combining vowel   suffix

DEFINITION: _____

7. esophagogastroduodenoscopy

_____
root   combining vowel   suffix

DEFINITION: _____

8. gastroscopy

_____
root   combining vowel   suffix

DEFINITION: _____

9. laparoscopy

_____
root   combining vowel   suffix

DEFINITION: _____

10. proctoscopy

_____
root   combining vowel   suffix

DEFINITION: _____

11. sigmoidoscopy

_____
root   combining vowel   suffix

DEFINITION: _____

EXERCISE 19

Replace the italicized phrase or abbreviation with the correct medical term.

1. Tom's *barium enema* revealed an obstruction in the descending colon.

    _____

2. The *microscopic screen for colorectal cancer* is usually ordered for all patients age 50 and older.

    _____

3. Elizabeth had a *barium swallow* that revealed no abnormalities.

    _____

4. The *x-ray examination of the small intestine* identified several hernias.

   _____

5. A patient is sedated but conscious during the *endoscopic examination of the entire large intestine.*

   _____

6. The *x-ray of the bile ducts* showed several large gallstones in the common bile duct.

   _____

7. Kwan was told not to eat or drink the night before his scheduled *ERCP.*

   _____

8. An upper GI series often includes an *SBF.*

   _____

Digestive System Surgery and Treatment Terms

Digestive system surgery and treatment terms cover a range of procedures, from an appendectomy to proctocolectomy (i.e., the surgical removal of the entire large intestine, including the rectum). Review the pronunciation and definition of the terms in Table 9-8 and complete the exercises.

TABLE 9-8   DIGESTIVE SYSTEM SURGERY AND TREATMENT TERMS

Term with Pronunciation	Definition
abdominoplasty (ab-**dom**-in-oh-**PLASS**-tee) abdomin/o = abdomen -plasty = surgical repair	surgical repair of the abdomen
anoplasty (**AY**-noh-**plass**-tee) an/o = anus -plasty = surgical repair	surgical repair of the anus
appendectomy (ap-en-**DEK**-toh-mee) append/o = appendix -ectomy = surgical removal	surgical removal of the appendix
bariatric surgery (bair-ee-**AT**-rik)	weight-loss surgical procedure accomplished by gastric bypass or adjustable gastric banding

(continues)

TABLE 9-8 DIGESTIVE SYSTEM SURGERY AND TREATMENT TERMS (continued)

Term with Pronunciation	Definition
celiotomy (see-lee-**OT**-oh-mee) celi/o = abdomen -(o)tomy = incision into	surgical incision into the abdominal cavity
cheiloplasty (**KIGH**-loh-**plass**-tee) cheil/o = lip -plastic = surgical, plastic repair	surgical repair of the lip
cheilorrhaphy (kigh-**LOR**-ah-fee) cheil/o = lip -(r)rhaphy = to suture	suturing the lip
cholecystectomy (**koh**-lee-sist-**EK**-toh-mee) cholecyst/o = gallbladder -ectomy = surgical removal	surgical removal of the gallbladder
choledocholithotomy (koh-leh-**doh**-koh-lith-**OT**-oh-mee) choledoch/o = bile duct lith/o = stones; calculi -(o)tomy = incision into	removal of gallstones through an incision into the common bile duct
choledocholithotripsy (koh-leh-**doh**-koh-**LITH**-oh-trip-see) choledoch/o = bile duct lith/o = stones; calculi -tripsy = crushing	crushing of gallstones in the common bile duct
colectomy (koh-**LEK**-toh-mee) col/o = colon; large intestine -ectomy = surgical removal	surgical removal of all or part of the colon or large intestine
colostomy (koh-**LOSS**-toh-mee) col/o = colon; large intestine -(o)stomy = creating a new or artificial opening	creation of a new or artificial opening for the colon through the abdominal wall to its outside surface
diverticulectomy (**digh**-ver-**tik**-yoo-**LEK**-toh-mee) diverticul/o = diverticulum -ectomy = surgical removal	surgical removal of diverticulum or diverticula

(continues)

TABLE 9-8   DIGESTIVE SYSTEM SURGERY AND TREATMENT TERMS (continued)

Term with Pronunciation	Definition
esophagogastroplasty (eh-**soff**-ah-goh-**GASS**-troh-plass-tee) esophag/o = esophagus gastr/o = stomach -plasty = surgical repair	surgical repair of the esophagus and stomach
extracorporeal shock wave lithotripsy (ESWL) (**eks**-trah-kor-**POR**-ee-al shock wave **LITH**-oh-trip-see) lith/o = stones; calculi -tripsy = crushing	crushing of gallstones using ultrasound and shock waves; nonsurgical treatment for gallstones
gastrectomy (gass-**TREK**-toh-mee) gastr/o = stomach -ectomy = surgical removal	surgical removal of all or a portion of the stomach; also known as gastric resection
gastric lavage (**GASS**-trik lah-**VAHZ**) gastr/o = stomach -ic = pertaining to	washing out the contents of the stomach; commonly called "pumping the stomach"

© 2016 Cengage Learning®

EXERCISE 20

Analyze each term by writing the root, combining vowel, and suffix separated by vertical slashes. Based on the meaning of the word parts, write a definition for each term. Check your definition in a medical dictionary.

1. abdominoplasty

   root   *combining vowel*   *suffix*

   DEFINITION: _____

2. anoplasty

   root   *combining vowel*   *suffix*

   DEFINITION: _____

3. appendectomy

   root   *combining vowel*   *suffix*

   DEFINITION: _____

4. cheilorrhaphy

   root   *combining vowel*   *suffix*

   DEFINITION: _____

5. cholecystectomy

root	*combining vowel*	*suffix*

DEFINITION: _____

6. choledocholithotomy

root	*combining vowel*	*suffix*

DEFINITION: _____

7. choledocholithotripsy

root	*combining vowel*	*suffix*

DEFINITION: _____

8. colectomy

root	*combining vowel*	*suffix*

DEFINITION: _____

9. colostomy

root	*combining vowel*	*suffix*

DEFINITION: _____

10. esophagogastroplasty

root	*combining vowel*	*suffix*

DEFINITION: _____

EXERCISE 21

Match the procedures in Column 1 with the descriptions in Column 2.

COLUMN 1

_____ 1. celiotomy

_____ 2. cheiloplasty

_____ 3. choledocholithotomy

_____ 4. choledocholithotripsy

_____ 5. colectomy

_____ 6. colostomy

_____ 7. diverticulectomy

_____ 8. ESWL

_____ 9. gastrectomy

_____ 10. gastric lavage

COLUMN 2

a. creation of a new or artificial opening for the colon

b. crushing of gallstones

c. excision of diverticula

d. incision into the abdomen or abdominal cavity

e. incision into the common bile duct to remove stones

f. pumping the stomach

g. removal of all or part of the large intestine

h. removal of all or part of the stomach

i. surgical repair of the lip

j. ultrasound crushing of gallstones

Review the pronunciation and definition of the terms in Table 9-9 and complete the exercises.

TABLE 9-9 DIGESTIVE SYSTEM SURGERY AND TREATMENT TERMS

Term with Pronunciation	Definition
gastric banding, bariatric	restrictive bariatric surgical procedure during which a silicone band is placed around a portion of the stomach to limit the volume of the contents of the stomach
gastric bypass, bariatric	weight-loss surgical procedure characterized by reducing the size of the stomach and connecting it to a portion of the small intestine; part of the stomach and the first segment of the small intestine are bypassed
gastroduodenostomy (**gass**-troh-doo-**wah**-den-**OSS**-toh-mee) gastr/o = stomach duoden/o = duodenum -(o)stomy = creation of a new or artificial opening	creation of a new or artificial opening between the stomach and the duodenum, usually after a portion of the stomach is removed
gavage (gah-**VAHZ**)	feeding through a stomach tube
gingivectomy (jin-jih-**VEK**-toh-mee gingiv/o = gingiva -ectomy = surgical removal	surgical removal of the gingiva (gums)
glossorrhaphy (gloss-**OR**-ah-fee) gloss/o = tongue -(r)rhaphy = to suture	suture of a wound of the tongue
herniorrhaphy (her-nee-**OR**-ah-fee)	suture repair of a hernia
ileostomy (ill-ee-**OSS**-toh-mee) ile/o = ileum -(o)stomy = creation of a new or artificial opening	surgical creation of a new or artificial opening for the ileum through the abdominal wall to its outside surface

(continues)

TABLE 9-9 DIGESTIVE SYSTEM SURGERY AND TREATMENT TERMS (continued)

Term with Pronunciation	Definition
laparoscopic adjustable gastric banding (LAGB) (**lap**-ah-roh-**SKAH**-pic) lapar/o = abdominal wall -scopy = process of viewing -ic = pertaining to gastr/o = stomach	bariatric surgical procedure in which a silicone band is placed around a portion of the stomach; the band, which is inserted via laparoscope, can be tightened or loosened
laparotomy (lap-ah-**ROT**-oh-mee) lapar/o = abdomen; abdominal wall -(o)tomy = incision into	surgical incision into the abdominal wall
nasogastric intubation (nay-zoh-**GASS**-trik in-too-**BAY**-nas/o = nose shun) gastr/o = stomach -ic = pertaining to	insertion of a tube through the nose into the stomach
palatoplasty (**PAL**-at-oh-plass-tee) palat/o = palate -plasty = surgical repair	surgical repair of the palate, usually to repair a cleft palate
polypectomy (pall-ih-**PEK**-toh-mee) polyp/o = polyp -ectomy = surgical removal	surgical removal of a polyp
proctocolectomy (**prock**-toh-koh-**LEK**-toh-mee) proct/o = rectum; anus col/o = colon; large intestine -ectomy = surgical removal	surgical removal of the large intestine and rectum
pyloroplasty (pigh-**LOR**-oh-plass-tee) pylor/o = pylorus -plasty = surgical repair	surgical procedure for enlarging the opening between the stomach and duodenum
Roux-en-Y gastric bypass (**ROO**-en-wigh) (RYGBP) gastr/o = stomach -ic = pertaining to	bariatric surgical procedure during which the size of the stomach is reduced and subsequently connected to a portion of the small intestine; also called proximal gastric bypass

(continues)

TABLE 9-9   DIGESTIVE SYSTEM SURGERY AND TREATMENT TERMS (continued)

Term with Pronunciation	Definition
total parenteral nutrition (TPN) (par-**EN**-ter-al)	provision of nutritional and caloric needs by an intravenous route in order to bypass the digestive tract
uvulopalatopharyngoplasty (UPPP) (**yoo**-vyoo-loh-**pal**-ah-toh-fah-**RING**-oh-plass-tee) uvul/o = uvula palat/o = palate pharyng/o = pharynx -plasty = surgical repair	surgical repair of the soft palate, uvula, and other structures of the oropharynx to correct sleep apnea

© 2016 Cengage Learning®

EXERCISE 22

Analyze each term by writing the root, combining vowel, and suffix separated by vertical slashes. Based on the meaning of the word parts, write a definition for each term. Check your definition in a medical dictionary.

1. gastroduodenostomy

   _____
   root   *combining vowel*   *suffix*
   DEFINITION: _____

2. gingivectomy

   _____
   root   *combining vowel*   *suffix*
   DEFINITION: _____

3. herniorrhaphy

   _____
   root   *combining vowel*   *suffix*
   DEFINITION: _____

4. ileostomy

   _____
   root   *combining vowel*   *suffix*
   DEFINITION: _____

5. palatoplasty

   _____
   root   *combining vowel*   *suffix*
   DEFINITION: _____

6. polypectomy

   _____
   root   *combining vowel*   *suffix*
   DEFINITION: _____

7. proctocolectomy

_____
root   combining vowel   suffix

DEFINITION: _____

8. uvulopalatopharyngoplasty

_____
root   combining vowel   suffix

DEFINITION: _____

EXERCISE 23

Replace the italicized phrase or abbreviation with the correct medical term or phrase.

1. Mrs. Wicket's nurse initiated _feeding through a stomach tube_ as the physician ordered.

   _____

2. After the anesthesia took effect, the surgical nurse proceeded with _the insertion of a tube through the nose into the stomach._

   _____

3. _Surgical incision into the abdominal wall_ might serve as a diagnostic or treatment procedure.

   _____

4. As a result of the accident, Jennifer underwent _surgical repair of the palate._

   _____

5. Caleb's physician recommended _the surgical removal of polyps_ to correct rectal bleeding.

   _____

6. Removal of the small intestine might result in the need for _TPN._

   _____

7. As a result of ulcerative colitis, Milton underwent a _removal of the colon, rectum, and anus._

   _____

8. Jeramiah's obstructive sleep apnea was corrected by _UPPP._

   _____

Abbreviations

Review the digestive system abbreviations in Table 9-10. Practice writing out the meaning of each abbreviation.

TABLE 9-10 ABBREVIATIONS

Abbreviation	Meaning
BE	barium enema
EGD	esophagogastroduodenoscopy
ERCP	endoscopic retrograde cholangiopancreatography
GERD	gastroesophageal reflux disease
GI	gastrointestinal
LAGBP	laparoscopic adjustable gastric bypass
NG	nasogastric
RYGBP	Roux-en-Y gastric bypass
SBF	small bowel follow-through
TPN	total parenteral nutrition
UGI	upper gastrointestinal
UPPP	uvulopalatopharyngoplasty

© 2016 Cengage Learning®

CHAPTER REVIEW

The Chapter Review can be used as a self-test. Go through each exercise and answer as many questions as you can without referring to previous exercises or earlier discussions within this chapter. Check your answers and fill in any blanks. Practice writing any terms you might have misspelled.

EXERCISE 24

Using your knowledge of roots, prefixes, and suffixes, write the medical term for each definition.

1. specialist in diseases and treatments of the stomach and intestines _____

2. study of the diseases and treatments of the stomach and intestines _____

3. pertaining to the ileum and cecum _____

4. pertaining to the nose and stomach _____

5. specialist in the diseases and treatments of the rectum and anus _____

6. study of the diseases and treatments of the rectum and anus _____

7. loss of the ability to swallow _____

8. inflammation of the gallbladder _____

9. abnormal condition of gallstones _____

10. inflammation of the diverticula _____

11. abnormal or difficult digestion _____

12. inflammation of the stomach and intestines   _____

13. vomiting blood   _____

14. x-ray examination of the bile ducts   _____

15. visualization of the colon with a scope   _____

16. surgical removal of the appendix   _____

17. surgical removal of the gallbladder   _____

18. creation of a new or artificial opening for the colon   _____

19. creation of a new or artificial opening for the ileum   _____

20. surgical removal of all or part of the stomach   _____

21. surgical removal of the gingiva   _____

22. surgical removal of the anus, colon, and rectum   _____

23. presence of diverticula in the colon   _____

24. surgical incision into the abdominal wall
    or abdomen   _____

25. abnormal condition of gallstones in the
    common bile duct   _____

EXERCISE 25

Write a brief definition for each term.

1. aphthous stomatitis _____

2. ascites _____

3. bulimia _____

4. cirrhosis _____

5. dysentery _____

6. emaciation _____

7. eructation _____

8. gastric lavage _____

9. hernia _____

10. herpetic stomatitis _____

11. ileus _____

12. melena _____

13. occult blood test _____

14. thrush _____

15. volvulus _____

EXERCISE 26

Read the following operative report excerpt. Write a brief definition for each italicized term or phrase.

> PREOPERATIVE DIAGNOSIS: Chronic (1) *cholecystitis* and (2) *cholelithiasis*.
> POSTOPERATIVE DIAGNOSIS: Cholecystitis, cholelithiasis, and common duct stone.
> OPERATION PERFORMED: (3) *Cholecystectomy* and common bile duct exploration.
> INDICATIONS: The patient is a 48-year-old female who was admitted to the hospital with a chronic history of right upper quadrant pain and with associated (4) *dyspepsia*.
> FINDINGS: Surgical intervention revealed numerous cholesterol stones. The initial (5) *cystic duct* (6) *cholangiogram* failed to reveal clear passage of dye into the (7) *duodenum*. There was a concentric defect in the terminal (8) *common bile duct*. After 1 mg of glucagon was given, cholangiograms were repeated and the common duct was open.

1. _____

2. _____

3. _____

4. _____

5. _____

6. _____

7. _____

8. _____

EXERCISE 27

Explain the difference between the following conditions.

1. choledocholithiasis and cholelithiasis

   _____

   _____

2. diarrhea and dysentery

   _____

   _____

3. diverticulitis and diverticulosis

   _____

   _____

4. dyspepsia and dysphagia

   _____

   _____

5. aphthous stomatitis and herpetic stomatitis

_____

_____

6. irritable bowel syndrome and inflammatory bowel disease

_____

_____

7. intussusception and volvulus

_____

_____

EXERCISE 28

Select the best answer for each question or statement.

1. Which term describes the wavelike movement of the gastrointestinal tract?
   a. bolus
   b. volvulus
   c. involuntary ileus
   d. peristalsis

2. Select the term for foodstuffs mixed with saliva.
   a. volvulus
   b. bolus
   c. chyme
   d. digestion

3. Which accessory organ produces bile?
   a. gallbladder
   b. pancreas
   c. liver
   d. spleen

4. Select the medical term for the "gums" of the oral cavity.
   a. gingiva
   b. buccal ridges
   c. glossorus
   d. hard palate

5. Which structure triggers the gag reflex and assists in the production of sound?
   a. hard palate
   b. soft palate
   c. tongue
   d. uvula

6. Select the area of the gastrointestinal tract where most digestion occurs.
   a. stomach
   b. oral cavity
   c. duodenum
   d. ileum

7. Which accessory organ stores the bile?
   a. liver
   b. common bile duct
   c. pancreatic duct
   d. gallbladder

8. Choose the name of the digestive system structure that secretes hydrochloric acid.
   a. liver
   b. stomach
   c. oral cavity
   d. duodenum

9. Select the structure chiefly responsible for the absorption of nutrients.
   a. stomach
   b. large intestine
   c. jejunum
   d. small intestine

10. Which muscular tube directs food to the stomach?
    a. appendix
    b. pharynx
    c. esophagus
    d. pyloric sphincter

CHALLENGE EXERCISE

Bariatric surgery, commonly called gastric bypass, was initially developed in the 1960s. The number of such surgeries performed has steadily increased. In 2005, approximately 140,000 bariatric procedures were performed in the United States for weight loss. Visit the American Society for Bariatric Surgery (ASBS) website at www.asbs.org to learn about this operation. What are the indications for bariatric surgery? What are the differences between a Roux-en-Y (RYGBP) and laparoscopic adjustable gastric banding (LAGB)? Review the advantages, disadvantages, and complications associated with these procedures.

Pronunciation Review

Review the terms in the chapter. Pronounce each term using the following phonetic pronunciations. Check off the term when you are comfortable saying it.

TERM	PRONUNCIATION
☐ abdominal	ab-**DOM**-ih-nal
☐ abdominocentesis	ab-**dom**-ih-noh-sen-**TEE**-sis
☐ abdominoplasty	ab-**dom**-in-oh-**PLASS**-tee
☐ achalasia	ak-ah-**LAY**-zee-ah
☐ anal	**AY**-nal
☐ anoplasty	**AY**-noh-**plass**-tee
☐ anorexia nervosa	an-oh-**REK**-see-ah ner-**VOH**-sah
☐ antrum; pylorus	**AN**-trum; pigh-**LOR**-us
☐ anus	**AY**-nus
☐ aphagia	ah-**FAY**-jee-ah
☐ aphthous stomatitis	**AFF**-thuss **stoh**-mah-**TIGH**-tis
☐ appendectomy	ap-en-**DEK**-toh-mee
☐ appendicitis	ah-**pen**-dih-**SIGH**-tis
☐ ascending colon	ascending **KOH**-lon
☐ ascites	ah-**SIGH**-teez
☐ bolus	**BOH**-lus
☐ buccal	**BUCK**-al
☐ bulimia	buh-**LIM**-ee-ah
☐ cecum	**SEE**-kum
☐ celiotomy	see-lee-**OT**-oh-mee
☐ cheilorrhaphy	kigh-**LOR**-ah-fee
☐ cholangiogram	kohl-**AN**-jee-oh-gram
☐ cholangiography	**kohl**-an-jee-**OG**-rah-fee
☐ cholecystectomy	**koh**-lee-sist-**EK**-toh-mee
☐ cholecystitis	**koh**-lee-sist-**EYE**-tis
☐ cholecystogram	**koh**-lee-**SISS**-toh-gram
☐ cholecystography	**koh**-lee-sist-**OG**-rah-fee
☐ choledocholithiasis	koh-leh-**doh**-koh-lih-**THIGH**-ah-sis
☐ choledocholithotomy	koh-leh-**doh**-koh-lith-**OT**-oh-mee
☐ choledocholithotripsy	koh-leh-**doh**-koh-**LITH**-oh-trip-see
☐ cholelithiasis	**koh**-lee-lih-**THIGH**-ah-sis
☐ cirrhosis	sih-**ROH**-sis
☐ colectomy	koh-**LEK**-toh-mee
☐ colonoscopy	koh-lon-**OSS**-koh-pee
☐ colorectal carcinoma	koh-loh-**REK**-tal kar-sin-**OH**-mah
☐ colostomy	koh-**LOSS**-toh-mee
☐ Crohn's disease	KROHNZ disease
☐ diarrhea	digh-ah-**REE**-ah
☐ diverticulectomy	**digh**-ver-**tik**- yoo-**LEK**-toh-mee
☐ diverticulitis	**digh**-ver-**tik**-yoo-**LIGH**-tis
☐ diverticulosis	**digh**-ver-**tik**-yoo-**LOH**-sis
☐ diverticulum	**digh**-ver-**TIK**-yoo-lum
☐ duodenal ulcer	doo-**OD**-eh-nal **ULL**-sir, doo-oh-**DEE**-nal **ULL**-sir
☐ duodenum	doo-**OD**-eh-num, doo-oh-**DEE**-num
☐ dysentery	**DISS**-en-ter-ee
☐ dyspepsia	diss-**PEP**-see-ah

☐ dysphagia	diss-**FAY**-jee-ah
☐ emaciation	ee-**may**-she-**AY**-shun
☐ endoscopic retrograde cholangiopancreatogram (ERCP)	en-doh-**SKOP**-ic **REH**-troh-grayd kohl-**an**-jee-oh-**PAN**-kree-ah-toh-gram en-doh-**SKOP**-ic **REH**-troh-grayd kohl-**an**-jee-oh-**pan**-kree-ah-**TOG**- rah-fee
☐ eructation	eh-ruk-**TAY**-shun
☐ esophagogastroduodenoscopy (EGD)	eh-**soff**-ah-goh-**gass**-troh-doo-**wah**-den-**OSS**-koh-pee
☐ esophagogastroplasty	eh-**soff**-ah-goh-**GASS**-troh-plass-tee
☐ esophagoscopy	eh-**soff**-ah-**GOSS**-koh-pee
☐ esophagus	eh-**SOFF**-ah-gus
☐ extracorporeal shock wave lithotripsy (ESWL)	**eks**-trah-kor-**POR**-ee-al shock wave **LITH**-oh-trip-see
☐ fecal	**FEE**-kal
☐ feces	**FEE**-seez
☐ flatus	**FLAY**-tus
☐ gastrectomy	gass-**TREK**-toh-mee
☐ gastric	**GASS**-trik
☐ gastric lavage	**GASS**-trik lah-**VAHZ**
☐ gastric ulcer	**GASS**-trik **ULL**-sir
☐ gastroduodenostomy	**gass**-troh-doo-**wah**-den-**OSS**-toh-mee
☐ gastrodynia	gass-troh-**DIN**-ee-ah
☐ gastroenteritis	**gass**-troh-**en**-ter-**EYE**-tis
☐ gastroenterologist	**gass**-troh-**en**-ter-**ALL**-oh-jist
☐ gastroenterology	**gass**-troh-**en**-ter-**ALL**-oh-jee
☐ gastroesophageal reflux disease (GERD)	**gass**-troh-eh-**soff**-oh-**JEE**-al reflux disease
☐ gastroscopy	gass-**TROSS**-koh-pee
☐ gavage	gah-**VAHZ**
☐ gingivectomy	jin-jih-**VEK**-toh-mee
☐ gingivitis	jin-jih-**VIGH**-tis
☐ glossorrhaphy	gloss-**OR**-ah-fee
☐ hard palate; soft palate	hard **PAL**-at; soft **PAL**-at
☐ *Helicobacter pylori* antibodies test	hee-lih-koh-**BAK**-ter pigh-**LOR**-eye antibodies test
☐ hematemesis	hem-at-**EM**-eh-sis
☐ hepatitis	hep-ah-**TIGH**-tis
☐ hernia	**HER**-nee-ah
☐ herniorrhaphy	her-nee-**OR**-ah-fee
☐ herpetic stomatitis	her-**PEH**-tik **stoh**-mah-**TIGH**-tis
☐ hiatal hernia	high-**AY**-tal **HER**-nee-ah
☐ ileocecal	**ill**-ee-oh-**SEE**-kal
☐ ileocecal valve	**ill**-ee-oh-**SEE**-kal valve
☐ ileostomy	ill-ee-**OSS**-toh-mee
☐ ileum	**ILL**-ee-um
☐ ileus	**ILL**-ee-us

☐ intussusception	in-**tuh**-suh-**SEP**-shun
☐ jejunum	jeh-**JOO**-num
☐ laparoscopy	lap-ah-**ROSS**-koh-pee
☐ laparotomy	lap-ah-**ROT**-oh-mee
☐ lower gastrointestinal series	**gass**-troh-in-**TESS**-tin-al series
☐ melena	**MELL**-eh-nah
☐ nasogastric	nay-zoh-**GASS**-trik
☐ nasogastric intubation	nay-zoh-**GASS**-trik in-too-**BAY**-shun
☐ nausea	**NAW**-zee-ah
☐ occult blood test	uh-**KULT** blood test
☐ oral	**OR**-al
☐ oral leukoplakia	**OR**-al loo-koh-**PLAY**-kee-ah
☐ palatoplasty	**PAL**-at-oh-**plass**-tee
☐ pancreas	**PAN**-kree-ass
☐ pancreatic	pan-kree-**AT**-ik
☐ pancreatitis	**pan**-kree-ah-**TIGH**-tis
☐ parotid glands	pah-**ROT**-id glands
☐ peristalsis	pair-ih-**STALL**-sis
☐ peritoneal	**pair**-ih-toh-**NEE**-al
☐ pharynx	**FAIR**-inks
☐ polyp	**PALL**-ip
☐ polypectomy	pall-ih-**PEK**-toh-mee
☐ polyposis, chronic	pall-ee-**POH**-sis, chronic
☐ proctocolectomy	**prock**-toh-koh-**LEK**-toh-mee
☐ proctologist	prok-**TALL**-oh-jist
☐ proctology	prok-**TALL**-oh-jee
☐ proctoscopy	prok-**TOSS**-koh-pee
☐ pruritus ani	proo-**RIGH**-tus **AN**-eye
☐ pyloric sphincter	pigh-**LOR**-ik **SFINGK**-ter
☐ pyloroplasty	pigh-**LOR**-oh-**plass**-tee
☐ saliva	sah-**LIGH**-vah
☐ salivary glands	**SAL**-ih-vair-ee glands
☐ sialolithiasis	**sigh**-ah-loh-lih-**THIGH**-ah-sis
☐ sigmoid colon	**SIG**-moyd colon
☐ sigmoidoscopy	sig-moyd-**OSS**-koh-pee
☐ sublingual glands	sub-**LING**-gwall glands
☐ submandibular glands	sub-man-**DIB**-yoo-lar glands
☐ total parenteral nutrition (TPN)	total par-**EN**-ter-al nutrition
☐ ulcerative colitis	**ULL**-ser-ah-tiv koh-**LIGH**-tis
☐ uvula	**YOO**-vyoo-lah
☐ uvulopalatopharyngoplasty	**yoo**-vyoo-loh-**pal**-ah-toh-fah-**RING**-oh-**plass**-tee
☐ volvulus	**VOL**-vyoo-lus

CHAPTER 10

Urinary System

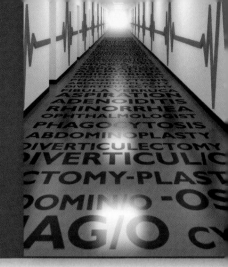

OBJECTIVES

At the completion of this chapter, the student should be able to:

1. Identify, define, and spell word roots associated with the urinary system.
2. Label the basic structures of the urinary system.
3. Discuss the functions of the urinary system.
4. Provide the correct spelling of urinary terms, given the definition of the terms.
5. Analyze urinary terms by defining the roots, prefixes, and suffixes of these terms.
6. Identify, define, and spell disease, disorder, and procedure terms related to the urinary system.

OVERVIEW

The urinary system is made up of the kidneys, ureters, urinary bladder, and urethra. The structures of the urinary system function together for the following purposes: (1) to filter the blood; (2) to maintain the proper balance of water, salts, and other substances found in our body fluids; and (3) to remove waste and excess fluids from the body. Each urinary system structure and its unique characteristics are presented individually.

Urinary System Word Roots

To understand and use urinary system medical terms, it is necessary to acquire a thorough knowledge of the associated word roots. Word roots associated with the urinary system structures are listed with the combining vowel. The suffix *-uria*, which means "urine," is included on the list. Review the word roots in Table 10-1 and complete the exercises that follow.

TABLE 10-1 URINARY SYSTEM WORD ROOTS

Word Root/Combining Form	Meaning
cyst/o	bladder; sac; urinary bladder
glomerul/o	glomerulus
meat/o	meatus (opening)
nephr/o	kidney
pyel/o	renal pelvis
ren/o	kidney
ur/o	urine; urinary system

(continues)

TABLE 10-1   URINARY SYSTEM WORD ROOTS (continued)

Word Root/Combining Form	Meaning
ureter/o	ureter
urethr/o	urethra
vesic/o	urinary bladder
Suffix	
-uria	urine; urination

© 2016 Cengage Learning®

EXERCISE 1

Write the meanings of the following word roots.

1. cyst/o _____

2. glomerul/o _____

3. meat/o _____

4. nephr/o _____

5. pyel/o _____

6. ren/o _____

7. ureter/o _____

8. urethr/o _____

9. vesic/o _____

EXERCISE 2

Write the word root and meaning.

1. cystectomy

   ROOT: _____ MEANING: _____

2. ureterocele

   ROOT: _____ MEANING: _____

3. nephritis

   ROOT: _____ MEANING: _____

4. renogram

   ROOT: _____ MEANING: _____

5. pyelogram

   ROOT: _____ MEANING: _____

6. meatotomy

   ROOT: _____ MEANING: _____

7. vesicocele

   ROOT: _____ MEANING: _____

8. glomerulonephritis

ROOT: _____   MEANING: _____

ROOT: _____   MEANING: _____

9. urethritis

ROOT: _____   MEANING: _____

EXERCISE 3

Write the correct word root(s) for the following definitions.

1. bladder; sac; urinary bladder   _____

2. glomerulus   _____

3. kidney   _____

4. meatus (opening)   _____

5. renal pelvis   _____

6. ureter   _____

7. urethra   _____

Structures of the Urinary System

The major structures of the urinary system include the kidneys, ureters, urinary bladder, and urethra. The (1) **kidneys** are responsible for filtering the blood and producing urine. The (2) **ureters** transport the urine from the kidney to the (3) **urinary bladder**, which is the storage sac for the urine. Urine leaves the body through the (4) **urethra** (yoo-**REE**-thrah). Figure 10-1 illustrates the major structures of the urinary system.

Kidneys

The kidneys are bean-shaped organs located on the posterior wall of the abdominal cavity. There is one kidney on each side of the spinal column. The kidneys are super-filters for the blood. They remove waste products from the bloodstream and help maintain the proper balance of water, salts, and other necessary substances found in body fluids.

The outer layer of the kidney is called the (1) **cortex** (**KOR**-tecks) and contains the **nephrons** (**NEFF**-ronz), or kidney cells. The inner layer of the kidney is called the (2) **medulla** (meh-**DULL**-ah). The (3) **renal pelvis** is the upper, expanded section of the ureters. Urine collects in the renal pelvis and then travels to the urinary bladder by way of the ureters. Figure 10-2 illustrates the major areas of the kidney and nephrons. Refer to this figure as you learn about these structures.

Nephrons are the filtering unit of the kidney. The nephrons filter blood to form urine and at the same time, reabsorb essential minerals and needed substances. There are two important parts of each nephron: the (4) **glomerulus** (glom-**AIR**-yoo-lus) and (5) **renal tubules** (**TOOB**-yoolz). The glomerulus is a cluster or ball of capillaries. The glomerulus is surrounded by a cup-shaped membrane called the (6) **Bowman's capsule**. The renal tubule has many loops and coils.

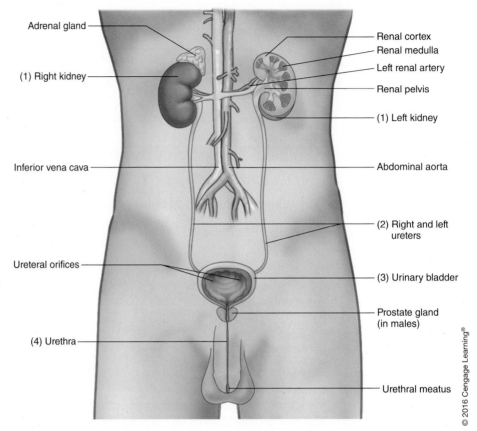

Figure 10-1 Primary structures of the urinary system.

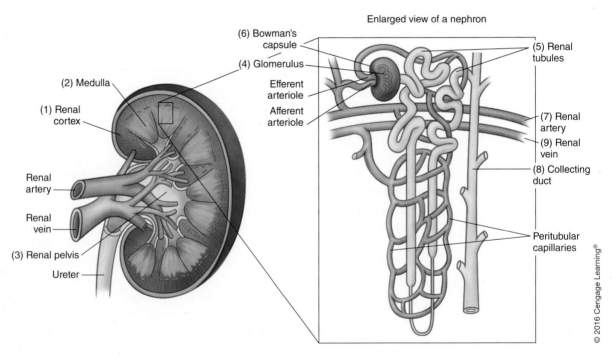

Figure 10-2 Areas and structures of the kidney and nephrons.

Blood enters the kidney via the (7) **renal artery** and passes through the **glomeruli** (glom-**AIR**-yoo-ligh) of the nephrons. The blood is filtered by the glomeruli. Capillaries carry the filtered blood around the renal tubules. The renal tubules capture water and waste products to form urine. The renal tubules eventually uncoil and become the (8) **collecting ducts**. The collecting ducts empty the urine into the renal pelvis. The filtered blood continues to flow through the blood vessels that surround the renal tubules. Essential minerals, proteins, and glucose are reabsorbed into the capillaries that surround the renal tubules. Waste products are passed into the venous blood that leaves the kidney via the (9) **renal vein**.

Urine is the liquid waste of the body. It is made up of 95% water and 5% of other substances. These substances, known as *waste products*, include urea (yoo-**REE**-ah), creatinine (kree-**AT**-in-in), ammonia, and mineral salts.

Ureters, Urinary Bladder, and Urethra

The ureters, urinary bladder, and urethra are responsible for moving urine out of the body. Figure 10-3 illustrates these structures in cross-sectional views of the male and female urinary organs.

The (1) **ureters** are narrow tubes and are about 10 to 12 inches in length. The upper ends of the ureters are located in the kidney. These sections of the ureters are called the renal pelvis. From the kidney, the ureters narrow and connect to the (2) **urinary bladder**.

The urinary bladder is a hollow, muscular organ or sac that temporarily stores urine. When the body is ready to release urine, the bladder contracts and expels the urine. *Urination*, *voiding*, and **micturition** (mick-too-**RIH**-shun) are terms that mean the normal process of expelling urine.

The (3) **urethra** is the tube leading from the urinary bladder to the outside of the body. The male urethra is about 7 to 8 inches long, and the female urethra is about 1.5 to 2 inches long. The male urethra is a passageway for both urine and semen through the penis, but not at the same time. Only urine passes through the female

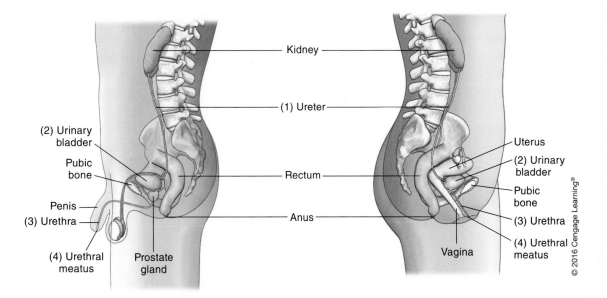

Figure 10-3 Cross sections of the male and female urinary systems.

urethra. The (4) **urethral meatus** (mee-**AY**-tus), also called the *urinary meatus*, is the external opening of the urethra. In the male, the urinary meatus is at the tip of the penis; in the female, it is located between the clitoris and the vaginal opening.

EXERCISE 4

Match the urinary system structures in Column 1 with the correct definition in Column 2.

COLUMN 1

_____ 1. glomerulus

_____ 2. nephron

_____ 3. renal pelvis

_____ 4. renal tubule

_____ 5. ureter

_____ 6. urethra

_____ 7. urinary bladder

_____ 8. urinary meatus

COLUMN 2

a. tube that leads to the urinary bladder

b. tube that leads to the outside of the body

c. filtering unit of the kidney

d. storage sac for urine

e. cluster of capillaries

f. external opening of the urethra

g. captures water and waste from blood

h. upper expanded end of the ureters

EXERCISE 5

Label the structures of the urinary system identified in Figure 10-4. Write your answers on the spaces provided.

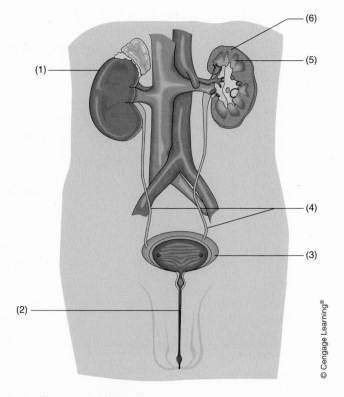

© Cengage Learning®

Figure 10-4 Labeling exercise.

Labeling exercise

1. _____
2. _____
3. _____
4. _____
5. _____
6. _____

EXERCISE 6

Write the name of the defined urinary system structure.

1. tube that leads to the outside of the body   _____

2. tubes that bring urine to the bladder   _____

3. outer area of the kidney   _____

4. inner area of the kidney   _____

5. microscopic filtration unit of the kidney   _____

6. cluster or ball of capillaries   _____

7. captures water and waste products   _____

Urinary System Medical Terminology

Urinary medical terms are organized into three main categories: (1) general medical terms; (2) disease and disorder terms; and (3) diagnostic procedure, surgery, and laboratory test terms. The roots, prefixes, and suffixes used in urinary system terms are listed in Table 10-2. Review these word parts and complete the exercises.

TABLE 10-2   COMBINING FORMS, PREFIXES, AND SUFFIXES FOR URINARY SYSTEM TERMS

Root	Meaning	Prefix	Meaning	Suffix	Meaning
hemat/o	blood	an-	without	-cele	hernia; protrusion
lith/o	stone	dys-	abnormal; painful; difficult	-gram	record; x-ray film
noct/o	night	poly-	many	-graph	instrument for recording
olig/o	few; diminished			-graphy	process of recording
py/o	pus			-pexy	surgical fixation
				-ptosis	drooping; sagging

(continues)

TABLE 10-2 COMBINING FORMS, PREFIXES, AND SUFFIXES FOR URINARY SYSTEM TERMS (continued)

Root	Meaning	Prefix	Meaning	Suffix	Meaning
				-scope	instrument for viewing
				-scopy	process of viewing
				-(o)stomy	creation of a new or artificial opening
				-(o)tomy	incision into
				-tripsy	crushing

© 2016 Cengage Learning®

EXERCISE 7

Write the root, prefix, suffix, and their meanings for each medical term. Based on the meanings of the word parts, write a definition for each term. Check your definition using a medical dictionary. Note: Not all terms have a root, prefix, and suffix.

1. pyuria

   ROOT: _____ MEANING: _____

   PREFIX: _____ MEANING: _____

   SUFFIX: _____ MEANING: _____

   DEFINITION: _____

2. anuria

   ROOT: _____ MEANING: _____

   PREFIX: _____ MEANING: _____

   SUFFIX: _____ MEANING: _____

   DEFINITION: _____

3. oliguria

   ROOT: _____ MEANING: _____

   PREFIX: _____ MEANING: _____

   SUFFIX: _____ MEANING: _____

   DEFINITION: _____

4. polyuria

   ROOT: _____ MEANING: _____

   PREFIX: _____ MEANING: _____

   SUFFIX: _____ MEANING: _____

   DEFINITION: _____

5. hematuria

    ROOT: _____ MEANING: _____

    PREFIX: _____ MEANING: _____

    SUFFIX: _____ MEANING: _____

    DEFINITION: _____

6. nocturia

    ROOT: _____ MEANING: _____

    PREFIX: _____ MEANING: _____

    SUFFIX: _____ MEANING: _____

    DEFINITION: _____

EXERCISE 8

Write the suffix associated with the following definitions.

1. cut into; incision   _____
2. drooping; sagging   _____
3. hernia; protrusion   _____
4. instrument for recording   _____
5. instrument for viewing   _____
6. process of recording   _____
7. record; x-ray film   _____
8. creation of a new or artificial opening   _____
9. surgical fixation   _____

Urinary System General Medical Terms

Review the pronunciation and meaning of each term in Table 10-3. Note that some terms are built from word parts and some are not. The exercises for these few terms are included with the exercises for urinary system disease terms.

TABLE 10-3 URINARY SYSTEM GENERAL MEDICAL TERMS

Term with Pronunciation	Definition
meatal (mee-**AY**-tal) meat/o = meatus -al = pertaining to	pertaining to the meatus
urine (**YOOR**-in)	liquid waste product

(continues)

TABLE 10-3   URINARY SYSTEM GENERAL MEDICAL TERMS (continued)

Term with Pronunciation	Definition
urologist (yoor-**ALL**-oh-jist) ur/o = urinary system -(o)logist = physician specialist	physician who specializes in the urinary system and male reproductive system
urology (yoor-**ALL**-oh-jee) ur/o = urinary system -(o)logy = study of	study of the urinary tract

© 2016 Cengage Learning®

Urinary System Disease and Disorder Terms

Urinary system diseases and disorders include familiar problems such as urinary tract infection (UTI) as well as other more complex and less familiar diagnoses such as glomerulonephritis. The disease and disorder terms are presented in alphabetical order in Table 10-4. Review the pronunciation and definition for each term and complete the exercises.

TABLE 10-4   URINARY SYSTEM DISEASE AND DISORDER TERMS

Term with Pronunciation	Definition
anuria (an-**YOO**-ree-ah) an- = lack of; without -uria = urine	absence of urine
azoturia (azz-oh-**TOO**-ree-ah)	an increase of urea in urine
cystitis (siss-**TIGH**-tis) cyst/o = urinary bladder -itis = inflammation	inflammation of the urinary bladder
cystocele (**SISS**-toh-seel) cyst/o = urinary bladder -cele = hernia; protrusion	hernia of the urinary bladder through the vaginal wall
diuresis (**digh**-yoo-**REE**-siss)	secretion of large amounts of urine
diuretic (**digh**-yoo-**RET**-ik)	increasing the secretion of urine; a substance that increases the secretion of urine

(continues)

TABLE 10-4   URINARY SYSTEM DISEASE AND DISORDER TERMS (continued)

Term with Pronunciation	Definition
dysuria (diss-**YOO**-ree-ah) dys- = abnormal; painful; difficult -uria = urine	painful or difficult urination
enuresis (en-yoo-**REE**-siss)	involuntary release of urine; bedwetting
epispadias (ep-ih-**SPAY**-dee-as)	congenital defect in which the urinary meatus is on the upper surface of the penis
glomerulonephritis (glom-**air**-yoo-loh-neh-**FRIGH**-tis) glomerul/o = glomerulus nephr/o = kidney -itis = inflammation	inflammation of the glomerulus of the kidneys
glycosuria (**gligh**-kohs-**YOO**-ree-ah) glycos/o = glucose -uria = urine	presence of glucose in the urine
hematuria (**hee**-mah-**TOO**-ree-ah) hemat/o = blood -uria = urine	presence of blood in the urine

© 2016 Cengage Learning®

EXERCISE 9

Analyze each term by writing the prefix, root, combining vowel, and suffix separated by vertical slashes. Based on the meaning of the word parts, write a definition for each term. Check the definition in a medical dictionary.

EXAMPLE: urologist:

	/ur	/o	/logist
prefix	*root*	*combining vowel*	*suffix*

DEFINITION: <u>specialist in the urinary and male reproductive systems</u>

1. anuria

prefix	*root*	*combining vowel*	*suffix*

DEFINITION: _____

2. cystitis

prefix	*root*	*combining vowel*	*suffix*

DEFINITION: _____

3. cystocele

prefix	root	combining vowel	suffix

DEFINITION: _____

4. dysuria

prefix	root	combining vowel	suffix

DEFINITION: _____

5. glycosuria

prefix	root	combining vowel	suffix

DEFINITION: _____

6. glomerulonephritis

prefix	root	combining vowel	suffix

DEFINITION: _____

7. hematuria

prefix	root	combining vowel	suffix

DEFINITION: _____

8. urologist

prefix	root	combining vowel	suffix

DEFINITION: _____

9. urology

prefix	root	combining vowel	suffix

DEFINITION: _____

EXERCISE 10

Replace the italicized phrase or word with the correct medical term.

1. Victoria's physician said that her history of *secretion of large amounts of urine* called for special kidney tests.

   _____

2. Thomas was relieved when he learned that *bedwetting* can be treated.

   _____

3. To relieve fluid overload, the physician might prescribe a *medication that increases the secretion of urine.*

   _____

4. *Increased urea in urine* is associated with kidney failure.

   _____

5. Surgical intervention might correct *a urinary meatus on the upper surface of the penis.*

_____

6. *The presence of glucose in the urine* is seen in uncontrolled diabetes mellitus.

_____

EXERCISE 11

Match the medical term in Column 1 with the correct definition in Column 2.

COLUMN 1	COLUMN 2
_____ 1. anuria	a. blood in the urine
_____ 2. azoturia	b. glucose in the urine
_____ 3. cystitis	c. herniation of the urinary bladder
_____ 4. cystocele	d. absence of urine
_____ 5. diuresis	e. painful urination
_____ 6. dysuria	f. inflammation of the urinary bladder
_____ 7. enuresis	g. pertaining to the meatus
_____ 8. glycosuria	h. increase of urea in the urine
_____ 9. hematuria	i. bedwetting
_____ 10. meatal	j. secretion of large amounts of urine

Review the pronunciation and definition for each term in Table 10-5 and complete the exercises.

TABLE 10-5 URINARY SYSTEM DISEASE AND DISORDER TERMS

Term with Pronunciation	Definition
hydronephrosis (**high**-droh-neh-**FROH**-sis) hydro- = water nephr/o = kidney -osis = condition	distention of the renal pelvis caused by the inability of the urine to leave the kidney (Figure 10-5)
hypospadias (**high**-poh-**SPAY**-dee-as)	a congenital defect in which the urinary meatus is on the under surface of the penis
incontinence (in-**KON**-tin-ents)	loss of urinary bladder control
nephritis (neh-**FRIGH**-tis) nephr/o = kidney -itis = inflammation	inflammation of the kidney

(continues)

TABLE 10-5 URINARY SYSTEM DISEASE AND DISORDER TERMS (continued)

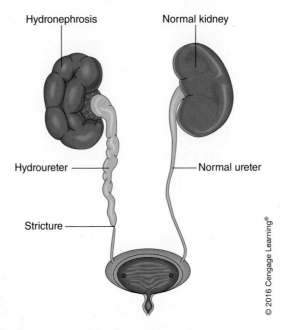

Figure 10-5 Hydroureter and hydronephrosis.

Term with Pronunciation	Definition
nephrolithiasis (**neh**-froh-lih-**THIGH**-ah-sis) nephr/o = kidney lith/o = stone -iasis = condition	presence of stones in the kidneys; kidney stones; also called renal calculi (Figure 10-6)
nephroma (neh-**FROH**-mah) nephr/o = kidney -oma = tumor	kidney tumor
nephromegaly (**neh**-froh-**MEG**-ah-lee) nephr/o = kidney -megaly = enlarged; enlargement	enlargement of one or both kidneys
nephroptosis (**neh**-frop-**TOH**-sis) nephr/o = kidney -ptosis = drooping; sagging	downward displacement of the kidney; falling, drooping kidney; also known as a *floating kidney*
nocturia (nok-**TOO**-ree-ah) noct/o = night -uria = urine	excessive urination at night

(continues)

TABLE 10-5 URINARY SYSTEM DISEASE AND DISORDER TERMS (continued)

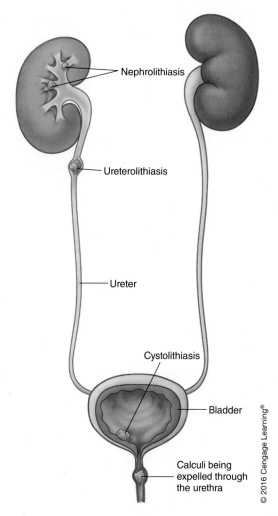

Figure 10-6 Nephrolithiasis, with stones (calculi) in the renal pelvis. Note: Stones (calculi) located in the ureter or bladder changes the name of the condition.

Term with Pronunciation	Definition
oliguria (all-ig-**YOO**-ree-ah) olig/o = few; diminished -uria = urine	diminished urine secretion
polycystic kidney (pall-ee-**SISS**-tik) poly- = many cyst/o = fluid-filled sac -ic = pertaining to	a hereditary kidney disorder in which fluid-filled cysts or sacs replace normal kidney tissue (Figure 10-7)

(continues)

TABLE 10-5 URINARY SYSTEM DISEASE AND DISORDER TERMS (continued)

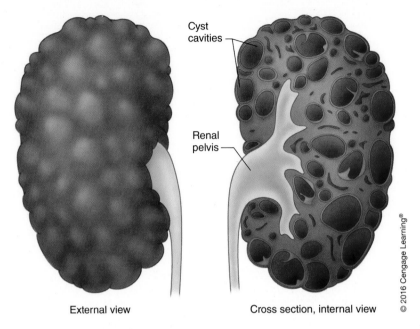

Cyst cavities

Renal pelvis

External view

Cross section, internal view

© 2016 Cengage Learning®

Figure 10-7 Polycystic kidney disease.

Term with Pronunciation	Definition
polyuria (pall-ee-**YOO**-ree-ah) poly- = many -uria = urine	excessive urination

© 2016 Cengage Learning®

EXERCISE 12

Analyze each term by writing the prefix, root, combining vowel, and suffix separated by vertical slashes. Based on the meaning of the word parts, write a definition for each term. Check the definition in a medical dictionary.

1. hydronephrosis

prefix	*root*	*combining vowel*	*suffix*

DEFINITION: _____

2. nephritis

prefix	*root*	*combining vowel*	*suffix*

DEFINITION: _____

3. nephrolithiasis

prefix	*root*	*combining vowel*	*suffix*

DEFINITION: _____

4. nephroptosis

prefix	root	combining vowel	suffix

DEFINITION: _____

5. nocturia

prefix	root	combining vowel	suffix

DEFINITION: _____

6. oliguria

prefix	root	combining vowel	suffix

DEFINITION: _____

7. polyuria

prefix	root	combining vowel	suffix

DEFINITION: _____

8. nephromegaly

prefix	root	combining vowel	suffix

DEFINITION: _____

9. nephroma

prefix	root	combining vowel	suffix

DEFINITION: _____

EXERCISE 13

Write the medical term for each definition.

1. fluid-filled cysts replace normal kidney tissue   _____

2. urinary meatus opens on the under surface
   of the penis   _____

3. loss of urinary bladder control   _____

4. kidney tumor   _____

5. excessive urination   _____

6. enlarged kidney   _____

7. diminished urine secretion   _____

Review the pronunciation and definition for each term in Table 10-6 and complete the exercises.

TABLE 10-6 URINARY SYSTEM DISEASE AND DISORDER TERMS

Term with Pronunciation	Definition
pyelitis (**pigh**-eh-**LIGH**-tis) pyel/o = renal pelvis -itis = inflammation	inflammation of the renal pelvis
pyelonephritis (**pigh**-eh-loh-neh-**FRIGH**-tis) pyel/o = renal pelvis nephr/o = kidney -itis = inflammation	inflammation of the renal pelvis and kidney
pyuria (pigh-**YOO**-ree-ah) py/o = pus -uria = urine	presence of pus in the urine
renal hypertension (**REE**-nal)	increased blood pressure caused by kidney disease
uremia (yoo-**REE**-mee-ah)	presence of urea and other waste products in the blood
ureteritis (yoo-**ree**-ter-**EYE**-tis) ureter/o = ureter -itis = inflammation	inflammation of the ureters
ureterocele (yoo-**REE**-ter-oh-seel) ureter/o = ureter -cele = hernia; protrusion	herniation or protrusion of the ureter into the urinary bladder
ureterolithiasis (yoo-**ree**-ter-oh-lih-**THIGH**-ah-sis) ureter/o = ureter lith/o = stone -iasis = condition	presence of stones in the ureter (Figure 10-6)
ureterostenosis (yoo-**ree**-ter-oh-sten-**OH**-sis) ureter/o = ureter -stenosis = narrowing	narrowing or stricture of the ureter
urethrocystitis (yoo-**ree**-throh-siss-**TIGH**-tis) urethr/o = urethra cyst/o = urinary bladder -itis = inflammation	inflammation of the urethra and urinary bladder

(continues)

TABLE 10-6   URINARY SYSTEM DISEASE AND DISORDER TERMS (continued)

Term with Pronunciation	Definition
urinary retention (**YOOR**-in-air-ee ree-**TEN**-shun) ur/o = urine -ary = pertaining to	inability to empty the urinary bladder
urinary tract infection (UTI) (**YOOR**-in-air-ee tract in-**FEK**-shun)	infection of the urinary tract that can include the urethra, urinary bladder, and ureters

© 2016 Cengage Learning®

EXERCISE 14

Analyze each term by writing the prefix, root, combining vowel, and suffix separated by vertical slashes. Based on the meaning of the word parts, write a definition for each term. Check the definition in a medical dictionary.

1. pyelitis

prefix	root	combining vowel	suffix

DEFINITION: _____

2. pyelonephritis

prefix	root	combining vowel	suffix

DEFINITION: _____

3. pyuria

prefix	root	combining vowel	suffix

DEFINITION: _____

4. ureteritis

prefix	root	combining vowel	suffix

DEFINITION: _____

5. ureterocele

prefix	root	combining vowel	suffix

DEFINITION: _____

6. ureterolithiasis

prefix	root	combining vowel	suffix

DEFINITION: _____

7. ureterostenosis

prefix	root	combining vowel	suffix

DEFINITION: _____

8. urethrocystitis

_____

prefix   *root*   *combining vowel*   *suffix*

DEFINITION: _____

EXERCISE 15

Replace the italicized phrase with the correct medical term.

1. Stavra's urinalysis revealed *the presence of pus in her urine.*

    _____

2. *Urea in the blood* is often associated with kidney failure.

    _____

3. *Increased blood pressure due to kidney disease* can be treated with antibiotics, diuretics, or surgical intervention.

    _____

4. *Inability to empty the urinary bladder* can be a postoperative complication of pelvic cavity surgery.

    _____

5. Dysuria can be caused by *the presence of stones in the ureters.*

    _____

6. *Narrowing of the ureter* can interfere with the ability to urinate.

    _____

7. An untreated urinary tract infection might lead to *inflammation of the renal pelvis and kidneys.*

    _____

Urinary System Diagnostic Terms

Review the pronunciation and definition of the diagnostic terms in Table 10-7. *Note:* In the urinary system diagnostic terms, the combining form *metr/o* means "to measure."

TABLE 10-7   URINARY SYSTEM DIAGNOSTIC TERMS

Term with Pronunciation	Definition
blood urea nitrogen (BUN) (yoo-**REE**-ah **NIGH**-tro-jen)	blood test that measures the amount of urea and nitrogen in the blood; urea and nitrogen are normally removed by the kidneys
creatinine clearance test (kree-**AT**-in-in)	blood test that measures the amount of creatinine in the blood; creatinine is normally removed by the kidneys

(continues)

TABLE 10-7 URINARY SYSTEM DIAGNOSTIC TERMS (continued)

Term with Pronunciation	Definition
cystography (siss-**TOG**-rah-fee) cyst/o = urinary bladder -graphy = process of recording	process of recording an x-ray of the urinary bladder
cystometrography (**siss**-toh-meh-**TROG**-rah-fee) cyst/o = urinary bladder metr/o = to measure -graphy = process of recording	process of measuring and recording bladder pressure during filling and voiding
cystoscopy (sist-**OSS**-koh-pee) cyst/o = urinary bladder -scopy = visual examination	visual examination of the interior of the urinary bladder using a cystoscope (Figure 10-8)

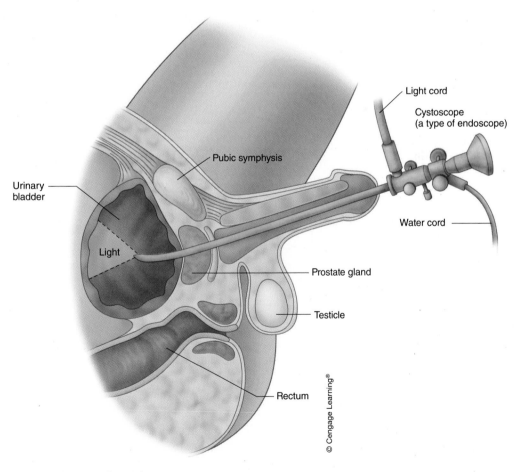

Figure 10-8 Cystoscopy.

(continues)

TABLE 10-7 URINARY SYSTEM DIAGNOSTIC TERMS (continued)

Term with Pronunciation	Definition
hemodialysis (**hee**-moh-digh-**AL**-ih-sis)	a treatment procedure to filter blood when the kidneys are unable to function; blood is circulated through a dialysis machine, filtered, and returned to the body (Figure 10-9)

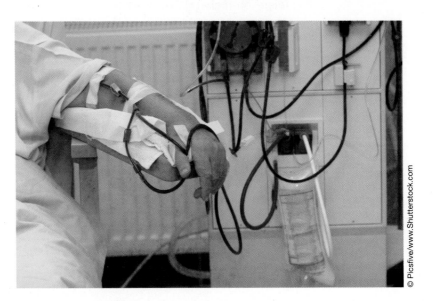

© Picsfive/www.Shutterstock.com

Figure 10-9 Hemodialysis.

Term with Pronunciation	Definition
intravenous pyelography (IVP) (in-trah-**VEE**-nus **pigh**-eh-**LOG**-rah-fee) intra- = within ven/o = vein -ous = pertaining to pyel/o = renal pelvis -graphy = process of recording	process of recording an x-ray picture of the internal structures of the kidneys, ureters, urinary bladder, and urethra after a contrast medium is injected into a vein; also called *intravenous urography*
kidneys, ureters, and bladder (KUB)	an x-ray of the lower abdomen that may be used as a screening test for kidney stones; also called a *scout film*

(continues)

TABLE 10-7   URINARY SYSTEM DIAGNOSTIC TERMS (continued)

Term with Pronunciation	Definition
peritoneal dialysis (**pair**-ih-toh-**NEE**-al digh-**AL**-ih-sis)	a treatment to filter blood when the kidneys are unable to function; the peritoneum, the membrane that lines the abdominal cavity, is the filter and blood does not leave the body; *continuous ambulatory peritoneal dialysis* (CAPD), gravity-assisted dialysis that requires three to five exchanges of solution during waking hours (Figure 10-10); *continuous cycler-assisted peritoneal dialysis* (CCPD), and *nocturnal intermittent peritoneal dialysis* (NIPD), machine-assisted dialysis that uses an automated cycler to perform three to five exchanges of solution during sleeping hours
retrograde pyelography (**REH**-troh-grayd **pigh**-eh-**LOG**-rah-fee) pyel/o = renal pelvis -graphy = process of recording	process of recording the internal structure of the ureters and renal pelvis; contrast medium is injected into the ureters and travels up the ureters into the renal pelvis
urinalysis (UA)	physical, chemical and microscopic analysis of urine
urinary catheterization (**YOOR**-in-air-ee **kath**-eh-ter-ih-**ZAY**-shun)	insertion of a catheter (i.e., a small tube) into the urinary bladder for the purpose of collecting urine
voiding cystourethrography (VCUG) (**siss**-toh-yoo-ree-**THROG**-rah-fee) cyst/o = urinary bladder urethr/o = urethra -graphy = process of recording	recording the activity and internal condition of the urinary bladder and urethra during the voiding process

(continues)

TABLE 10-7 URINARY SYSTEM DIAGNOSTIC TERMS (continued)

Peritoneal Dialysis

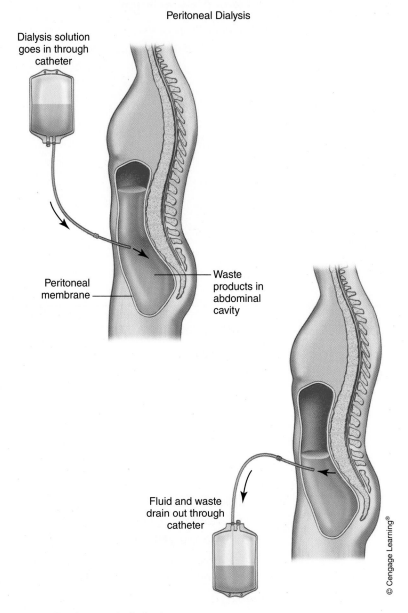

Dialysis solution
goes in through
catheter

Peritoneal
membrane

Waste
products in
abdominal
cavity

Fluid and waste
drain out through
catheter

© Cengage Learning®

Figure 10-10 Peritoneal dialysis.

© 2016 Cengage Learning®

EXERCISE 16

Analyze each term by writing the prefix, root, combining vowel, and suffix separated by vertical slashes. Based on the meaning of the word parts, write a definition for each term. Check the definition in a medical dictionary.

1. cystography

_____

prefix   *root*   *combining vowel*   *suffix*

DEFINITION: _____

2. cystometrography

prefix	*root*	*combining vowel*	*suffix*

DEFINITION: _____

3. cystoscopy

prefix	*root*	*combining vowel*	*suffix*

DEFINITION: _____

4. intravenous pyelography

prefix	*root*	*combining vowel*	*suffix*

DEFINITION: _____

5. retrograde pyelography

prefix	*root*	*combining vowel*	*suffix*

DEFINITION: _____

6. voiding cystourethrography

prefix	*root*	*combining vowel*	*suffix*

DEFINITION: _____

EXERCISE 17

Change the suffix -graphy to -gram. Rewrite the medical term and the new definition.

EXAMPLE: cardiography
TERM: cardiogram
DEFINITION: x-ray film of the heart

1. cystography

   TERM: _____

   DEFINITION: _____

2. cystometrography

   TERM: _____

   DEFINITION: _____

3. intravenous pyelography

   TERM: _____

   DEFINITION: _____

4. retrograde pyelography

   TERM: _____

   DEFINITION: _____

5. voiding cystourethrography

TERM: _____

DEFINITION: _____

EXERCISE 18

Replace the italicized phrase or abbreviation with the correct medical term.

1. Matt went to the treatment center three days a week for *a procedure to filter blood through a machine.*

   _____

2. Unrelenting lower back pain, radiating both left and right, was justification for an *IVP.*

   _____

3. The *test to measure the amount of creatinine in the blood* provides information about the kidneys' ability to filter blood.

   _____

4. *Filtering blood through the peritoneum* is an alternative to hemodialysis.

   _____

5. A *VCUG* requires the patient to drink substantial amounts of water.

   _____

6. A *microscopic examination of urine* is a screening test for urinary system diseases and disorders.

   _____

7. *Collecting urine with a catheter* is a common postoperative physician's order.

   _____

8. A *BUN* is often ordered to assess kidney function.

   _____

Urinary System Procedure Terms

Review the pronunciation and definition of the urinary system procedure terms in Table 10-8.

TABLE 10-8 URINARY SYSTEM PROCEDURE TERMS

Term with Pronunciation	Definition
cystectomy (siss-**TEK**-toh-mee) cyst/o = urinary bladder -ectomy = surgical removal	surgical removal of the bladder; excision of the bladder

(continues)

TABLE 10-8 URINARY SYSTEM PROCEDURE TERMS (continued)

Term with Pronunciation	Definition
cystolithotomy (**siss**-toh-lith-**OT**-oh-mee) cyst/o = urinary bladder lith/o = stone -(o)tomy = incision into	incision into the bladder to remove a stone
cystopexy (**SISS**-toh-**pek**-see) cyst/o = urinary bladder -pexy = surgical fixation	surgical fixation of the urinary bladder
cystoplasty (**SISS**-toh-**plass**-tee) cyst/o = urinary bladder -plasty = surgical repair	surgical repair of the urinary bladder
cystorrhaphy (sist-**OR**-ah-fee) cyst/o = urinary bladder -(r)rhaphy = suturing	suturing of the urinary bladder
cystostomy (sist-**OSS**-toh-mee) cyst/o = urinary bladder -(o)stomy = surgical creation of a new or artificial opening	surgical creation of a new or artificial opening between the urinary bladder and the surface of the body
kidney transplant	replacing a failed kidney with a donated kidney; also called *renal transplant*; the nonfunctioning kidney may be left in place; the donor kidney with associated structures are sutured in place at a lower point in the abdominopelvic cavity (Figure 10-11)
lithotripsy (**LITH**-oh-trip-see) lith/o = stone -tripsy = crushing	intentional crushing of stones for the purpose of removal
meatotomy (mee-ah-**TOT**-oh-mee) meat/o = urinary meatus -(o)tomy = incision into	incision into the urinary meatus to enlarge the opening
nephrectomy (neh-**FREK**-toh-mee) nephr/o = kidney -ectomy = surgical removal	surgical removal of a kidney; excision of a kidney

(continues)

TABLE 10-8 URINARY SYSTEM PROCEDURE TERMS (continued)

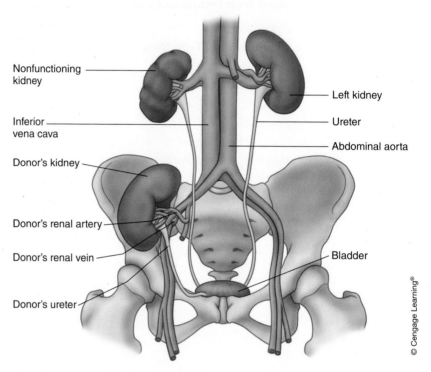

Figure 10-11 Kidney transplant.

Term with Pronunciation	Definition
nephrolithotomy (**neh**-froh-lith-**OT**-oh-mee) nephr/o = kidney lith/o = stone -(o)tomy = incision into	surgical incision into a kidney to remove stones
nephropexy (**NEFF**-roh-pek-see) nephr/o = kidney -pexy = surgical fixation	surgical fixation of a fallen or prolapsed kidney
pyelolithotomy (**pigh**-eh-loh-lith-**OT**-oh-mee) pyel/o = renal pelvis lith/o = stone -(o)tomy = incision into	incision into the renal pelvis to remove stones
ureterectomy (yoo-**ree**-ter-**ECK**-toh-mee) ureter/o = ureter -ectomy = surgical removal	surgical removal of a ureter; excision of a ureter

(continues)

TABLE 10-8　URINARY SYSTEM PROCEDURE TERMS (continued)

Term with Pronunciation	Definition
urethropexy (yoo-**REE**-throh-pek-see) urethr/o = urethra -pexy = surgical fixation	surgical fixation of the urethra
urethroplasty (yoo-**REE**-throh-plass-tee) urethr/o = urethra -plasty = surgical repair	surgical repair of the urethra
urethrostomy (**yoo**-reh-**THROSS**-toh-mee) urethr/o = urethra -(o)stomy = surgical creation of a new or artificial opening	surgical creation of a new or artificial opening between the urethra and surface of the body
vesicourethral suspension (**vess**-ih-koh-yoo-**REETH**-ral)	surgical suspension of a drooping or prolapsed urinary bladder and urethra

© 2016 Cengage Learning®

EXERCISE 19

Analyze each term by writing the prefix, root, combining vowel, and suffix separated by vertical slashes. Based on the meaning of the word parts, write a definition for each term. Check the definition in a medical dictionary.

1. cystectomy

prefix	*root*	*combining vowel*	*suffix*

DEFINITION: _____

2. urethroplasty

prefix	*root*	*combining vowel*	*suffix*

DEFINITION: _____

3. cystolithotomy

prefix	*root*	*combining vowel*	*suffix*

DEFINITION: _____

4. urethropexy

prefix	*root*	*combining vowel*	*suffix*

DEFINITION: _____

5. cystopexy

prefix	*root*	*combining vowel*	*suffix*

DEFINITION: _____

6. ureterectomy

prefix	*root*	*combining vowel*	*suffix*

DEFINITION: _____

7. cystoplasty

prefix	*root*	*combining vowel*	*suffix*

DEFINITION: _____

8. pyelolithotomy

prefix	*root*	*combining vowel*	*suffix*

DEFINITION: _____

9. cystorrhaphy

prefix	*root*	*combining vowel*	*suffix*

DEFINITION: _____

10. nephropexy

prefix	*root*	*combining vowel*	*suffix*

DEFINITION: _____

11. cystostomy

prefix	*root*	*combining vowel*	*suffix*

DEFINITION: _____

12. lithotripsy

prefix	*root*	*combining vowel*	*suffix*

DEFINITION: _____

13. nephrolithotomy

prefix	*root*	*combining vowel*	*suffix*

DEFINITION: _____

14. meatotomy

prefix	*root*	*combining vowel*	*suffix*

DEFINITION: _____

15. nephrectomy

prefix	*root*	*combining vowel*	*suffix*

DEFINITION: _____

EXERCISE 20

Circle the medical term that best fits the definition.

DEFINITION	CIRCLE ONE TERM
1. incision into the urinary bladder to remove a stone	*cystotomy* OR *cystolithotomy*
2. surgical repair of the urinary bladder	*cystoplasty* OR *cystorrhaphy*
3. surgical fixation of the kidney	*nephroplasty* OR *nephropexy*
4. surgical creation of a new or artificial opening for the urinary meatus	*meatostomy* OR *meatotomy*
5. surgical excision of the urethra	*urethrectomy* OR *ureterectomy*
6. surgical fixation of the urinary bladder	*cystoplasty* OR *cystopexy*
7. surgical repair of the ureter	*ureteroplasty* OR *ureteropexy*
8. creating a new or artificial opening for the urethra	*urethrotomy* OR *urethrostomy*

Abbreviations

Review the urinary system abbreviations in Table 10-9. Practice writing out the meaning of each abbreviation.

TABLE 10-9   ABBREVIATIONS

Abbreviation	Meaning
BUN	blood urea nitrogen
CAPD	continuous ambulatory peritoneal dialysis
CCPD	continuous cycler-assisted peritoneal dialysis
IVP	intravenous pyelography
KUB	kidneys, ureters, and bladder
NIPD	nocturnal intermittent peritoneal dialysis
UA	urinalysis
UTI	urinary tract infection
VCUG	voiding cystourethrography

© 2016 Cengage Learning®

CHAPTER REVIEW

The Chapter Review can be used as a self-test. Go through each exercise and answer as many questions as you can without referring to previous exercises or earlier discussions within this chapter. Check your answers and fill in any blanks. Practice writing any terms you might have misspelled.

EXERCISE 21

Fill in the blanks with the correct urinary system medical term.

1. Painful urination, called _____, can be a sign of a urinary tract infection.

2. A/An _____ is a physician who specializes in the study of the urinary tract.

3. The medical term for bedwetting is _____.

4. Marilyn was concerned when she learned that _____ meant blood in the urine.

5. Excessive urination at night is called _____.

6. Victoria told her sister that the official name for her floating kidney is

   _____.

7. Roger was less than enthusiastic when he realized that he was scheduled for a/an _____, a visual examination of the urinary bladder.

8. A/An _____ is performed to enlarge the opening of the urinary meatus.

9. Urinalysis can identify _____, the presence of glucose in the urine.

10. The condition called _____ indicates that urine is unable to leave the kidney.

EXERCISE 22

Carefully read the following case history. Replace each italicized phrase with the correct medical term. For extra practice, rewrite the case history using the correct medical terms.

CASE HISTORY

Jeneesha is a 6-year-old female who came to the walk-in clinic with her mother. Mom states that her daughter has been treated for (1) *inflammation of the urinary bladder* three times in the past year and she was again complaining about (2) *pain during urination*. A urine sample was sent to the lab for (3) *physical, chemical,* and *microscopic examination*. The results indicated that Jeneesha had a (4) *UTI*, as evidenced by (5) *pus in the urine*. I discussed the implications of recurrent urinary tract infections. Problems such as (6) *inflammation of the ureters*, scarring of the ureters, and (7) *inflammation of the renal pelvis* can be triggered by recurrent urinary tract infections.

1. _____

2. _____

3. _____

4. _____

5. _____

6. _____

7. _____

EXERCISE 23

Read the discharge summary and write a brief definition for each italicized medical term.

DISCHARGE SUMMARY

The patient was admitted on 11/15/xx for a scheduled (1) *nephropexy*. The indications for surgery are based on the results of the (2) *intravenous pyelography* that was done last week. The IVP demonstrated (3) *nephroptosis* and (4) *hydronephrosis*. The patient's preoperative course was uneventful. He tolerated the procedure and was returned to his unit in good condition. On the fifth postoperative day, he developed (5) *urinary retention*, which necessitated (6) *urinary catheterization*. Urinary output continued to be diminished. The (7) *KUB* was negative for (8) *ureterostenosis* and (9) *ureterolithiasis*. The patient was encouraged to increase fluids, and by the ninth postoperative day, urinary output was normal. The patient was discharged home on restricted activity for six weeks. He is scheduled for a follow-up office visit next week.

1. _____

2. _____

3. _____

4. _____

5. _____

6. _____

7. _____

8. _____

9. _____

EXERCISE 24

With your knowledge of urinary system roots, prefixes, and suffixes, build medical terms for each statement.

1. physician who specializes in the urinary
   and male reproductive systems   _____

2. inflammation of the glomeruli of the kidneys   _____

3. inflammation of the urinary bladder   _____

4. blood in the urine   _____

5. enlargement of the kidneys   _____

6. incision into the urinary bladder to remove
   stones

   _____

7. distention of the renal pelvis due to retained
   urine in the urinary bladder

   _____

8. hernia of the urinary bladder through the
   vaginal wall

   _____

9. presence of stones in the kidney; kidney stones   _____

10. kidney tumor   _____

11. downward displacement of the kidney; drooping
    kidney

    _____

12. creation of a new or artificial opening between
    the urethra and the surface of the body

    _____

13. diminished urine secretion   _____

14. excessive urination   _____

15. surgical repair of the urethra   _____

16. intentional crushing of stones   _____

17. surgical fixation of the kidney   _____

18. absence of urine   _____

19. surgical removal of a ureter   _____

20. excessive urination at night   _____

EXERCISE 25

Select the best answer to each statement.

1. The medical term for bedwetting is
   a. incontinence
   b. diuresis
   c. enuresis
   d. nocturia

2. Which term best describes a substance that increases urine secretion?
   a. diuretic
   b. uremic
   c. polyuretic
   d. dialysis

3. Loss of urinary bladder control is called
   a. incontinence
   b. diuresis
   c. enuresis
   d. nocturia

4. Uremia is best defined as
   a. urine in blood
   b. blood in urine
   c. urea in blood
   d. a normal condition of urine

5. Filtering blood through a machine is known as
   a. dialysis
   b. peritoneal dialysis
   c. retrograde dialysis
   d. hemodialysis

CHALLENGE EXERCISE

Write a report comparing the advantages and disadvantages of hemodialysis and peritoneal dialysis. Use at least three references or resources, which may include interviewing a dialysis patient or dialysis nurse. Search the Internet, using the keywords hemodialysis and peritoneal dialysis, for websites that might be helpful to students and patients.

Pronunciation Review

Review the terms in this chapter. Pronounce each term using the following phonetic pronunciations. Check off the term when you are comfortable saying it.

TERM	PRONUNCIATION
☐ anuria	an-**YOO**-ree-ah
☐ azoturia	azz-oh-**TOO**-ree-ah
☐ blood urea nitrogen	blood yoo-**REE**-ah **NIGH**-tro-jen
☐ cortex	**KOR**-teks
☐ creatinine clearance test	kree-**AT**-in-in clearance test
☐ cystectomy	siss-**TEK**-toh-mee
☐ cystitis	siss-**TIGH**-tis
☐ cystocele	**SISS**-toh-seel
☐ cystography	siss-**TOG**-roh-fee
☐ cystolithotomy	**siss**-toh-lith-**OT**-oh-mee
☐ cystometrography	**siss**-toh-meh-**TROG**-rah-fee
☐ cystopexy	**SISS**-toh-**pek**-see
☐ cystoplasty	**SISS**-toh-**plass**-tee
☐ cystorrhaphy	sist-**OR**-ah-fee
☐ cystoscopy	sist-**OSS**-koh-pee
☐ cystostomy	sist-**OSS**-toh-mee
☐ diuresis	**digh**-yoo-**REE**-siss
☐ diuretic	**digh**-yoo-**RET**-ik
☐ dysuria	diss-**YOO**-ree-ah
☐ enuresis	en-yoo-**REE**-siss
☐ epispadias	ep-ih-**SPAY**-dee-as
☐ glomeruli	glom-**AIR**-yoo-ligh

☐ glomerulonephritis	glom-**air**-yoo-loh-neh-**FRIGH**-tis
☐ glomerulus	glom-**AIR**-yoo-lus
☐ glycosuria	**gligh**-kohs-**YOO**-ree-ah
☐ hematuria	**hee**-mah-**TOO**-ree-ah
☐ hemodialysis	**hee**-moh-digh-**AL**-ih-sis
☐ hydronephrosis	**high**-droh-neh-**FROH**-sis
☐ hypospadias	**high**-poh-**SPAY**-dee-as
☐ incontinence	in-**KON**-tin-ents
☐ intravenous pyelography	in-trah-**VEE**-nus pigh-eh-**LOG**-rah-fee
☐ lithotripsy	**LITH**-oh-trip-see
☐ meatotomy	mee-ah-**TOT**-oh-mee
☐ medulla	meh-**DULL**-ah
☐ micturition	mick-too-**RIH**-shun
☐ nephrectomy	neh-**FREK**-toh-mee
☐ nephritis	neh-**FRIGH**-tis
☐ nephrolithiasis	**neh**-froh-lih-**THIGH**-ah-sis
☐ nephrolithotomy	**neh**-froh-lith-**OT**-oh-mee
☐ nephroma	neh-**FROH**-mah
☐ nephromegaly	**neh**-froh-**MEG**-ah-lee
☐ nephron	**NEFF**-ron
☐ nephropexy	**NEFF**-roh-pek-see
☐ nephroptosis	neh-frop-**TOH**-sis
☐ nocturia	nok-**TOO**-ree-ah
☐ oliguria	oh-lig-**YOO**-ree-ah
☐ peritoneal dialysis	**pair**-ih-toh-**NEE**-al digh-**AL**-ih-sis
☐ polycystic kidney disease	**pall**-ee-**SISS**-tik kidney disease
☐ polyuria	**pall**-ee-**YOO**-ree-ah
☐ pyelitis	**pigh**-eh-**LIGH**-tis
☐ pyelolithotomy	**pigh**-eh-loh-lith-**OT**-oh-mee
☐ pyelonephritis	**pigh**-eh-loh-neh-**FRIGH**-tis
☐ pyuria	pigh-**YOO**-ree-ah
☐ renal hypertension	**REE**-nal hypertension
☐ renal pelvis	**REE**-nal **PELL**-viss
☐ renal tubules	**REE**-nal **TOOB**-yoolz
☐ retrograde pyelography	**REH**-troh-grayd **pigh**-eh-**LOG**-rah-fee
☐ uremia	yoo-**REE**-mee-ah
☐ ureter	**YOO**-reh-ter
☐ ureterectomy	yoo-**ree**-ter-**EK**-toh-mee
☐ ureteritis	yoo-**ree**-ter-**EYE**-tis
☐ ureterocele	yoo-**REE**-ter-oh-seel
☐ ureterolithiasis	yoo-**ree**-ter-oh-lih-**THIGH**-ah-sis
☐ ureterostenosis	yoo-**ree**-ter-oh-sten-**OH**-sis
☐ urethra	yoo-**REE**-thrah
☐ urethrocystitis	yoo-**ree**-throh-siss-**TIGH**-tis
☐ urethropexy	yoo-**REE**-throh-pek-see
☐ urethroplasty	yoo-**REE**-throh-plass-tee
☐ urethrostomy	**yoo**-reh-**THROSS**-toh-mee
☐ urinalysis	yoor-in-**AL**-ih-sis

☐ urinary bladder   **YOOR**-in-air-ee bladder
☐ urinary catheterization   **YOOR**-in-air-ee **kath**-eh-ter-ih-**ZAY**-shun
☐ urinary meatus   **YOOR**-in-air-ee mee-**AY**-tus
☐ urinary retention   **YOOR**-in-air-ee ree-**TEN**-shun
☐ urinary tract infection   **YOOR**-in-air-ee tract in-**FEK**-shun
☐ urine   **YOOR**-in
☐ urologist   yoor-**ALL**-oh-jist
☐ urology   yoor-**ALL**-oh-jee
☐ vesicourethral suspension   **vess**-ih-koh-yoo-**REETH**-ral suspension
☐ voiding cystourethrography   voiding **siss**-toh-yoo-ree-**THROG**- rah-fee

11

Endocrine System

OBJECTIVES

At the completion of this chapter, the student should be able to:

1. Identify, define, and spell word roots associated with the endocrine system.
2. Label the basic structures of the endocrine system.
3. Discuss the functions of the endocrine system.
4. Provide the correct spelling of endocrine terms, given the definition of the terms.
5. Analyze endocrine terms by defining the roots, prefixes, and suffixes of these terms.
6. Identify, define, and spell disease, disorder, and procedure terms related to the endocrine system.

OVERVIEW

The endocrine system is made up of the pituitary gland, pineal gland, thyroid gland, parathyroid glands, thymus, adrenal gland, pancreas, ovaries, and testes. Endocrine glands are ductless and release their hormones directly into the bloodstream. Hormones are chemicals that maintain and regulate the growth and activity of specific organs and the body as a whole. For example, hormones from the thyroid gland regulate metabolism, adrenal gland hormones help maintain the body's fluid balance, and the hormones from the testes and ovaries are important to the development of secondary sex characteristics. In fact, every single aspect of human growth and development is affected by the hormones of the endocrine system.

Endocrine System Word Roots

To understand and use endocrine system medical terms, it is necessary to acquire a thorough knowledge of the associated word roots. The word roots are listed with the combining vowel. Review the word roots in Table 11-1 and complete the exercises that follow.

TABLE 11-1 ENDOCRINE SYSTEM WORD ROOTS

Word Root/Combining Form	Meaning
acr/o	extremities
aden/o	gland
adren/o; adrenal/o	adrenal glands
andr/o	male; man

(continues)

TABLE 11-1   ENDOCRINE SYSTEM WORD ROOTS (continued)

Word Root/Combining Form	Meaning
calc/i	calcium
cortic/o	cortex
endocrin/o	endocrine
gonad/o	sex glands
gluc/o; glyc/o	glucose; sugar; sweet
kal/i	potassium
lact/o	milk
natr/o	sodium
pancreat/o	pancreas
parathyroid/o	parathyroid glands
somat/o	body
toxic/o	poison
thym/o	thymus gland
thyr/o; thyroid/o	thyroid gland

EXERCISE 1

Write the meanings for the following word roots.

1. adrenal/o   _____
2. thym/o   _____
3. calc/i   _____
4. kal/i   _____
5. cortic/o   _____
6. pancreat/o   _____
7. somat/o   _____
8. natr/o   _____
9. andr/o   _____
10. lact/o   _____
11. toxic/o   _____
12. aden/o   _____
13. thyr/o   _____

EXERCISE 2

Write the root and meaning on the spaces provided.

1. hypoglycemia

   ROOT: _____ MEANING: _____

2. adrenalectomy

   ROOT: _____ MEANING: _____

3. hypercalcemia

   ROOT: _____ MEANING: _____

4. toxicology

   ROOT: _____ MEANING: _____

5. adrenocortical

   ROOT: _____ MEANING: _____

6. cortisol

   ROOT: _____ MEANING: _____

7. acromegaly

   ROOT: _____ MEANING: _____

8. hyperkalemia

   ROOT: _____ MEANING: _____

9. pancreatitis

   ROOT: _____ MEANING: _____

EXERCISE 3

Write the correct word root(s) for the following definitions.

1. body _____
2. thymus gland _____
3. gland _____
4. sex glands _____
5. parathyroid glands _____
6. thyroid gland _____
7. sweet _____
8. adrenal glands _____
9. calcium _____
10. poisons _____
11. pancreas _____

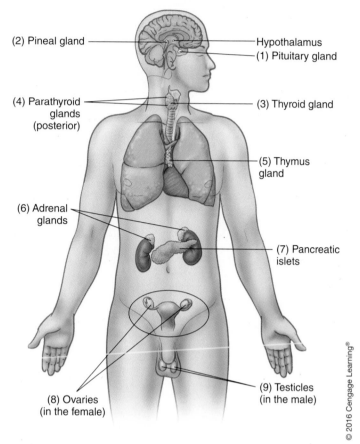

Figure 11-1 Endocrine system glands.

© 2016 Cengage Learning®

Structures of the Endocrine System

The major structures of the endocrine system include the (1) **pituitary gland**, (2) **pineal gland**, (3) **thyroid gland**, (4) **parathyroid glands**, (5) **thymus**, (6) **adrenal glands**, (7) **pancreas**, (8) **ovaries**, and (9) **testes**. The endocrine system structures are located throughout the body. Figure 11-1 illustrates the location of these structures.

Pituitary Gland

The pituitary gland, often called the *master gland*, is a pea-sized structure located at the base of the brain. Figure 11-2 illustrates the pituitary gland and the organs or structures targeted by pituitary gland hormones.

The pituitary gland has two lobes, (1) **anterior** and (2) **posterior**, that secrete specific hormones. Table 11-2 identifies the hormones of the anterior and posterior lobes of the pituitary gland. The function and targeted organs or structures are included in Table 11-2.

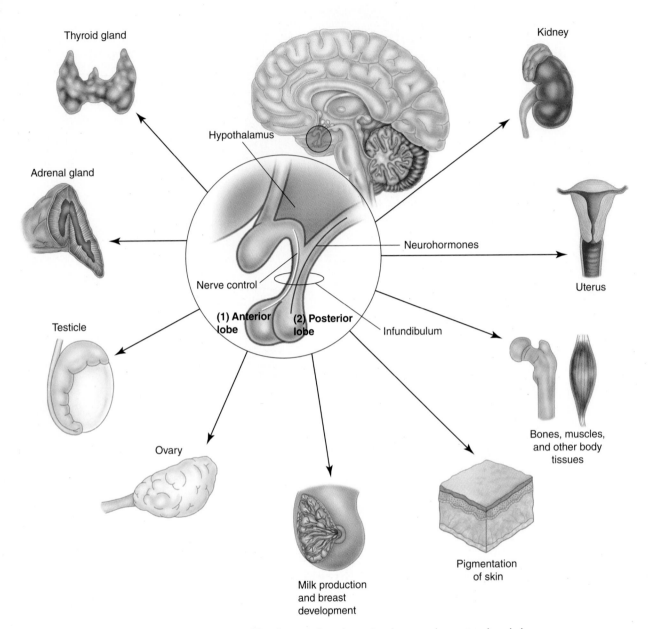

Thyroid gland

Kidney

Hypothalamus

Adrenal gland

Neurohormones

Nerve control

Uterus

Testicle

(1) Anterior lobe

(2) Posterior lobe

Infundibulum

Ovary

Bones, muscles, and other body tissues

Milk production and breast development

Pigmentation of skin

Figure 11-2   Pituitary gland, anterior and posterior lobes, and target organs.

TABLE 11-2   PITUITARY GLAND HORMONES

Anterior Lobe Hormones	Function
adrenocorticotropic hormone (ACTH)	stimulates the adrenal cortex
follicle-stimulating hormone (FSH)	stimulates estrogen secretion, ovum production, and sperm production
growth hormone (GH), or somatotropic hormone (STH)	regulates the growth of body tissues (i.e., muscles and bones)
lactogenic hormone, or prolactin	stimulates breast development and milk production
luteinizing hormone (LH)	stimulates ovulation and testosterone production
melanocyte-stimulating hormone (MSH)	controls the pigmentation of skin cells
thyroid-stimulating hormone (TSH)	stimulates the thyroid gland
Posterior Lobe Hormones	**Function**
antidiuretic hormone (ADH) or vasopressin	regulates urine secretion
oxytocin	stimulates uterine contractions and release of breast milk

© 2016 Cengage Learning®

Pituitary gland hormones affect nearly all body functions.

Pineal Gland

The pineal gland is a pinecone-shaped gland located in the midbrain. The pineal gland secretes **melatonin** (mell-ah-**TOH**-nin), a hormone that seems to have a role in promoting sleep. Figure 11-1 illustrates the location of the pineal gland. Although the precise function of the pineal gland is not clearly understood, evidence suggests that this gland helps regulate our biological clock.

Thyroid Gland and Parathyroid Glands

The thyroid gland is located in the neck and attached to the trachea. The thyroid gland has two lobes, one on either side of the trachea, that are connected by a strip of tissue called the *isthmus*. The parathyroid glands are four round bodies of tissue on the back of the thyroid gland, two on each thyroid lobe. Figure 11-3 illustrates the (1) **thyroid gland** and the (2) **parathyroid glands**.

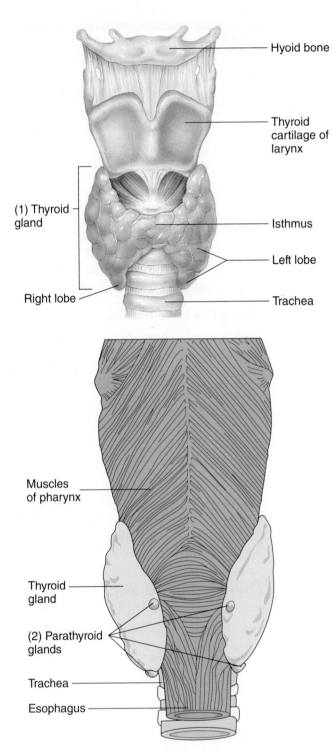

Figure 11-3 Thyroid and parathyroid glands.

Thyroid gland hormones include **triiodothyronine** (try-**eye**-oh-doh-**THIGH**-roh-neen) (**T**$_3$), **thyroxine** (thigh-**ROCKS**-in) (**T**$_4$), and **calcitonin** (**kal**-sih-**TOH**-nin). T$_3$ and T$_4$ regulate growth and control body temperature and metabolism. Calcitonin helps regulate the amount of calcium in the blood. The parathyroid glands secrete **parathyroid hormone (PTH)**. This hormone, in partnership with calcitonin, regulates the amount of calcium in the blood.

Thymus Gland

The thymus gland is located in the middle of the pleural cavity. It is large in infants and shrinks as the body ages. The thymus gland is primarily responsible for the development of the immune system. Figure 11-4 illustrates the location of this important gland.

Thymus gland hormones include **thymosin** (thigh-**MOH**-sin) and **thymopoietin** (**thigh**-moh-**POY**-eh-tin), which stimulate the production of T cells. T cells are specialized lymphocytes and are part of the immune system.

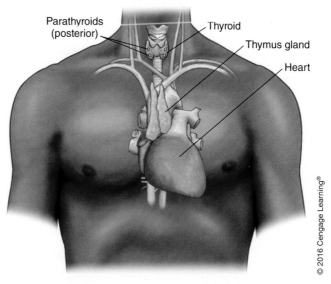

Parathyroids (posterior)
Thyroid
Thymus gland
Heart

© 2016 Cengage Learning®

Figure 11-4   Thymus gland.

Adrenal Glands

The (1) **adrenal glands** are two small glands that sit on top of each kidney. The adrenal gland consists of two parts: the (2) **adrenal cortex** (outer part) and the (3) **adrenal medulla** (inner part). Figure 11-5 illustrates the location and sections of the adrenal glands.

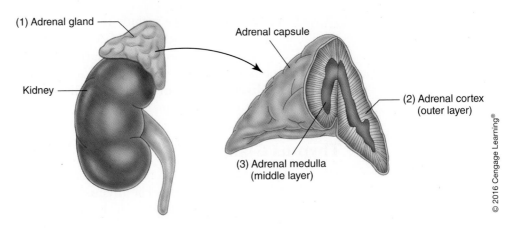

Figure 11-5 Adrenal gland.

Each part of the adrenal gland secretes different hormones. Table 11-3 lists and describes the adrenal gland hormones. The adrenal cortex hormones are classified as steroid hormones, and the adrenal medulla hormones are classified as nonsteroid hormones.

TABLE 11-3 ADRENAL GLAND HORMONES

Steroid Hormones of the Adrenal Cortex

Mineralocorticoids: regulate the fluid and electrolyte balance in the body	**Aldosterone** is the primary mineralocorticoid of the adrenal cortex.
Glucocorticoids: influence the metabolism of carbohydrates, fats, and proteins; maintain normal blood pressure; have an anti-inflammatory effect during times of stress	**Cortisol**, also called **hydrocortisone**, is the primary glucocorticoid of the adrenal cortex.
Gonadocorticoids: sex hormones that contribute to the secondary sex characteristics in males and females	**Androgen** is one of the gonadocorticoid hormones secreted by the adrenal cortex.

Nonsteroid Hormones of the Adrenal Medulla

Epinephrine or **adrenaline**: increases heart rate; dilates the bronchioles; raises blood glucose levels	This hormone plays an important role in the body's response to stress by increasing the availability of oxygen and glucose in the blood.
Norepinephrine or **noradrenaline**: causes the blood vessels to constrict and thereby raises the blood pressure	This hormone also plays an important role in the body's response to stress by raising the individual's blood pressure.

Pancreas

The pancreas is a gland that is located in the upper-left quadrant of the abdomen, under the stomach. Figure 11-6 illustrates the pancreas.

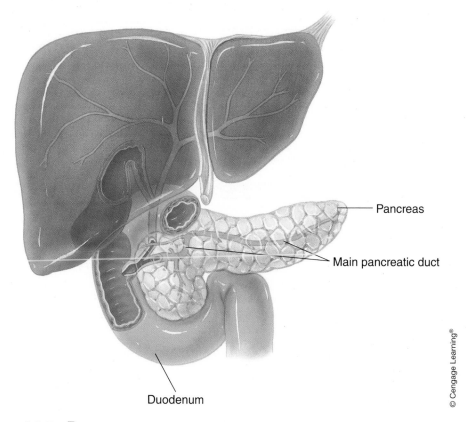

Pancreas

Main pancreatic duct

Duodenum

Figure 11-6   Pancreas.

Specialized pancreatic cells called the **islets** (**EYE**-lets) **of Langerhans** (**LONG**-er-honz) produce **insulin** and **glucagon** (**GLOO**-kah-gon), the pancreatic hormones. Insulin is responsible for decreasing the amount of glucose in the blood. Glucagon is responsible for increasing the amount of glucose in the blood.

Ovaries and Testes

The ovaries are female sex glands or gonads. There are two ovaries, one on each side of the pelvic cavity. The ovaries produce the hormones **estrogen** (**ESS**-troh-jen) and **progesterone** (proh-**JESS**-ter-ohn). Estrogen promotes the maturation of the ovum (egg) and prepares the uterus for implantation of a fertilized ovum. Estrogen is necessary for the development of female secondary sex characteristics. Progesterone also helps prepare the uterus for implantation and is responsible for the growth and development of the placenta.

Testes are the male sex organs, or gonads, and are contained in the scrotum. The testes produce **testosterone** (tess-**TOSS**-ter-ohn), the hormone responsible for the maturation of sperm and the development of male secondary sex characteristics. A complete discussion of the functions of the ovaries and testes is presented in Chapters 12 and 13.

EXERCISE 4

Match the endocrine gland in Column 1 with the correct definition in Column 2.

COLUMN 1

_____ 1. thyroid gland

_____ 2. pancreas

_____ 3. testes

_____ 4. parathyroid glands

_____ 5. pituitary gland

_____ 6. adrenal glands

_____ 7. thymus

_____ 8. ovaries

COLUMN 2

a. produce male hormones

b. primarily functions during childhood

c. produces insulin

d. secrete adrenaline

e. produce female hormones

f. four round bodies

g. secretes T_3 and T_4

h. the master gland

EXERCISE 5

Label the structures of the endocrine system identified in Figure 11-7. Write your answer on the spaces provided.

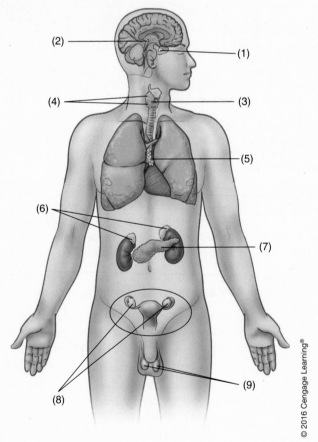

© 2016 Cengage Learning®

Figure 11-7 Labeling exercise.

1. _____
2. _____
3. _____
4. _____
5. _____
6. _____
7. _____
8. _____
9. _____

EXERCISE 6

Match the hormone in Column 1 with the endocrine gland in Column 2. Note that some endocrine glands will be used more than once.

COLUMN 1

_____ 1. adrenocorticotropic hormone

_____ 2. androgen

_____ 3. antidiuretic hormone

_____ 4. calcitonin

_____ 5. cortisol

_____ 6. epinephrine

_____ 7. estrogen

_____ 8. glucagon

_____ 9. growth hormone

_____ 10. insulin

_____ 11. testosterone

_____ 12. PTH

_____ 13. T_3, T_4

_____ 14. thymopoietin

_____ 15. thyroid-stimulating hormone

COLUMN 2

a. adrenal cortex

b. adrenal medulla

c. anterior lobe of the pituitary gland

d. ovaries

e. pancreas

f. parathyroid glands

g. posterior lobe of the pituitary gland

h. testes

i. thymus gland

j. thyroid gland

Endocrine System Medical Terminology

Endocrine system medical terms are organized into three main categories: (1) general medical terms; (2) disease and condition terms; and (3) diagnostic procedure, surgery, and laboratory test terms. The roots, prefixes, and suffixes associated with endocrine system terms are listed in Table 11-4. Review these word parts and complete the related exercises.

TABLE 11-4   ROOTS, PREFIXES, AND SUFFIXES FOR ENDOCRINE
SYSTEM TERMS

Root	Meaning	Prefix	Meaning	Suffix	Meaning
acid/o	sour; bitter	eu-	same; normal	-crine	secrete
dips/o	thirst	ex-	out; outward	-dipsia	thirst
				-ectomy	surgical removal
ket/o	ketone bodies	oxy-	sharp; quick	-emia	blood condition
ophthalm/o	eye	poly-	excessive	-tropin	stimulating effect of a hormone

© 2016 Cengage Learning®

EXERCISE 7

Write the root, prefix, suffix, and their meanings on the spaces provided.

1. endocrine

   ROOT: _____ MEANING: _____

   PREFIX: _____ MEANING: _____

   SUFFIX: _____ MEANING: _____

2. polydipsia

   ROOT: _____ MEANING: _____

   PREFIX: _____ MEANING: _____

   SUFFIX: _____ MEANING: _____

3. somatotropin

   ROOT: _____ MEANING: _____

   PREFIX: _____ MEANING: _____

   SUFFIX: _____ MEANING: _____

4. acromegaly

   ROOT: _____ MEANING: _____

   PREFIX: _____ MEANING: _____

   SUFFIX: _____ MEANING: _____

5. thyrotoxicosis

   ROOT: _____ MEANING: _____

   PREFIX: _____ MEANING: _____

   SUFFIX: _____ MEANING: _____

6. hypoglycemia

   ROOT: _____ MEANING: _____

   PREFIX: _____ MEANING: _____

   SUFFIX: _____ MEANING: _____

EXERCISE 8

Based on the meaning of the word parts, write a definition for each term.

1. euthyroid _____

2. adrenomegaly _____

3. polydipsia _____

4. hyperglycemia _____

5. somatotropin _____

6. pancreatitis _____

7. thyroidectomy _____

Endocrine System General Medical Terms

Review the pronunciation and meaning of each term in Table 11-5. Note that some terms are built from word parts and some are not. Complete the exercises for these terms.

TABLE 11-5   ENDOCRINE SYSTEM GENERAL MEDICAL TERMS

Term with Pronunciation	Definition
cortical (**KOR**-tih-kal)	pertaining to the cortex
corticoid (**KOR**-tih-koyd)	pertaining to the hormones of the adrenal cortex
endocrinologist (**en**-doh-krin-**ALL**-oh-jist) endocrin/o = endocrine -(o)logist = specialist	physician who specializes in the diseases and disorders of the endocrine system
endocrinology (**en**-doh-krin-**ALL**-oh-jee) endocrin/o = endocrine -(o)logy = study of	study and treatment of endocrine system diseases and disorders
euthyroid (**YOO**-thigh-royd) eu- = normal	normal thyroid function
hormone (**HOR**-mohn)	chemical substance that affects the function of a specific organ or body tissue
isthmus (**ISS**-mus)	a narrow structure connecting two parts
metabolism (meh-**TAB**-oh-lizm)	the sum of all the chemical changes that take place in the body

EXERCISE 9

Write the medical term for each definition.

1. chemical that affects the function of a specific body structure or organ _____

2. narrow structure that connects two parts _____

3. normal thyroid function _____

4. pertaining to the cortex _____

5. pertaining to the hormones of the adrenal cortex _____

6. physician who specializes in the endocrine system _____

7. study and treatment of endocrine system diseases and disorders _____

8. sum of all chemical changes in the body _____

Endocrine System Disease and Disorder Terms

Endocrine system diseases and disorders include familiar problems such as diabetes as well as more complex and less familiar diagnoses such as virilism. The medical terms are presented in alphabetical order in Table 11-6. Review the pronunciation and definition for each term and complete the exercises.

TABLE 11-6   ENDOCRINE SYSTEM DISEASE AND DISORDER TERMS

Term with Pronunciation	Definition
acidosis (ass-ih-**DOH**-sis) acid/o = sour; bitter -osis = condition	excessive acidity of body fluids
acromegaly (ak-roh-**MEG**-ah-lee) acr/o = extremities -megaly = enlargement	enlargement of the bones of the extremities and face
Addison's disease (**AD**-ih-sons)	deficiency in the secretion of adrenal cortex hormones
adrenalitis (ah-**dree**-nah-**LIGH**-tis) adren/o = adrenal gland -itis = inflammation	inflammation of the adrenal gland
adrenomegaly (ah-**dree**-no-**MEG**-ah-lee) adren/o = adrenal gland -megaly = enlargement	enlargement of the adrenal gland

(continues)

TABLE 11-6   ENDOCRINE SYSTEM DISEASE AND DISORDER TERMS
(continued)

Term with Pronunciation	Definition
cretinism (**KREE**-tin-izm)	congenital condition related to the lack of thyroid hormone secretion
Cushing's syndrome (**CUSH**-ings **SIN**-drohm)	hypersecretion of adrenal cortex glucocorticoids
diabetes insipidus (**digh**-ah-**BEE**-teez in-**SIP**-ih-dus)	disorder of the pituitary gland due to a deficiency in the secretion of antidiuretic hormone (ADH)
diabetes mellitus (**digh**-ah-**BEE**-teez **MELL**-ih-tus)	disorder of carbohydrate metabolism due to insufficient insulin secretion; diabetes mellitus can be insulin-dependent (IDDM), which means the individual must inject insulin to control blood glucose levels, or non-insulin-dependent (NIDDM); in NIDDM blood glucose may be controlled by diet and exercise or may also require diabetes medications or insulin therapy
dwarfism	congenital condition characterized by abnormal underdevelopment due to a deficiency of human growth hormone
exophthalmia (**eks**-off-**THAL**-me-ah) ex- = outward ophthalm/o = eye -ia = condition	abnormal outward protrusion of the eyeball; also called *exophthalmos*
gigantism (**JIGH**-gan-tism)	excessive size and height caused by excessive secretion of growth hormone
goiter (**GOY**-ter)	hyperplasia of the thyroid gland due to a lack of dietary iodine; iodine is necessary for the production of thyroid hormones T_3 and T_4
Graves' disease	hyperthyroidism characterized by excessive secretion of thyroid hormone and exophthalmia
Hashimoto's thyroiditis (**HASH**-ee-moh-toz **thigh**-royd-**EYE**-tis) thyr/o = thyroid gland -itis = inflammation	an autoimmune disease in which the immune system produces antibodies that target thyroid cells; often results in hypothyroidism
hirsutism (**HER**-soot-izm)	excessive body hair, especially on a female in a male distribution pattern

EXERCISE 10

Analyze each term by writing the prefix, root, combining vowel, and suffix separated by vertical slashes. Based on the meaning of the word parts, write a definition for each term. Check the definition in your medical dictionary.

EXAMPLE: *endocrinologist:*

	/endocrin	/o	/logist
prefix	*root*	*combining vowel*	*suffix*

DEFINITION: physician who specializes in the endocrine system

1. acromegaly

prefix	*root*	*combining vowel*	*suffix*

DEFINITION: _____

2. acidosis

prefix	*root*	*combining vowel*	*suffix*

DEFINITION: _____

3. adrenalitis

prefix	*root*	*combining vowel*	*suffix*

DEFINITION: _____

4. adrenomegaly

prefix	*root*	*combining vowel*	*suffix*

DEFINITION: _____

5. exophthalmia

prefix	*root*	*combining vowel*	*suffix*

DEFINITION: _____

EXERCISE 11

Replace the italicized medical term with its definition.

1. Gina was recently diagnosed with *diabetes mellitus*.

   _____

2. Maintaining iodine in the diet prevents the development of a *goiter*.

   _____

3. Roberta's *hirsutism* was corrected after she began hormone replacement therapy.

   _____

4. *Cretinism* is usually accompanied by arrested physical and mental development.

   _____

5. *Cushing's syndrome* is usually caused by an adrenal tumor.

_____

6. Adrenal gland hemorrhage might result in *Addison's disease*.

_____

EXERCISE 12

Match the medical term in Column 1 with the correct definition in Column 2.

COLUMN 1

_____ 1. acidosis
_____ 2. acromegaly
_____ 3. Addison's disease
_____ 4. adrenomegaly
_____ 5. diabetes insipidus
_____ 6. diabetes mellitus
_____ 7. exophthalmos
_____ 8. gigantism
_____ 9. goiter
_____ 10. Graves' disease

COLUMN 2

a. abnormal eyeball protrusion
b. deficient secretion of adrenal cortex hormones
c. disorder of the pituitary gland
d. excessive acidity of body fluids
e. enlarged thyroid gland
f. enlarged adrenal gland
g. excessive size and height
h. enlargement of the extremities
i. hyperthyroidism with exophthalmia
j. insufficient insulin secretion

Review the pronunciation and definition for each term in Table 11-7 and complete the exercises.

TABLE 11-7   ENDOCRINE SYSTEM DISEASE AND DISORDER TERMS

Term with Pronunciation	Definition
hypercalcemia (**high**-per-kal-**SEE**-mee-ah) hyper- = excessive calc/o = calcium -emia = blood condition	excessive amount of calcium in the blood
hyperglycemia (**high**-per-gligh-**SEE**-mee-ah) hyper- = excessive glyc/o = glucose; sugar; sweet -emia = blood condition	excessive amount of glucose in the blood
hyperkalemia (**high**-per-kal-**EE**-mee-ah) hyper- = excessive kal/i = potassium -emia = blood condition	excessive amount of potassium in the blood

(continues)

TABLE 11-7 ENDOCRINE SYSTEM DISEASE AND DISORDER TERMS
(continued)

Term with Pronunciation	Definition
hyperthyroidism (**high**-per-**THIGH**-royd-izm) hyper- = excessive thyroid/o = thyroid gland -ism = condition	overactivity of the thyroid gland
hypocalcemia (**high**-poh-kal-**SEE**-mee-ah) hypo- = decreased calc/o = calcium -emia = blood condition	decreased amount of calcium in the blood
hypoglycemia (**high**-poh-gligh-**SEE**-mee-ah) hypo- = decreased glyc/o = glucose; sugar; sweet -emia = blood condition	decreased amount of glucose in the blood
hypokalemia (**high**-poh-kal-**EE**-mee-ah) hypo- = decreased kal/i = potassium -emia = blood condition	decreased amount of potassium in the blood
hyponatremia (**high**-poh-nah-**TREE**-mee-ah) hypo- = decreased natr/o = sodium -emia = blood condition	decreased amount of sodium in the blood
hypothyroidism (**high**-poh-**THIGH**-royd-izm) hypo- = decreased thyroid/o = thyroid gland -ism = condition	decreased activity of the thyroid gland
ketoacidosis (**kee**-toh-**ass**-ih-**DOH**-sis) ket/o = ketone bodies acid/o = sour; bitter -osis = condition	an accumulation of toxic acids called ketones (or ketone bodies) in the blood, accompanied by increased acidity of the blood; often seen as a complication of diabetes
myxedema (miks-eh-**DEE**-mah)	the most severe form of adult hypothyroidism
pancreatitis (**pan**-kree-ah-**TIGH**-tis) pancreat/o = pancreas -itis = inflammation	inflammation of the pancreas

(continues)

TABLE 11-7   ENDOCRINE SYSTEM DISEASE AND DISORDER TERMS
(continued)

Term with Pronunciation	Definition
polydipsia (pall-ee-**DIP**-see-ah) poly- = excessive dips/o = thirst -ia = condition	excessive thirst
thyroiditis (**thigh**-royd-**EYE**-tis) thyr/o = thyroid gland -itis = inflammation	chronic inflammation and enlargement of the thyroid gland
thyrotoxicosis (**thigh**-roh-toks-ih-**KOH**-sis) thyr/o = thyroid toxic/o = poison -osis = condition	toxic condition caused by hyperactivity of the thyroid gland
virilism (**VEER**-il-izm)	development of masculine physical traits in a female

© 2016 Cengage Learning®

EXERCISE 13

Analyze each term by the prefix, root, combining vowel, and suffix separated by vertical slashes. Based on the meaning of the word parts, write a definition for each term. Check the definition in a medical dictionary.

1. hypercalcemia

prefix	*root*	*combining vowel*	*suffix*

DEFINITION: _____

2. hyperglycemia

prefix	*root*	*combining vowel*	*suffix*

DEFINITION: _____

3. hyperkalemia

prefix	*root*	*combining vowel*	*suffix*

DEFINITION: _____

4. hyperthyroidism

prefix	*root*	*combining vowel*	*suffix*

DEFINITION: _____

5. hypocalcemia

prefix	*root*	*combining vowel*	*suffix*

DEFINITION: _____

6. hypoglycemia

_____

| prefix | root | combining vowel | suffix |

DEFINITION: _____

7. hypokalemia

_____

| prefix | root | combining vowel | suffix |

DEFINITION: _____

8. hyponatremia

_____

| prefix | root | combining vowel | suffix |

DEFINITION: _____

9. hypothyroidism

_____

| prefix | root | combining vowel | suffix |

DEFINITION: _____

10. pancreatitis

_____

| prefix | root | combining vowel | suffix |

DEFINITION: _____

11. polydipsia

_____

| prefix | root | combining vowel | suffix |

DEFINITION: _____

12. thyrotoxicosis

_____

| prefix | root | combining vowel | suffix |

DEFINITION: _____

EXERCISE 14

Replace the italicized phrase with the correct medical term.

1. Uncontrolled diabetes mellitus might result in _an accumulation of ketone bodies and increased acidity in the blood._

   _____

2. _The most severe form of adult hypothyroidism_ is a life-threatening endocrine disease.

   _____

3. Lack of female hormones might contribute to *the development of masculine traits in a female.*

_____

4. *Excessive thirst* is a symptom of diabetes mellitus.

_____

5. A *decreased amount of potassium in the blood* has serious implications for heart function.

_____

6. Insufficient insulin secretion leads to *excessive amounts of glucose in the blood.*

_____

7. *Inflammation of the pancreas* might interfere with adequate hormone secretion.

_____

8. Weight control is an issue for individuals who have *decreased activity of the thyroid gland.*

_____

Endocrine System Diagnostic, Laboratory, and Treatment Terms

Review the pronunciation and definition of the diagnostic, laboratory, and treatment terms in Table 11-8 and complete the exercise.

TABLE 11-8   ENDOCRINE SYSTEM DIAGNOSTIC, LABORATORY, AND TREATMENT TERMS

Laboratory/Diagnostic Tests	Definition
fasting blood sugar (FBS)	blood test that measures the amount of glucose in the blood; screening test for diabetes mellitus
glucose tolerance test (GTT)	blood test that measures blood glucose levels over a period of time, usually 2 to 3 hours
hemoglobin A1c (HgA1c)	blood test that evaluates and measures blood glucose levels for the preceding two or three months; used to monitor blood glucose control in individuals with diabetes
radioactive iodine uptake (RAIU)	thyroid function test that measures thyroid activity by determining the amount of radioactive iodine taken up by the thyroid gland
thyroid function tests	blood tests that measure the blood levels of the thyroid hormones T_3 and T_4
thyroid scan	nuclear medicine imaging scan to determine the size, shape, and function of the thyroid gland

(continues)

TABLE 11-8 ENDOCRINE SYSTEM DIAGNOSTIC, LABORATORY, AND TREATMENT TERMS (continued)

Laboratory/Diagnostic Tests	Definition
thyroid-stimulating hormone test	blood test that measures the concentration of thyroid-stimulating hormone in the blood
adrenalectomy (ah-**dreen**-al-**EK**-toh-mee) adrenal/o = adrenal gland -ectomy = surgical removal	surgical removal of one or both of the adrenal glands
parathyroidectomy (**pair**-ah-**thigh**-royd-**EK**-toh-mee) parathyroid/o = parathyroid gland -ectomy = surgical removal	surgical removal of one or all of the parathyroid glands
thyroidectomy (**thigh**-royd-**EK**-toh-mee) thyroid/o = thyroid gland -ectomy = surgical removal	surgical removal of all or part of the thyroid

© 2016 Cengage Learning®

EXERCISE 15

Match the diagnostic and treatment terms in Column 1 with the definitions in Column 2.

COLUMN 1

_____ 1. adrenalectomy

_____ 2. fasting blood sugar

_____ 3. glucose tolerance test

_____ 4. parathyroidectomy

_____ 5. radioactive iodine uptake

_____ 6. thyroid function tests

_____ 7. thyroid scan

_____ 8. thyroid-stimulating hormone test

_____ 9. thyroidectomy

COLUMN 2

a. excision of all or part of the thyroid gland

b. measures blood levels of thyroid-stimulating hormone

c. measures the level of T_3 and T_4 in the blood

d. screening test for diabetes mellitus

e. removal of one or both of the adrenal glands

f. nuclear medicine imaging scan of the thyroid

g. measures blood glucose levels over a period of time

h. surgical removal of one or all of the parathyroid glands

i. measures thyroid activity using iodine

Abbreviations

Review the endocrine system abbreviations in Table 11-9. Practice writing out the meaning of each abbreviation.

TABLE 11-9 ABBREVIATIONS

Abbreviation	Meaning
ACTH	adrenocorticotropic hormone
ADH	antidiuretic hormone
FBS	fasting blood sugar
FSH	follicle-stimulating hormone
GH	growth hormone
GTT	glucose tolerance test
IDDM	insulin-dependent diabetes mellitus
LH	luteinizing hormone
MSH	melanocyte-stimulating hormone
NIDDM	non-insulin-dependent diabetes mellitus
PTH	parathyroid hormone
RAIU	radioactive iodine uptake test
STH	somatotropin hormone
T_3	triiodothyronine
T_4	thyroxine
TSH	thyroid-stimulating hormone

© 2016 Cengage Learning®

CHAPTER REVIEW

The Chapter Review can be used as a self-test. Go through each exercise and answer as many questions as you can without referring to previous exercises or earlier discussions within this chapter. Check your answers and fill in any blanks. Practice writing any terms you might have misspelled.

EXERCISE 16

Write the medical term for each definition.

1. excessive acidity of body fluids _____

2. enlargement of the bones of the extremities and face _____

3. inflammation of the adrenal gland _____

4. enlargement of the adrenal gland _____

5. abnormal outward protrusion of the eyeball _____

6. overactivity of the thyroid gland _____

7. increased glucose in the blood _____

8. most severe form of adult hypothyroidism _____

9. inflammation of the pancreas _____

10. excessive thirst _____

11. toxic condition due to hyperactivity of the thyroid gland _____

12. development of masculine physical traits in a female _____

13. male-pattern hair distribution in a female _____

14. surgical removal of the thyroid gland _____

15. enlarged thyroid gland due to hypertrophy of thyroid cells and tissue _____

EXERCISE 17

Write the names of the following hormones next to the endocrine gland that secretes the hormone.

ACTH	cortisol	insulin	PTH
androgen	epinephrine	noradrenaline	testosterone
aldosterone	FSH	oxytocin	T_3, T_4
antidiuretic hormone	glucagon	prolactin	TSH
calcitonin	growth hormone	progesterone	thymopoietin

1. pituitary gland _____

2. thyroid gland _____

3. parathyroid glands _____

4. thymus _____

5. pancreas _____

6. adrenal glands _____

7. ovaries _____

8. testes _____

EXERCISE 18

Read the following progress notes. For progress notes A and B, define each italicized term in the space provided; for progress note C, write the medical term for the italicized phrase.

PROGRESS NOTE A

Viola was seen today for a (1) *glucose tolerance test.* Her (2) *fasting blood sugar,* which was done two days ago, indicated hyperglycemia, which might indicate diabetes mellitus. The results of the GTT will confirm or rule out that diagnosis.

1. _____

2. _____

PROGRESS NOTE B

Gerald has recent complaints of fatigue, lack of energy, and weight gain. His initial (3) *thyroid function test* showed a decreased level of T_3 and T_4. A follow-up (4) *thyroid-stimulating hormone test* ruled out pituitary malfunction. A (5) *thyroid scan* is scheduled for tomorrow.

3. _____

4. _____

5. _____

PROGRESS NOTE C

Alonzo is seen today for a complete evaluation of endocrine gland function. He is very concerned because his family history is positive for the following: Paternal grandfather underwent (6) *the surgical removal of adrenal glands* at age 54; his mother had a (7) *surgical removal of the thyroid gland* at age 45; and his father, age 62, recently was treated for hyperparathyroidism with (8) *a surgical removal of the parathyroid glands.*

6. _____

7. _____

8. _____

EXERCISE 19

Write out the following endocrine system abbreviations.

1. FBS _____

2. ADH _____

3. GTT _____

4. IDDM _____

5. NIDDM _____

6. FSH _____

7. TSH _____

8. GH _____

9. MSH _____

10. LH _____

EXERCISE 20

Select the best answer for each statement or question.

1. Which endocrine gland has two lobes that secrete different hormones?
   a. parathyroid gland
   b. thyroid gland
   c. pineal gland
   d. pituitary gland

2. Select the hormone that is responsible for stimulating the release of breast milk.
   a. oxytocin
   b. luteinizing hormone
   c. prolactin
   d. follicle-stimulating hormone

3. Choose the hormone that stimulates breast development and milk production.
    a. oxytocin
    b. prolactin
    c. luteinizing hormone
    d. follicle-stimulating hormone

4. Which term means development of masculine physical traits in a female?
    a. hirsutism
    b. testosteronism
    c. virilism
    d. myxedema

5. Select the disease associated with insufficient insulin secretion.
    a. diabetes insipidus
    b. diabetes mellitus
    c. pancreatitis
    d. acromegaly

6. Which term means excessive body hair on a female in a male pattern?
    a. virilism
    b. acromegaly
    c. testosteronism
    d. hirsutism

7. Select the term for an enlarged thyroid gland.
    a. goiter
    b. Graves' disease
    c. exophthalmia
    d. thyroidosis

8. Which disease is caused by an insufficient secretion of ADH?
    a. diabetes mellitus
    b. Graves' disease
    c. acromegaly
    d. diabetes insipidus

9. Select the blood test that is a screening test for diabetes mellitus.
    a. glucose tolerance test
    b. fasting blood sugar
    c. insulin secretion test
    d. pancreatic hormone screening test

10. Which term is defined as the most severe form of adult hypothyroidism?
    a. cretinism
    b. Cushing's syndrome
    c. myxedema
    d. acromegaly

CHALLENGE EXERCISE

Diabetes mellitus is a serious health problem that can affect many organs in the body, especially the eyes and kidneys. Research how this disease affects one of these organ pairs. Information should be available from the local public health department, the local hospital's patient education department, or the American Diabetic Association's website. If you search the Internet, keywords are diabetes mellitus *or* American Diabetes Association.

Pronunciation Review

Review the terms in this chapter. Pronounce each term using the following phonetic pronunciations. Check off the term when you are comfortable saying it.

TERM	PRONUNCIATION
☐ acidosis	ass-ih-**DOH**-sis
☐ acromegaly	ak-roh-**MEG**-ah-lee
☐ Addison's disease	**AD**-ih-sons disease
☐ adrenalectomy	ah-**dree**-nal-**EK**-toh-mee
☐ adrenal gland	ah-**DREE**-nal gland
☐ adrenalitis	ah-**dree**-nah-**LIGH**-tis
☐ adrenomegaly	ah-**dree**-noh-**MEG**-ah-lee
☐ calcitonin	**kal**-sih-**TOH**-nin
☐ cortical	**KOR**-tih-kal
☐ cretinism	**KREE**-tin-izm
☐ Cushing's syndrome	**CUSH**-ings **SIN**-drohm
☐ diabetes insipidus	**digh**-ah-**BEE**-teez in-**SIP**-ih-dus
☐ diabetes mellitus	**digh**-ah-**BEE**-teez **MELL**-ih-tus
☐ dwarfism	**DWARF**-ism
☐ endocrinologist	**en**-doh-krin-**ALL**-oh-jist
☐ endocrinology	**en**-doh-krin-**ALL**-oh-jee
☐ estrogen	**ESS**-troh-jen
☐ euthyroid	**YOO**-thigh-royd
☐ exophthalmia	**eks**-off-**THAL**-mee-ah
☐ exophthalmos	**eks**-off-**THAL**-mohs
☐ gigantism	**JIGH**-gan-tizm
☐ glucagon	**GLOO**-kah-gon
☐ glucose tolerance test (GTT)	**GLOO**-kohs **TALL**-er-ans test
☐ goiter	**GOY**-ter
☐ Hashimoto's thyroiditis	**HASH**-ee-moh-toz **thigh**-royd-**EYE**-tis
☐ hirsutism	**HER**-soot-izm
☐ hormone	**HOR**-mohn
☐ hypercalcemia	**high**-per-kal-**SEE**-mee-ah
☐ hyperglycemia	**high**-per-gligh-**SEE**-mee-ah
☐ hyperkalemia	**high**-per-kal-**EE**-mee-ah
☐ hyperthyroidism	**high**-per-**THIGH**-royd-izm
☐ hypocalcemia	**high**-poh-kal-**SEE**-mee-ah
☐ hypoglycemia	**high**-poh-gligh-**SEE**-mee-ah
☐ hypokalemia	**high**-poh-kal-**EE**-mee-ah

TERM	**PRONUNCIATION**
☐ hyponatremia	**high**-poh-nah-**TREE**-mee-ah
☐ hypothyroidism	**high**-poh-**THIGH**-royd-izm
☐ insulin	**IN**-suh-lin
☐ islets of Langerhans	**EYE**-lets of **LONG**-er-honz
☐ isthmus	**ISS**-mus
☐ ketoacidosis	**kee**-toh-ass-ih-**DOH**-sis
☐ melatonin	mell-ah-**TOH**-nin
☐ metabolism	meh-**TAB**-oh-lizm
☐ myxedema	miks-eh-**DEE**-mah
☐ ovaries	**OH**-vah-reez
☐ pancreas	**PAN**-kree-as
☐ pancreatitis	pan-kree-ah-**TIGH**-tis
☐ parathyroidectomy	**pair**-ah-**thigh**-royd-**EK**-toh-me
☐ parathyroid gland	**pair**-ah-**THIGH**-royd gland
☐ parathyroid hormone	**pair**-ah-**THIGH**-royd **HOR**-mohn
☐ pineal gland	**PIN**-ee-al gland
☐ pituitary gland	pih-**TOO**-ih-tair-ee gland
☐ polydipsia	pall-ee-**DIP**-see-ah
☐ progesterone	proh-**JESS**-ter-ohn
☐ testes	**TESS**-teez
☐ testosterone	tess-**TOSS**-ter-ohn
☐ thymopoietin	**thigh**-moh-**POY**-eh-tin
☐ thymosin	thigh-**MOH**-sin
☐ thymus	**THIGH**-mus
☐ thyroidectomy	**thigh**-royd-**EK**-toh-mee
☐ thyroiditis	**thigh**-royd-**EYE**-tis
☐ thyrotoxicosis	**thigh**-roh-toks-ih-**KOH**-sis
☐ thyroxine (T4)	thigh-**ROKS**-in
☐ triiodothyronine	try-**eye**-oh-doh-**THIGH**-roh-neen
☐ virilism	**VEER**-il-izm

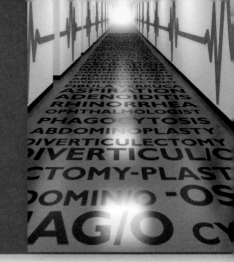

OBJECTIVES

At the completion of this chapter, the student should be able to:

1. Identify, define, and spell word roots associated with the male reproductive system.
2. Label the basic structures of the male reproductive system.
3. Discuss the functions of the male reproductive system.
4. Provide the correct spelling of male reproductive system terms, given the definition of the terms.
5. Analyze the male reproductive system terms by defining the roots, prefixes, and suffixes of these terms.
6. Identify, define, and spell disease, disorder, and procedure terms related to the male reproductive system.
7. Describe the characteristics of sexually transmitted infections.

OVERVIEW

The structures of the male reproductive system include the testes, epididymis, vas deferens, seminal vesicle, ejaculatory duct, prostate gland, Cowper's gland, urethra, and penis. These structures function to produce male hormones and to produce, sustain, and transport **spermatozoa** (sper-**mat**-oh-**ZOH**-ah), usually called *sperm*. The reproductive structures are collectively known as the male **genitalia** (jen-ih-**TAY**-lee-ah).

This chapter also covers sexually transmitted infections and diseases. Information includes the characteristics, lesions, and symptoms associated with the infections.

Male Reproductive System Word Roots

To understand and use male reproductive system medical terms, it is necessary to acquire a thorough knowledge of the associated word roots. Word roots associated with the male reproductive system are listed with the combining vowel. Review the word roots in Table 12-1 and complete the exercises that follow.

TABLE 12-1 MALE REPRODUCTIVE SYSTEM WORD ROOTS

Word Root/Combining Form	Meaning
andr/o	male
balan/o	glans penis
hydr/o	water

(continues)

TABLE 12-1   MALE REPRODUCTIVE SYSTEM WORD ROOTS (continued)

Word Root/Combining Form	Meaning
orch/o; orchi/o; orchid/o	testis; testicle
prostat/o	prostate gland
semin/i	semen
sperm/o; spermat/o	sperm; spermatic cord
test/o; testicul/o	testes; testis; testicle
vas/o	vessel

© 2016 Cengage Learning®

EXERCISE 1

Write the definitions of the following word roots.

1. spermat/o   _____

2. orchid/o   _____

3. prostat/o   _____

4. vas/o   _____

5. test/o   _____

6. crypt/o   _____

7. orch/o   _____

8. epididym/o   _____

9. semin/i   _____

10. andr/o   _____

11. hydr/o   _____

EXERCISE 2

Write the word root and its meaning on the spaces provided.

1. hydrocele

    ROOT: _____   MEANING: _____

2. vasectomy

    ROOT: _____   MEANING: _____

3. android

    ROOT: _____   MEANING: _____

4. prostatectomy

    ROOT: _____   MEANING: _____

5. epididymitis

    ROOT: _____   MEANING: _____

6. balanitis

ROOT: _____   MEANING: _____

7. cryptorchidism

ROOT: _____   MEANING: _____

8. seminal vesicles

ROOT: _____   MEANING: _____

9. orchidectomy

ROOT: _____   MEANING: _____

EXERCISE 3

Write the correct word root(s) for the following definitions.

1. testicle   _____

2. epididymis   _____

3. male   _____

4. hidden   _____

5. prostate gland   _____

6. semen   _____

7. vessel   _____

8. sperm   _____

Structures of the Male Reproductive System

The male reproductive system is made up of the (1) **testes** (**TESS**-teez) (pl.), (2) **scrotum** (**SKROH**-tum), (3) **epididymis** (ep-ih-**DID**-ih-miss), (4) **vas deferens** (**VAZ DEFF**-er-enz), (5) **seminal vesicle** (**SEM**-ih-nall **VESS**-ih-kal), (6) **ejaculatory** (ee-**JACK**-yoo-lah-**tor**-ee) **duct**, (7) **prostate** (**PROSS**-tayt) **gland**, (8) **Cowper's** (**COW**-perz) **glands**, (9) **urethra**, and (10) **penis**. Figure 12-1 illustrates the structures of the male reproductive system in a lateral cross-section view. The structures of this system are discussed individually. Figure 12-2 shows some of the structures in an anterior cross-section view.

Testes, Epididymis, and Vas Deferens

The (1) testes, also called *testicles*, are the male gonads, or sex organs. They develop in the abdominal cavity and eventually descend into the scrotum, the sac that houses the testes. Figure 12-3 illustrates a testis and related structures. Refer to this figure as you learn about the testes.

The (1) testes are composed of tiny, coiled tubules called (2) **seminiferous tubules** (sem-ih-**NIFF**-er-us **TOO**-byools), which are responsible for sperm production. The tissue between the tubules secretes the male sex hormone testosterone.

The (3) epididymis, which is a continuation of the seminiferous tubules, is a tightly coiled tube on the testes. Sperm mature and become motile (i.e., able to

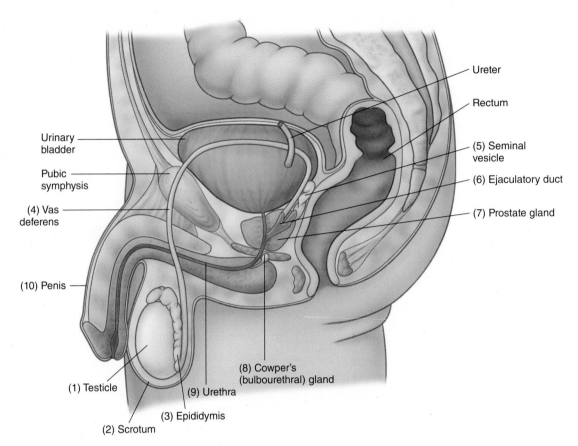

Figure 12-1 Male reproductive system.

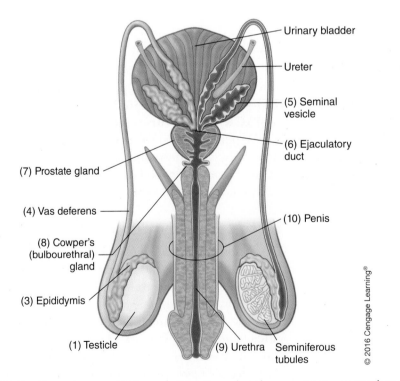

Figure 12-2 Structures of the male reproductive system, anterior cross-section view.

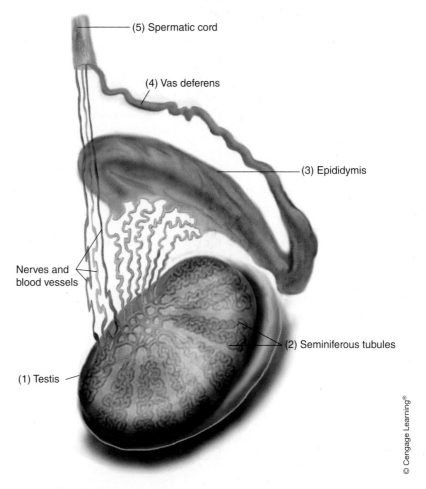

(5) Spermatic cord

(4) Vas deferens

(3) Epididymis

Nerves and
blood vessels

(2) Seminiferous tubules

(1) Testis

© Cengage Learning®

Figure 12-3   Testis (testes, pl.).

move) in the epididymis. The (4) vas deferens, which is a continuation of the epididy-mis, leaves the scrotum, passes around the urinary bladder, and eventually connects with the urethra. Refer to Figure 12-1 for an illustration of the entire vas deferens.

Each testicle is suspended by a (5) **spermatic cord** that contains blood and lymph vessels, nerves, and the vas deferens.

Seminal Vesicles, Ejaculatory Duct, and Cowper's Gland

Refer to Figures 12-1 and 12-2 for an illustration of the seminal vesicles, ejaculatory duct, and Cowper's glands. The (5) seminal vesicles, two glands located behind the urinary bladder, open into the vas deferens and secrete a thick fluid called seminal fluid. Seminal fluid is part of the **semen**, which is the substance discharged from the penis.

The seminal vesicles narrow into a straight duct that joins with the vas deferens to form the (6) ejaculatory duct. The ejaculatory duct passes through the (7) prostate gland and joins with the urethra.

The (8) Cowper's glands, also called the **bulbourethral** (**bull**-boh-yoo-**REE**-thrall) **glands**, are a pair of glands that lie just below the prostate gland. The Cowper's glands secrete a mucus like fluid into the urethra. The fluid, which is a component of semen, provides lubrication during intercourse.

Prostate Gland

The (7) prostate gland lies at the base of the bladder and surrounds the urethra. Refer to Figures 12-1 and 12-2 for an illustration of the prostate gland. The prostate gland secretes a milky-colored fluid that enhances sperm motility and helps neutralize vaginal secretions. Prostate fluid is added to the semen via ducts that open into the urethra. During ejaculation, the muscular action of the prostate gland helps propel semen through the urethra into the vagina.

Penis

The (10) penis consists of a base that attaches the penis to the pubic region, a shaft or body that becomes engorged with blood during arousal, and a tip or head called the (11) **glans penis**. Refer to Figures 12-1 and 12-2 for an illustration of the penis. A retractable fold of skin called the **prepuce** (**PREE**-pus), or foreskin, covers the glans penis. The prepuce may be removed by a procedure known as **circumcision**.

EXERCISE 4

Label the structures of the male reproductive system as shown in Figure 12-4. Write your answer in the spaces provided.

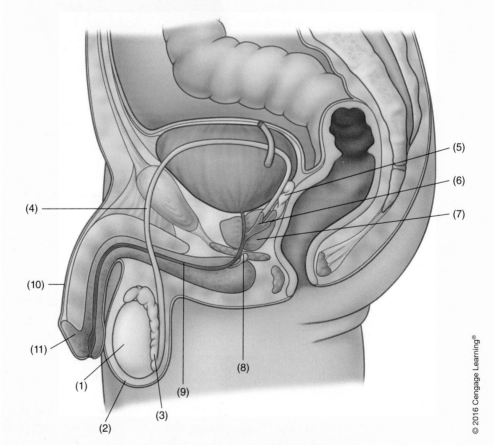

© 2016 Cengage Learning®

Figure 12-4 Male reproductive system labeling exercise.

1. _____
2. _____
3. _____
4. _____
5. _____
6. _____
7. _____
8. _____
9. _____
10. _____
11. _____

EXERCISE 5

Match the male reproductive system structures in Column 1 with the correct definition in Column 2.

COLUMN 1

_____ 1. Cowper's glands

_____ 2. epididymis

_____ 3. glans penis

_____ 4. penis

_____ 5. prepuce

_____ 6. prostate gland

_____ 7. scrotum

_____ 8. seminal vesicle

_____ 9. sperm

_____ 10. testes

_____ 11. vas deferens

COLUMN 2

a. assists in the ejaculation of semen

b. continuation of the epididymis

c. fold of retractable skin; foreskin

d. gonads; male sex glands

e. male sex cell

f. male sex organ

g. provides lubrication during intercourse

h. secretes seminal fluid

i. sac containing the testicles

j. tightly coiled tubules; sperm mature here

k. tip of the penis

Male Reproductive System Medical Terminology

Male reproductive system medical terms are organized into three main categories: (1) general medical terms; (2) disease and condition terms; and (3) diagnostic procedure, surgery, and laboratory test terms. The word roots *olig/o*, which means "few" or "diminished," and *varic/o*, which means "twisted veins," are used in a few male reproductive system medical terms. The roots, prefixes, and suffixes associated with the male reproductive system are listed in Table 12-2. Review these word parts and complete the related exercises.

TABLE 12-2   ROOTS, PREFIXES, AND SUFFIXES FOR MALE REPRODUCTIVE SYSTEM

Root	Meaning	Prefix	Meaning	Suffix	Meaning
cry/o	cold	a-	lack of; without	-cele	hernia; protrusion
olig/o	few; diminished	carcin-	cancer; malignant	-genesis	Producing
				-oma	tumor
varic/o	twisted veins	epi-	upon; on	-pexy	surgical fixation
		hypo-	beneath; below	-plasty	surgical repair
				-(r)rhea	flow; discharge
				-trophy	growth; development

EXERCISE 6

Each term has either a prefix, suffix, or both. Write the prefix and suffix and its meaning on the spaces provided.

1. aspermia

   PREFIX: _____ MEANING: _____

   SUFFIX: _____ MEANING: _____

2. hypertrophy

   PREFIX: _____ MEANING: _____

   SUFFIX: _____ MEANING: _____

3. epispadias

   PREFIX: _____ MEANING: _____

   SUFFIX: _____ MEANING: _____

4. gonorrhea

   PREFIX: _____ MEANING: _____

   SUFFIX: _____ MEANING: _____

5. spermatocele

   PREFIX: _____ MEANING: _____

   SUFFIX: _____ MEANING: _____

6. spermatogenesis

   PREFIX: _____ MEANING: _____

   SUFFIX: _____ MEANING: _____

7. orchidopexy

   PREFIX: _____ MEANING: _____

   SUFFIX: _____ MEANING: _____

8. orchidoplasty

PREFIX: _____   MEANING: _____

SUFFIX: _____   MEANING: _____

Male Reproductive System General Medical Terms

Review the pronunciation and meaning of each term in Table 12-3. Complete the exercise for these terms.

TABLE 12-3   MALE REPRODUCTIVE SYSTEM GENERAL MEDICAL TERMS

Term with Pronunciation	Definition
ejaculation (ee-**jack**-yoo-**LAY**-shun)	expulsion of semen from the penis
genitalia (jen-ih-**TAY**-lee-ah)	male and female reproductive structures
sexually transmitted disease (STD) sexually transmitted infection (STI)	any disease that is spread from one person to another during any type of sexual contact; STD refers to the actual disease; STI may be used to indicate that an individual is infected with an organism, but does not exhibit symptoms of the disease; STD and STI are often used interchangeably
spermatogenesis (**sperm**-at-oh-**JEN**-eh-sis) spermat/o = sperm -genesis = formation	formation of mature sperm
testosterone (tess-**TOSS**-ter-ohn)	male hormone
urologist (yoor-**ALL**-oh-jist) ur/o = urine -(o)logist = specialist	physician who specializes in the study of the male reproductive and urinary systems

© 2016 Cengage Learning®

EXERCISE 7

Replace the italicized phrase with the correct medical term.

1. Chlamydia is classified as a *disease acquired as a result of sexual intercourse.*

_____

2. Sperm are deposited in the vagina when *the expulsion of semen* occurs.

_____

3. *The male hormone* is necessary for the development of male secondary sex characteristics.

_____

4. After experiencing testicular pain, Roger made an appointment with a *physician specialist for the male reproductive system.*

_____

5. Healthy *formation of mature sperm* is a necessary component of male fertility.

_____

6. The *male reproductive structures* include both internal and external organs and glands.

_____

Male Reproductive System Disease and Disorder Terms

Male reproductive system diseases and disorders include familiar problems such as prostate cancer as well as more complex and less familiar diagnoses such as priapism. Medical terms related specifically to the male reproductive system are discussed first. Sexually transmitted infections, which affect both male and female reproductive structures, are discussed second. In both cases, the terms are presented in alphabetical order in Table 12-4. Review the pronunciation and definition for each term and complete the exercises.

TABLE 12-4   MALE REPRODUCTIVE SYSTEM DISEASE AND DISORDER TERMS

Term with Pronunciation	Definition
anorchism (an-**ORK**-izm) an- = without orch/i = testes -ism = condition	absence of one or both testes
aspermia (ah-**SPERM**-ee-ah) a- = lack of; without sperm/o = sperm -ia = condition	lack or absence of sperm
balanitis (bal-ah-**NIGH**-tis) balan/o = glans penis -itis = inflammation	inflammation of the glans penis

(continues)

TABLE 12-4 MALE REPRODUCTIVE SYSTEM DISEASE AND
DISORDER TERMS (continued)

Term with Pronunciation	Definition
benign prostatic hypertrophy (BPH) (bee-**NIGHN** pross-**TAT**-ik high-**PER**-troh-fee) prostat/o = prostate -ic = pertaining to hyper- = excessive -trophy = growth; development	noncancerous enlargement of the prostate gland
cryptorchidism (kript-**OR**-kid-izm) crypt/o = hidden orchid/o = testes -ism = condition	undescended testicle; failure of one or both testes to descend into the scrotum
epididymitis (**ep**-ih-**did**-ih-**MIGH**-tis) epididym/o = epididymis -itis = inflammation	inflammation of the epididymis
epispadias (**ep**-ih-**SPAY**-dee-as)	congenital condition in which the urethra opens on the upper side of the penis (Figure 12-5)

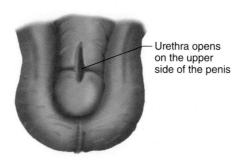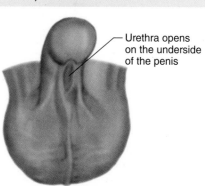

Urethra opens on the upper side of the penis

Urethra opens on the underside of the penis

© Cengage Learning®

Figure 12-5 Epispadias and hypospadias.

erectile dysfunction	inability to achieve or maintain an erection; impotence
hydrocele (**HIGH**-droh-seel) hydr/o = water -cele = hernia; protrusion	accumulation of fluid in the scrotum or along the spermatic cord
hypospadias (**high**-poh-**SPAY**-dee-as)	congenital condition in which the urethra opens on the underside of the penis (Figure 12-5)

(continues)

TABLE 12-4 MALE REPRODUCTIVE SYSTEM DISEASE AND
DISORDER TERMS (continued)

Term with Pronunciation	Definition
impotence (**IM**-poh-tens)	inability to achieve or maintain an erection; erectile dysfunction (ED)
indirect inguinal hernia (**ING**-gwih-nal **HER**-nee-ah)	protrusion of the intestine through the internal inguinal ring, possibly descending into the scrotum
oligospermia (**all**-ih-goh-**SPER**-mee-ah) olig/o = few; deficient sperm/o = sperm -ia = condition	deficient number of sperm present in semen
orchitis (or-**KIGH**-tis) orch/i = testes -itis = inflammation	inflammation of the testes
phimosis (fih-**MOH**-sis)	tightness of the prepuce, or foreskin, that prevents it from being pulled back from the glans penis
premature ejaculation	expulsion of semen before complete erection or immediately after vaginal penetration
priapism	abnormal, painful, and prolonged erection of the penis not related to sexual arousal
prostate cancer	malignant tumor or neoplasm of the prostate gland
prostatitis (**pross**-tah-**TIGH**-tis) prostat/o = prostate gland -itis = inflammation	inflammation of the prostate gland
spermatolysis (sper-mah-**TALL**-ih-sis) spermat/o = sperm -lysis = destruction; break down	destruction, dissolution, or break down of sperm
testicular carcinoma (tess-**TICK**-yoo-lar **kar**-sin-**OH**-ma) testicul/o = testes; testicles -ar = pertaining to carcin- = cancer; malignant -oma = tumor	malignant tumor of one or both testes

(continues)

**TABLE 12-4   MALE REPRODUCTIVE SYSTEM DISEASE AND
DISORDER TERMS** (continued)

Term with Pronunciation	Definition
varicocele (**VAIR**-ih-koh-seel) varic/o = enlarged; twisted veins -cele = hernia; protrusion	enlarged, twisted, and swollen veins of the spermatic cord

EXERCISE 8

Analyze each term by writing the prefix, root, combining vowel, and suffix separated by vertical slashes. Based on the meaning of the word parts, write a definition for each term. Check the definition in a medical dictionary. Note that some terms may have more than one root.

EXAMPLE: urologist

	/ ur	/ o	/ logist
prefix	*root*	*combining vowel*	*suffix*

DEFINITION: specialist in the male reproductive and urinary system

1. anorchism

prefix	*root*	*combining vowel*	*suffix*

DEFINITION: _____

2. aspermia

prefix	*root*	*combining vowel*	*suffix*

DEFINITION: _____

3. balanitis

prefix	*root*	*combining vowel*	*suffix*

DEFINITION: _____

4. cryptorchidism

prefix	*root*	*combining vowel*	*suffix*

DEFINITION: _____

5. epididymitis

prefix	*root*	*combining vowel*	*suffix*

DEFINITION: _____

6. hydrocele

prefix	*root*	*combining vowel*	*suffix*

DEFINITION: _____

7. oligospermia

_____
prefix   _root_   _combining vowel_   _suffix_

DEFINITION: _____

8. orchitis

_____
prefix   _root_   _combining vowel_   _suffix_

DEFINITION: _____

9. prostatitis

_____
prefix   _root_   _combining vowel_   _suffix_

DEFINITION: _____

10. spermatolysis

_____
prefix   _root_   _combining vowel_   _suffix_

DEFINITION: _____

EXERCISE 9

Replace the italicized phrase with the correct medical term.

1. Calhoun's diagnosis was _noncancerous enlargement of the prostate gland._

   _____

2. _Urethral opening on the underside of the penis_ is a congenital condition that may require surgery.

   _____

3. The _inability to achieve or maintain an erection_ may be caused by a physical or psychological condition.

   _____

4. Baby boy Smith was born with _a urethral opening on the upper side of the penis._

   _____

5. A _protrusion of the intestine through the internal inguinal ring_ can be corrected with surgery.

   _____

6. _Tightness of the foreskin_ prevents proper cleansing of the penis.

   _____

7. Ziad sought treatment for _abnormal, painful, and prolonged erection of the penis._

   _____

8. Surgical intervention or radiation may be used to treat *a malignant tumor of one or both testes.*

_____

9. *Enlargement of the veins of the spermatic cord* may lead to male infertility.

_____

Match the medical terms in Column 1 with the descriptions in Column 2.

COLUMN 1

_____ 1. BPH

_____ 2. epispadias

_____ 3. hydrocele

_____ 4. hypospadias

_____ 5. impotence

_____ 6. phimosis

_____ 7. priapism

_____ 8. prostate cancer

_____ 9. spermatolysis

_____ 10. varicocele

COLUMN 2

a. abnormal, prolonged, and painful penile erection

b. accumulation of fluid in the scrotum or spermatic cord

c. congenital condition; urethra on the underside of the penis

d. destruction or breakdown of sperm

e. enlarged veins of the spermatic cord

f. erectile dysfunction

g. malignant tumor of the prostate

h. noncancerous tumor of the prostate

i. tightness of the prepuce, or foreskin

j. urethral opening on the upper side of the penis

Sexually Transmitted Infection Terms

Sexually transmitted infections (STIs) are usually named for the bacteria or virus that cause the infection. Review the pronunciation and description for each term in Table 12-5 and complete the exercises. Note that symptoms might not be present, especially during the early stages of the infection. Because STIs affect men and women, the figures in this section include male and female genitalia.

TABLE 12-5   SEXUALLY TRANSMITTED INFECTION TERMS

Term with Pronunciation	Definition
chancre (**SHANG**-ker)	highly contagious pustule or lesion located on the penis, characteristic of primary syphilis (Figure 12-6)

(continues)

TABLE 12-5   SEXUALLY TRANSMITTED INFECTION TERMS (continued)

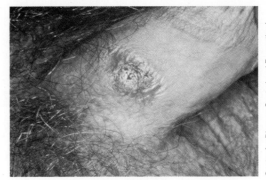

Figure 12-6   Chancre in primary syphilis.

Term with Pronunciation	Definition
chlamydia (klah-**MID**-ee-ah)	sexually transmitted infection caused by the bacteria *Chlamydia trachomatis*; symptoms are usually mild or absent and might include abnormal discharge from the penis or cervix, and a burning sensation during urination; bacteria can infect the urinary tract or cervix causing epididymitis in men and cervicitis in women (Figure 12-7)

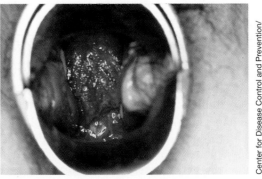

Figure 12-7   Chlamydia, cervix.

(continues)

TABLE 12-5   SEXUALLY TRANSMITTED INFECTION TERMS (continued)

Term with Pronunciation	Definition
genital herpes (**JEN**-ih-tal **HER**-peez)	sexually transmitted infection caused by herpes simplex virus (HSV), type 2; symptoms are called *outbreaks*, which appear two weeks after infection; outbreaks are characterized by small blisters in the genital area, penis, cervix, vagina, or in the urethra; blisters rupture, leaving an ulceration (sore) that heals without leaving a scar; genital herpes can recur spontaneously once the virus has been acquired; also called venereal herpes (Figure 12-8)

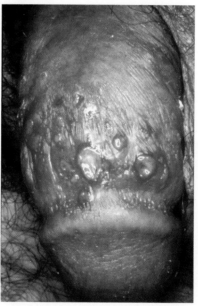

Center for Disease Control and Prevention/ Dr. N. J. Flumara, Dr. Gavin Hart

Figure 12-8   Genital herpes.

genital human papilloma virus (HPV)	the most common sexually transmitted infection (STI); includes more than 40 types of human papilloma virus that can infect the genital area; specific types of HPV cause different diseases, such as genital warts or cervical cancer

(continues)

TABLE 12-5   SEXUALLY TRANSMITTED INFECTION TERMS (continued)

Term with Pronunciation	Definition
genital warts (**JEN**-ih-tal)	sexually transmitted infection caused by the human papillomavirus (HPV), characterized by small, cauliflowerlike, fleshy growths usually seen along the penis and in or near the vagina or anus; also called venereal warts (Note: The HPV virus that causes genital warts is not the same virus associated with cervical cancer.) (Figure 12-9)

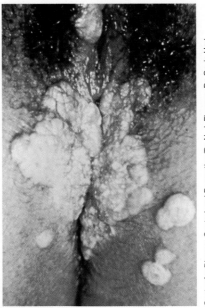

Center for Disease Control and Prevention/Dr. N. J. Flumara, Dr. Gavin Hart

Figure 12-9   Genital warts.

gonorrhea (gon-oh-**REE**-ah)	sexually transmitted infection caused by bacteria (*Neisseria gonorrhoeae*) that infect male and female genitalia; symptoms, which typically appear within 2 to 10 days after sexual contact with an infected individual, include yellow or bloody vaginal discharge; white, yellow, or green painful discharge from the penis; painful or burning sensations during urination; and swollen testicles; untreated, gonorrhea can lead to infection of the entire reproductive tract of both men and women

(continues)

TABLE 12-5   SEXUALLY TRANSMITTED INFECTION TERMS (continued)

Term with Pronunciation	Definition
sexually transmitted infection (STI)	an infection that is spread from one person to another during any type of sexual contact
syphilis (**SIFF**-ih-lis)	sexually transmitted disease that has three distinct stages, each more serious than the previous stage; lesions may involve any organ or tissue
trichomoniasis (**trik**-oh-moh-**NIGH**-ah-sis)	sexually transmitted infection caused by the protozoa *Trichomonas vaginalis*; men are usually asymptomatic, but might experience dysuria, urinary frequency, or urethritis; symptoms in women include itching, burning, and a strong-smelling, frothy, greenish-yellow vaginal discharge (Figure 12-10 shows the "strawberry cervix" that is associated with trichomoniasis.)

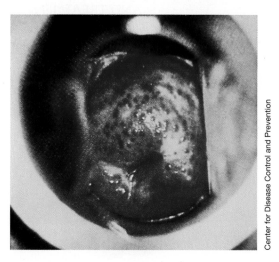

Center for Disease Control and Prevention

Figure 12-10   Trichomoniasis, strawberry cervix.

© 2016 Cengage Learning®

EXERCISE 11

Write the name of the sexually transmitted disease for each description.

1. cauliflowerlike, fleshy growths _____

2. bacterial infection of genital mucous membranes _____

3. caused by herpes simplex virus type 2 _____

4. parasitic infection of the genitourinary tract _____

5. disease with three distinct stages _____

EXERCISE 12

Rewrite the misspelled terms.

1. shancre
2. chlamydia
3. gonnorrhea
4. syphillis
5. trichomoniasis
6. venerial herpes

Male Reproductive System Surgical, Diagnostic and Treatment Terms

Review the pronunciation and definition of the diagnostic and treatment terms in Table 12-6 and complete the exercises.

TABLE 12-6   MALE REPRODUCTIVE SYSTEM SURGICAL, DIAGNOSTIC AND TREATMENT TERMS

Term with Pronunciation	Definition
circumcision (sir-kum-**SIH**-shun)	surgical removal of the foreskin (prepuce) of the penis (Figure 12-11)

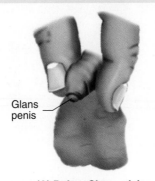

Glans penis

(A) Before Circumcision

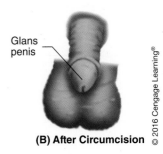

Glans penis

(B) After Circumcision

© 2016 Cengage Learning®

Figure 12-11   Circumcision.

| epididymectomy (**ep**-ih-**did**-ih-**MEK**-toh-mee) epididym/o = epididymis -ectomy = surgical removal | surgical removal of the epididymis |

(continues)

TABLE 12-6 MALE REPRODUCTIVE SYSTEM SURGICAL, DIAGNOSTIC
AND TREATMENT TERMS (continued)

Term with Pronunciation	Definition
orchidectomy (or-kid-**ECK**-toh-mee) orchid/o = testes -ectomy = surgical removal	surgical removal of one or both testes
orchidopexy; orchiopexy (**OR**-kid-oh-**pek**-see; **or**-kee-oh-**PEK**-see) orchid/o; orchi/o = testes -pexy = surgical fixation	surgical fixation of one or both testes
orchidoplasty; orchioplasty (**OR**-kid-oh-**plass**-tee; **OR**-kee-oh-**plass**-tee) orchid/o; orchi/o = testes -plasty = surgical repair	surgical repair of one or both testes; placement of undescended testes into the scrotum
prostatectomy (**pross**-tah-**TEK**-toh-mee) prostat/o = prostate gland -ectomy = surgical removal	surgical removal of all or part of the prostate
prostatic acid phosphatase (PAP) (pross-**STAT**-ic acid **FOSS**-fah-tays) prostat/o = prostate gland -ic = pertaining to	laboratory test that measures the level of acid phosphatase, an enzyme present in prostate cells and in the blood; elevated levels indicate prostate cancer
prostate-specific antigen (PSA) (**PROSS**-tayt specific **AN**-tih-jen) prostat/o = prostate gland -ic = pertaining to	laboratory test that measures the blood levels of PSA, a protein produced by the prostate gland; elevated PSA levels indicate benign prostatic hypertrophy or prostate cancer; a screening test for prostate cancer
semen analysis	laboratory analysis of the physical and chemical components of semen
sterilization	any procedure that renders a male incapable of producing sperm or impregnating a woman

(continues)

TABLE 12-6   MALE REPRODUCTIVE SYSTEM SURGICAL, DIAGNOSTIC AND TREATMENT TERMS (continued)

Term with Pronunciation	Definition
suprapubic prostatectomy (**soo**-prah-**PYOO**-bic **pross**-tah-**TEK**-toh-mee) supra- = above pub/o = pubis, pubic bone -ic = pertaining to prostat/o = prostate gland -ectomy = surgical removal of	surgical removal of all or part of the prostate gland through an incision just above the pubic bone
transurethral resection of the prostate (TURP) (**tranz**-yoo-**REE**-thral) trans- = through urethr/o = urethra -al = pertaining to	surgical removal of all or part of the prostate gland by passing an instrument into and through the urethra (Figure 12–12)

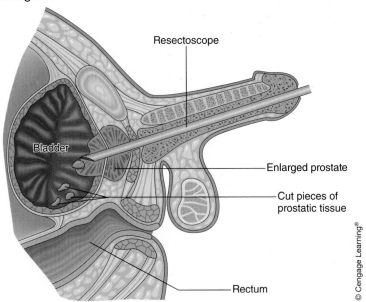

Resectoscope

Bladder

Enlarged prostate

Cut pieces of prostatic tissue

Rectum

© Cengage Learning®

Figure 12-12   Transurethral resection of the prostate.

varicocelectomy (**vair**-ih-koh-see-**LEK**-toh-mee) varic/o = twisted veins -cele = hernia; protrusion -ectomy = surgical removal	surgical removal of a varicocele by excision of a portion of the scrotum and tying off (ligation) of the enlarged, twisted veins

(continues)

TABLE 12-6   MALE REPRODUCTIVE SYSTEM SURGICAL, DIAGNOSTIC
AND TREATMENT TERMS (continued)

Term with Pronunciation	Definition
vasectomy (vas-**EK**-toh-mee) vas/o = vas deferens -ectomy = surgical removal	surgical removal of all or a portion of the vas deferens; male sterilization (Figure 12-13)

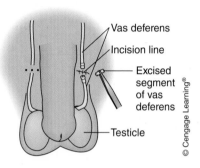

Figure 12-13   Vasectomy.

© 2016 Cengage Learning®

EXERCISE 13

Analyze each term by writing the prefix, root, combining vowel, and suffix separated by vertical slashes. Based on the meaning of the word parts, write a definition for each term. Check the definition in a medical dictionary. Note that some terms might have more than one root.

1. epididymectomy

prefix	*root*	*combining vowel*	*suffix*

    DEFINITION: _____

2. orchidectomy

prefix	*root*	*combining vowel*	*suffix*

    DEFINITION: _____

3. orchidopexy

prefix	*root*	*combining vowel*	*suffix*

    DEFINITION: _____

4. orchioplasty

prefix	*root*	*combining vowel*	*suffix*

    DEFINITION: _____

5. prostatectomy

prefix	root	combining vowel	suffix

DEFINITION: _____

6. suprapubic prostatectomy

prefix	root	combining vowel	suffix

prefix	root	combining vowel	suffix

DEFINITION: _____

7. varicocelectomy

prefix	root	combining vowel	suffix

DEFINITION: _____

EXERCISE 14

Replace the italicized phrase or abbreviation with the correct medical term.

1. Due to recurrent balanitis, Malcolm underwent *the removal of the foreskin.*

    _____

2. The *PAP test* is used to rule out prostate cancer.

    _____

3. The *PSA* laboratory blood test is a screening test for prostate cancer.

    _____

4. A *TURP* may result in an inability to achieve or sustain an erection.

    _____

5. *Surgical removal of all or part of the vas deferens* is a procedure for male sterilization.

    _____

Abbreviations

Review the male reproductive system abbreviations in Table 12-7. Practice writing out the meaning of each abbreviation.

TABLE 12-7 ABBREVIATIONS

Abbreviation	Meaning
BPH	benign prostatic hypertrophy
HPV	human papillomavirus
HSV	herpes simplex virus
PAP	prostatic acid phosphatase

(continues)

TABLE 12-7 ABBREVIATIONS (continued)

Abbreviation	Meaning
PSA	prostate specific antigen
STI	sexually transmitted infection
TURP	transurethral resection of the prostate

© 2016 Cengage Learning®

CHAPTER REVIEW

The Chapter Review can be used as a self-test. Go through each exercise and answer as many questions as you can without referring to previous exercises or earlier discussions within this chapter. Check your answers and fill in any blanks. Practice writing any terms you might have misspelled.

EXERCISE 15

Write the medical term for each definition.

1. expulsion of semen from the penis   _____

2. formation or development of mature sperm   _____

3. male hormone   _____

4. physician who specializes in the study
   of the male reproductive system   _____

5. lack or absence of sperm   _____

6. undescended testicle(s)   _____

7. inflammation of the epididymis   _____

8. few, diminished, or deficient number of
   sperm present in semen   _____

9. inflammation of the prostate gland   _____

10. destruction or breakdown of sperm   _____

11. enlargement of the veins of the spermatic cord   _____

12. removal of one or both of the testes   _____

13. surgical fixation of one or both of the testes   _____

14. surgical repair of one or both of the testes   _____

15. surgical removal of all or part
    of the prostate gland   _____

EXERCISE 16

Read the following operative report and write a brief definition for each italicized medical term.

OPERATIVE REPORT
PREOPERATIVE DIAGNOSIS: (1) *Cryptorchidism.*
POSTOPERTIVE DIAGNOSIS: Cryptorchidism.
OPERATION: (2) *Orchiopexy.*
HISTORY: This 4-year-old Native American male presented with undescended (3) *testes*, nonresponsive to hormone treatment. His parents have consented to surgical intervention and were advised of the risks and benefits of the procedure.
PROCEDURE: After adequate general anesthesia, the patient was prepped and draped in the usual manner. He was placed in the supine position, and an incision was made in the inguinal canal. The testes were freed with sharp dissection. The (4) *spermatic cord* was stripped, and the (5) *vas deferens* and spermatic vessels were left intact. The testes were placed away from the operative site. A channel for each (6) *testis* was created from the inguinal incision to the bottom of the (7) *scrotum.* Each testis was delivered through the respective channels, and the scrotal wound was closed. Sponge and needle counts were reported as correct, and the patient was returned to the recovery room in good condition.

1. _____

2. _____

3. _____

4. _____

5. _____

6. _____

7. _____

EXERCISE 17

Match the medical term in Column 1 with the description in Column 2.

COLUMN 1

_____ 1. balanitis

_____ 2. chancre

_____ 3. circumcision

_____ 4. genital warts

_____ 5. genitalia

_____ 6. impotence

_____ 7. phimosis

_____ 8. priapism

_____ 9. semen analysis

_____ 10. syphilis

COLUMN 2

a. abnormal, prolonged, painful erection

b. cauliflowerlike, fleshy growths along the penis

c. disease with three distinct stages

d. highly contagious pustule or lesion on the penis

e. identifies the components of semen

f. inflammation of the glans penis

g. inability to achieve or sustain an erection

h. male and female reproductive structures

i. parasitic sexually transmitted infection

j. removal of the prepuce

_____ 11. trichomoniasis   k. STI caused by herpes simplex virus type 2

_____ 12. venereal herpes   l. tightness of the foreskin

EXERCISE 18

Select the best answer to each statement or question.

1. Choose the term that means formation of mature sperm.
   a. spermatolysis
   b. spermatogenesis
   c. spermatosis
   d. spermatopoiesis

2. Which term means absence of one or both testes?
   a. aspermia
   b. anaorchidism
   c. anorchidism
   d. oligospermia

3. Select the term for urethral opening on the upper side of the penis.
   a. hypospadias
   b. perispadias
   c. hyperspadias
   d. epispadias

4. Choose the term for enlarged veins of the spermatic cord.
   a. varicocele
   b. spermatocele
   c. hydrocele
   d. inguinocele

5. Which term means surgical fixation of the testes?
   a. orchidoplasty
   b. orchidorrhaphy
   c. orchidopexy
   d. orchidodesis

6. Select the term for a procedure that results in male sterilization.
   a. epididymectomy
   b. prostatectomy
   c. orchidectomy
   d. vasectomy

7. Which term means undescended testicles?
   a. anorchism
   b. cryptorchidism
   c. orchidiasis
   d. orchiocele

8. Select the term for diminished number of sperm in the semen.
   a. oligospermia
   b. aspermia
   c. hypospermia
   d. spermatolysis

9. Which term means the placement of testes into the scrotum?
   a. orchidopexy
   b. orchidotomy
   c. orchidoplasty
   d. orchidectomy

10. Select the abbreviation that means a screening test for prostate cancer.
    a. PSA
    b. PAP
    c. TURP
    d. SPC

CHALLENGE EXERCISE

Human papillomavirus (HPV) is one of the most common sexually transmitted infections (STIs). Health experts believe there are more cases of genital HPV infection than any other STI in the United States. Approximately 5.5 million new cases of sexually transmitted HPV infections are reported every year. Search the Internet for information about HPV. Use the keywords human papillomavirus *or* HPV. *Prepare a handout that answers these questions: What is the difference between high-risk and low-risk HPV? What role does a PAP smear play in identifying HPV infections? How does HPV affect pregnancy and childbirth? How can HPV infection be prevented? (Note: The National Institute of Allergy and Infectious Diseases [NIAID], a division of the National Institutes of Health [NIH], maintains an excellent website at www. niaid.nih.gov.)*

Pronunciation Review

Review the terms in the chapter. Pronounce each term using the following phonetic pronunciations. Check off the term when you are comfortable saying it.

TERM	PRONUNCIATION
☐ anorchidism	an-**ORK**-id-izm
☐ anorchism	an-**ORK**-izm
☐ aspermia	ah-**SPERM**-ee-ah
☐ balanitis	bal-ah-**NIGH**-tis
☐ benign prostatic hypertrophy	bee-**NIGHN** pross-**TAT**-ik high-**PER**-troh-fee
☐ chancre	**SHANG**-ker
☐ chlamydia	klah-**MID**-ee-ah
☐ circumcision	sir-kom-**SIH**-shun
☐ Cowper's gland	**COW**-perz gland

☐ cryptorchidism — kript-**OR**-kid-izm
☐ ejaculation — ee-**jack**-yoo-**LAY**-shun
☐ ejaculatory duct — ee-**JACK**-yoo-lah-**tor**-ee duct
☐ epididymectomy — **ep**-ih-**did**-ih-**MEK**-toh-me
☐ epididymis — **ep**-ih-**DID**-ih-miss
☐ epididymitis — **ep**-ih-**did**-ih-**MIGH**-tis
☐ epispadias — **ep**-ih-**SPAY**-dee-as
☐ genital herpes — **JEN**-ih-tal **HER**-peez
☐ genital warts — **JEN**-ih-tal warts
☐ genitalia — jen-ih-**TAY**-lee-ah
☐ glans penis — **GLANZ** penis
☐ gonorrhea — gon-oh-**REE**-ah
☐ hydrocele — **HIGH**-droh-seel
☐ hypospadias — **high**-poh-**SPAY**-dee-as
☐ impotence — **IM**-poh-tens
☐ indirect inguinal hernia — indirect **ING**-gwih-nal **HER**-nee-ah
☐ oligospermia — **all**-ih-goh-**SPER**-mee-ah
☐ orchidectomy — or-kid-**ECK**-toh-mee
☐ orchidopexy — **OR**-kid-oh-**pek**-see
☐ orchioplasty — **OR**-kee-oh-**plass**-tee
☐ orchitis — or-**KIGH**-tis
☐ penis — **PEE**-nis
☐ phimosis — fih-**MOH**-sis
☐ prepuce — **PREE**-pus
☐ priapism — **PRIGH**-ah-pizm
☐ prostate cancer — **PROSS**-tayt cancer
☐ prostate gland — **PROSS**-tayt gland
☐ prostate-specific antigen — **PROSS**-tayt-specific **AN**-tih-jen
☐ prostatectomy — **pross**-tah-**TEK**-toh-mee
☐ prostatitis — **pross**-tah-**TIGH**-tis
☐ scrotum — **SKROH**-tum
☐ semen — **SEE**-men
☐ semen analysis — **SEE**-men analysis
☐ seminal vesicle — **SEM**-ih-nall **VESS**-ih-kal
☐ seminiferous tubules — sem-ih-**NIH**-fer-us **TOO**-byools

☐ spermatic cord — sper-**MAT**-ik cord
☐ spermatogenesis — **sperm**-at-oh-**JEN**-eh-sis
☐ spermatolysis — sper-mah-**TALL**-ih-sis
☐ spermatozoa — sper-**mat**-oh-**ZOH**-ah
☐ suprapubic prostatectomy — **soo**-prah-**PYOO**-bik **pross**-tah-**TEK**-toh-mee

☐ syphilis — **SIFF**-ih-lis
☐ testes — **TESS**-teez
☐ testicular carcinoma — tess-**TICK**-yoo-lar **kar**-sin-**OH**-ma
☐ testosterone — tess-**TOSS**-ter-ohn
☐ transurethral resection of the prostate — **tranz**-yoo-**REE**-thral resection of the prostate

☐ trichomoniasis   **trik**-oh-moh-**NIGH**-ah-sis
☐ urethra   yoo-**REE**-thrah
☐ urologist   yoor-**ALL**-oh-jist
☐ urology   yoor-**ALL**-oh-jee
☐ varicocele   **VAIR**-ih-koh-seel
☐ varicocelectomy   **vair**-ih-koh-see-**LEK**-toh-mee
☐ vas deferens   **VAZ DEFF**-er-enz
☐ vasectomy   vas-**EK**-toh-mee

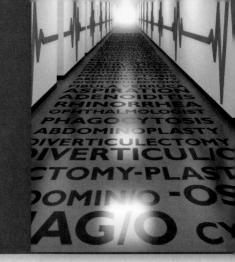

OBJECTIVES

At the completion of this chapter, the student should be able to:

1. Identify, define, and spell word roots associated with the female reproductive system and pregnancy.
2. Label the structures of the female reproductive system and structures relating to pregnancy.
3. Discuss the functions of the female reproductive system.
4. Provide the correct spelling of female reproductive system and pregnancy terms, given the definition of the terms.
5. Analyze female reproductive system and pregnancy terms by defining the roots, prefixes, and suffixes of these terms.
6. Identify, define, and spell disease, disorder, and procedure terms related to the female reproductive system and pregnancy.

OVERVIEW

The female reproductive system consists of external and internal genitalia (jen-ih-**TAY**-lee-ah). The internal genitalia function together to produce female hormones and provide an environment for the development and birth of a baby. The external genitalia function as a protective covering for internal female reproductive organs. General information about the female reproductive system is presented in the first section of this chapter. Specific information about the female reproductive system during pregnancy is presented in the second section of this chapter.

Female Reproductive System Word Roots

To understand and use female reproductive system medical terms, it is necessary to acquire a thorough knowledge of the associated word roots. The roots are listed with the combining vowel. Review the word roots in Table 13-1 and complete the exercises that follow.

TABLE 13-1   FEMALE REPRODUCTIVE SYSTEM WORD ROOTS

Word Root/Combining Form	Meaning
cervic/o	cervix
colp/o	vagina
epis/o	vulva
gyn/o; gynec/o	woman
hyster/o	uterus

(continues)

437

TABLE 13-1 FEMALE REPRODUCTIVE SYSTEM WORD ROOTS (continued)

Word Root/Combining Form	Meaning
mamm/o; mast/o	breast
men/o	menses; menstruation
metr/o; metr/i	uterus
oophor/o	ovary
ov/o	ovum; egg
ovari/o	ovary
salping/o	fallopian tubes; oviducts
uter/o	uterus
vagin/o	vagina
vulv/o	vulva

© 2016 Cengage Learning®

EXERCISE 1

Write the definitions of the following word roots.

1. uter/o _____
2. men/o _____
3. gynec/o _____
4. colp/o _____
5. cervic/o _____
6. mast/o _____
7. vagin/o _____
8. oophor/o _____
9. hyster/o _____
10. mamm/o _____

EXERCISE 2

Write the word root and its meaning.

1. dysmenorrhea

   ROOT: _____ MEANING: _____

2. mammography

   ROOT: _____ MEANING: _____

3. uterotomy

   ROOT: _____ MEANING: _____

4. oophoritis

   ROOT: _____ MEANING: _____

5. ovulation

ROOT: _____ MEANING: _____

6. hysterectomy

ROOT: _____ MEANING: _____

7. mastectomy

ROOT: _____ MEANING: _____

8. endometriosis

ROOT: _____ MEANING: _____

9. salpingitis

ROOT: _____ MEANING: _____

10. menarche

ROOT: _____ MEANING: _____

EXERCISE 3

Write the correct word root(s) for the following definitions.

1. woman _____

2. uterus _____

3. ovary _____

4. egg _____

5. cervix _____

6. menstruation _____

7. fallopian tubes _____

8. vulva _____

9. vagina _____

External Genitalia

The external genitalia includes the (1) **mons pubis** (**MONS PYOO**-bis), (2) **labia majora** (**LAY**-bee-ah mah-**JOR**-ah), (3) **clitoris** (**KLIT**-oh-ris), (4) **labia minora** (min-**OR**-ah), (5) **vaginal orifice**, (6) **hymen**, (7) **Bartholin's glands**, and (8) **perineum** (pair-ih-**NEE**-um). These structures, collectively called the *vulva*, are illustrated in Figure 13-1.

The mons pubis, which is covered with hair in adult women, is a pad of fatty tissue that covers the symphysis pubis. The labia majora are two folds of fatty tissue, one on each side of the vaginal opening. The labia minora are two thinner folds of tissue that are located within the labia majora.

The clitoris, located above the urethral orifice, is made of highly sensitive, erectile tissue. The urethral orifice is the external opening for the urethra. The vaginal orifice, which is surrounded by a thin layer of elastic connective tissue called the *hymen*, is the opening to the vagina. Bartholin's glands, located on each side of the vaginal opening, secrete a mucous substance that lubricates the vagina. The perineum is the area between the vaginal orifice and the anus.

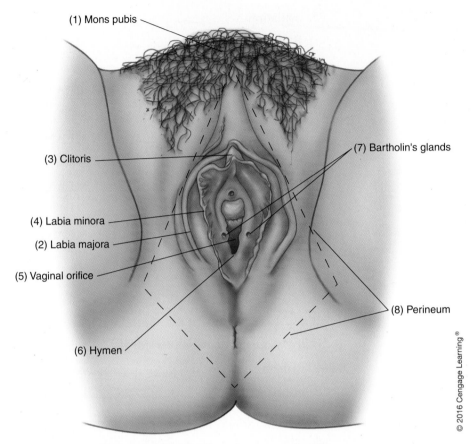

Figure 13-1 External genitalia, female reproductive system.

(1) Mons pubis

(3) Clitoris

(7) Bartholin's glands

(4) Labia minora

(2) Labia majora

(5) Vaginal orifice

(8) Perineum

(6) Hymen

© 2016 Cengage Learning®

Internal Genitalia

The internal genitalia of the female reproductive system include the (1) **vagina**, (2) **uterus**, (3) **fallopian tubes**, and (4) **ovaries**. These structures are illustrated in Figure 13-2. Refer to the figure as you learn about the structures.

Vagina

The vagina, commonly called the *birth canal*, is a muscular, elastic tube, about three inches long, that expands during childbirth. The vagina receives the penis during intercourse and is the outlet for the menstrual flow.

Uterus

The uterus is a hollow, pear-shaped, muscular organ commonly called the *womb*. It holds the fertilized ovum as it develops during pregnancy. The uterus has three distinct areas that are called the (5) **fundus**, the rounded upper section; the (6) **body**, the central section; and the (7) **cervix**, the lower end of the uterus. The walls of the uterus consist of the (8) **perimetrium** (pair-ih-**MEE**-tree-um), the outer layer; the (9) **myometrium** (my-oh-**MEE**-tree-um), the thick muscular layer; and the (10) **endometrium** (en-doh-**MEE**-tree-um), the inner layer or lining.

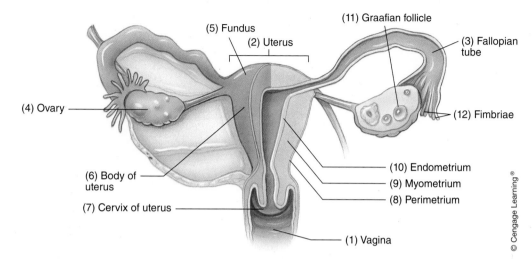

Figure 13-2   Internal genitalia, female reproductive system.

The endometrium thickens each month in preparation for implantation of a fertilized egg. When implantation does not occur, the endometrium is shed in a bloody discharge called **menses** (**MEN**-seez) or menstrual flow.

Ovaries and Fallopian Tubes

The ovaries are two small, almond-shaped organs located in the pelvic cavity on either side of the uterus. The fallopian tubes, also called *uterine tubes* and *oviducts*, are attached to the uterus and lie close to the ovaries. The ovaries and fallopian tubes are collectively known as the **adnexa** (add-**NECKS**-ah).

The ovaries are the female gonads and are responsible for producing mature **ovum**. Ova, commonly called *eggs*, are the female sex cells. Immature ova are stored in the microscopic sacs of the ovaries, called (11) **graafian follicles** (**GRAFF**-ee-an **FALL**-ih-kals). During the menstrual cycle, the ovum and graafian follicles mature. The graafian follicles move to the surface of the ovary and release the mature ovum. The release of a mature ovum is called **ovulation**.

The ovum is coaxed toward the (3) **fallopian tube** by the (12) **fimbriae** (**FIM**-bree-ay), fingerlike projections of the fallopian tubes that are very near the ovaries. The ovum travels through the fallopian tube and enters the uterus. If the ovum is not fertilized or does not implant in the endometrium, the ovum passes out of the body as part of the menstrual flow. The onset of menstruation is called **menarche** (men-**AR**-kee).

Mammary Glands

The mammary glands, or breasts, are responsible for the production of milk. This process is called **lactation** (lak-**TAY**-shun). Figure 13-3 illustrates the basic parts of the breast. Refer to this figure as you learn about the mammary glands.

Each breast consists of a (1) **nipple** that is surrounded by a pigmented area called the (2) **areola** (air-ee-**OH**-lah). Areolar pigmentation can range from

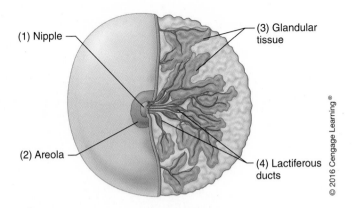

Figure 13-3 Structures of the breast.

pink-flesh tones to a dark brown. The main internal structures of the breasts include the (3) **glandular tissue** and the (4) **lactiferous** (lak-**TIFF**-er-us) **ducts**. The glandular tissue produces milk that moves through the lactiferous ducts to the nipple.

EXERCISE 4

Write the name of the female reproductive system structures illustrated in Figure 13-4. Write your answer on the spaces provided.

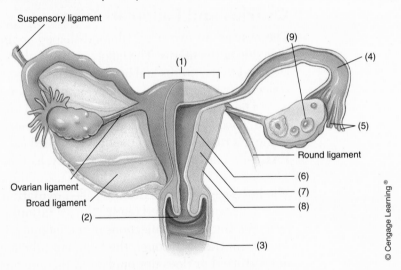

Figure 13-4 Labeling exercise.

1. _____

2. _____

3. _____

4. _____

5. _____

6. _____

7. _____

8. _____

9. _____

EXERCISE 5

Write the name of the defined female reproductive system structure.

1. pad of fatty tissue; covers the symphysis pubis _____

2. folds of fatty tissue surrounding the vaginal opening _____

3. thinner folds of tissue around the vaginal opening _____

4. highly sensitive erectile tissue _____

5. secretes a lubricating substance _____

6. produces ova _____

7. storage sacs for the ova _____

8. fingerlike projections _____

9. near the ovaries and connected to the uterus _____

Female Reproductive System Medical Terminology

Female reproductive system medical terms are organized into three main categories: (1) general medical terms; (2) disease and condition terms; and (3) diagnostic procedure, surgery, and laboratory test terms. The roots, prefixes, and suffixes associated with the female reproductive system are listed in Table 13-2. Review these word parts and complete the related exercises.

TABLE 13-2   ROOTS, PREFIXES, AND SUFFIXES FOR FEMALE REPRODUCTIVE SYSTEM TERMS

Root	Meaning	Prefix	Meaning	Suffix	Meaning
cry/o	cold	ante-	before; forward	-arche	beginning; onset
*cyst/o	cyst; sac	dys-	abnormal; painful; difficult	-cele	herniation; protrusion
fibr/o	fibrous tissue	endo-	within; inner	-ectomy-	surgical removal
lapar/o	abdominal wall	pre-	before	graphy	process of recording
olig/o	few; diminished	retro-	behind; backward; upward	-oma	tumor
				-osis	condition
				-pexy	surgical fixation
				-(r)rhagia	hemorrhage
				-(r)rhea	flow; discharge
				-version	to turn

* *cyst/o* also means urinary bladder.

EXERCISE 6

Write the root, prefix, suffix, and their meanings for the following medical terms.

1. cryosurgery

   ROOT: _____ MEANING: _____

   PREFIX: _____ MEANING: _____

   SUFFIX: _____ MEANING: _____

2. oligomenorrhea

   ROOT: _____ MEANING: _____

   PREFIX: _____ MEANING: _____

   SUFFIX: _____ MEANING: _____

3. dysmenorrhea

   ROOT: _____ MEANING: _____

   PREFIX: _____ MEANING: _____

   SUFFIX: _____ MEANING: _____

4. premenstrual

   ROOT: _____ MEANING: _____

   PREFIX: _____ MEANING: _____

   SUFFIX: _____ MEANING: _____

5. laparoscopy

   ROOT: _____ MEANING: _____

   PREFIX: _____ MEANING: _____

   SUFFIX: _____ MEANING: _____

6. fibrocystic

   ROOT: _____ MEANING: _____

   PREFIX: _____ MEANING: _____

   SUFFIX: _____ MEANING: _____

7. anteflexion

   ROOT: _____ MEANING: _____

   PREFIX: _____ MEANING: _____

   SUFFIX: _____ MEANING: _____

8. endocervical

   ROOT: _____ MEANING: _____

   PREFIX: _____ MEANING: _____

   SUFFIX: _____ MEANING: _____

9. hysterectomy

ROOT: _____   MEANING: _____

PREFIX: _____   MEANING: _____

SUFFIX: _____   MEANING: _____

EXERCISE 7

Write the suffix for each word or phrase.

1. hemorrhage _____

2. condition _____

3. discharge; flow _____

4. herniation or protrusion _____

5. process of recording _____

6. surgical fixation _____

7. surgical removal _____

8. to turn _____

9. tumor _____

Female Reproductive System General Medical Terms

Review the pronunciation and meaning of each term in Table 13-3. Note that some terms are built from word parts and some are not. Complete the exercises for these terms.

TABLE 13-3 FEMALE REPRODUCTIVE SYSTEM GENERAL MEDICAL TERMS

Term with Pronunciation	Definition
gynecologist (gigh-neh-**KALL**-oh-jist, jin-eh-**KALL**-oh-jist) gynec/o = woman -(o)logist = specialist in the study of	physician who specializes in the study and treatment of diseases related to the female
gynecology (gigh-neh-**KALL**-oh-jee, jin-eh-**KALL**-oh-jee) gynec/o = woman -(o)logy = study of	study of diseases and disorders related to the female
menarche (men-**ARK**-ee) men/o = menses; menstruation -arche = onset; beginning	onset of menstruation, first menstrual cycle

(continues)

TABLE 13-3 FEMALE REPRODUCTIVE SYSTEM GENERAL MEDICAL TERMS (continued)

Term with Pronunciation	Definition
menopause (**MEN**-oh-pawz) men/o = menses; menstruation	time frame that marks the permanent cessation of menstrual activity
menses (**MEN**-seez) men/o = menses; menstruation	bloody discharge associated with menstruation
menstruation (men-stroo-**AY**-shun) men/o = menses; menstruation	periodic flow of bloody fluid from the uterine lining
ovulation (ahv-yoo-**LAY**-shun) ov/o = ovum; egg	periodic release of a mature ovum from a graafian follicle

© 2016 Cengage Learning®

EXERCISE 8

Replace the italicized phrase with the correct medical term.

1. Rebecca was prepared for the *onset of menstruation.*

   _____

2. Shenesia completed a residency in the *study of the diseases and disorders related to the female.*

   _____

3. *The periodic discharge from the uterine lining* begins during puberty.

   _____

4. *Permanent cessation of menstrual activity* may take several years.

   _____

5. Sanitary pads or tampons are needed to dispose of the *bloody discharge of menstruation.*

   _____

6. A *physician who specializes in diseases and disorders related to the female* is able to diagnose cervical cancer.

   _____

7. *The periodic release of a mature ovum* usually occurs on a cyclical schedule.

   _____

Female Reproductive System Disease and Disorder Terms

Female reproductive system, including the breast, diseases and disorders include familiar problems such as vaginitis as well as more complex and less familiar diagnoses such as endometriosis. The medical terms are presented in alphabetical order in Table 13-4. Review the pronunciation and definition for each term and complete the exercises.

TABLE 13-4 FEMALE REPRODUCTIVE SYSTEM DISEASE AND DISORDER TERMS

Term with Pronunciation	Definition
amenorrhea (**ah**-men-oh-**REE**-ah) a- = lack of; without men/o = menses; menstrual flow -(r)rhea = flow; discharge	absence or lack of menstrual flow
anteflexion of the uterus (an-tee-**FLEK**-shun) ante- = before; forward	forward displacement of the uterus
carcinoma of the breast (**kar**-sin-**OH**-mah)	malignant tumor of the breast tissue
cervical carcinoma (**SER**-vih-kal **kar**-sin-**OH**-mah) cervic/o = cervix -al = pertaining to carcin- = cancer; malignant -oma = tumor	malignant tumor of the cervix, also called cervical cancer (Figure 13-5)

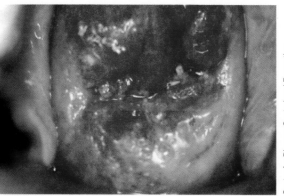

Center for Disease Control and Prevention

Figure 13-5 Cervical carcinoma.

cervicitis (ser-vih-**SIGH**-tis) cervic/o = cervix -itis = inflammation	inflammation of the cervix

(continues)

**TABLE 13-4   FEMALE REPRODUCTIVE SYSTEM DISEASE
AND DISORDER TERMS** (continued)

Term with Pronunciation	Definition
cystocele (**SISS**-toh-seel) cyst/o = urinary bladder -cele = hernia; protrusion	herniation or downward protrusion of the urinary bladder into the wall of the vagina
dysmenorrhea (**diss**-men-oh-**REE**-ah) dys- = abnormal; painful; difficult men/o = menses; menstruation -(r)rhea = flow; discharge	painful menstrual flow
endometriosis (**en**-doh-**mee**-tree-**OH**-sis) endo- = inner metr/i = uterus -osis = condition	presence and growth of endometrial tissue in areas outside the uterus
fibrocystic breast disease (**figh**-broh-**SISS**-tik) fibr/o = fibrous tissue cyst/o = cyst; sac -ic = pertaining to	presence of single or multiple fluid-filled cysts in the breasts
genital warts	a sexually transmitted infection caused by a low-risk human papillomavirus (HPV)
menometrorrhagia (**men**-oh-**met**-roh-**RAY**-jee-ah) men/o = menses; menstruation metr/o = uterus -(r)rhagia = hemorrhage	excessive uterine bleeding during and between the normal menstrual period
menorrhagia (men-oh-**RAY**-jee-ah) men/o = menses; menstruation -(r)rhagia = hemorrhage	excessive bleeding during the menstrual period
menorrhea (men-oh-**REE**-ah) men/o = menses; menstruation -(r)rhea = flow; discharge	normal menstrual flow

(continues)

TABLE 13-4   FEMALE REPRODUCTIVE SYSTEM DISEASE
AND DISORDER TERMS (continued)

Term with Pronunciation	Definition
metrorrhagia (meh-troh-**RAY**-jee-ah) metr/i = uterus -(r)rhagia = hemorrhage	excessive uterine bleeding at times other than during the menstrual period
oligomenorrhea (**oh**-lig-oh-**men**-oh-**REE**-ah) olig/o = few; diminished men/o = uterus -(r)rhea = flow; discharge	abnormally light or infrequent menstruation

© 2016 Cengage Learning®

EXERCISE 9

Analyze each term by writing the prefix, root, combining vowel, and suffix separated by vertical slashes. Based on the meaning of the word parts, write a definition for each term. Check the definition in a medical dictionary. Note that some terms might have more than one root.

EXAMPLE: gynecologist

	/ gynec	/o	/ logist
prefix	*root*	*combining vowel*	*suffix*

DEFINITION: specialist in the female reproductive system

1. amenorrhea

prefix	*root*	*combining vowel*	*suffix*

DEFINITION: _____

2. cervicitis

prefix	*root*	*combining vowel*	*suffix*

DEFINITION: _____

3. cystocele

prefix	*root*	*combining vowel*	*suffix*

DEFINITION: _____

4. dysmenorrhea

prefix	*root*	*combining vowel*	*suffix*

DEFINITION: _____

5. endometriosis

prefix	root	combining vowel	suffix

DEFINITION: _____

6. menorrhagia

prefix	root	combining vowel	suffix

DEFINITION: _____

7. metrorrhagia

prefix	root	combining vowel	suffix

DEFINITION: _____

8. menorrhea

prefix	root	combining vowel	suffix

DEFINITION: _____

9. oligomenorrhea

prefix	root	combining vowel	suffix

DEFINITION: _____

10. menometrorrhagia

prefix	root	combining vowel	suffix

DEFINITION: _____

EXERCISE 10

Replace the italicized phrase with the correct medical term.

1. The results of Maria's breast x-ray revealed *multiple fluid-filled cysts.*

    _____

2. After three abnormal evaluations, the final diagnosis was *a malignant tumor of the cervix.*

    _____

3. *Forward displacement* of the uterus might affect a woman's ability to become pregnant.

    _____

4. Athletes sometimes exhibit *abnormally light or infrequent menstruation.*

    _____

5. *Painful menstrual flow* might be alleviated with pain relievers.

    _____

6. *Excessive bleeding during the menstrual period* might be a symptom of uterine polyps.

   _____

7. Marlena informed her family physician that both her mother and sister had *malignant tumors of the breast* before they were 45 years of age.

   _____

8. *Normal menstrual flow* does not interfere with activities of daily living.

   _____

   Review the pronunciation and definition for each term in Table 13-5 and complete the exercises.

TABLE 13-5 FEMALE REPRODUCTIVE SYSTEM DISEASE AND DISORDER TERMS

Term with Pronunciation	Definition
oophoritis (oh-**off**-or-**EYE**-tis) oophor/o = ovary -itis = inflammation	inflammation of the ovaries
ovarian carcinoma (oh-**VAY**-ree-an kar-sin-**OH**-ma)	malignant tumor of the ovary
ovarian cyst (oh-**VAY**-ree-an **SIST**) ovari/o = ovary -an = pertaining to	fluid-filled, multichambered sac in the ovary
pelvic inflammatory disease (PID)	inflammation of the vagina, cervix, fallopian tubes, and broad ligament; often a result of untreated sexually transmitted infections such as chlamydia, gonorrhea, or genital herpes
polycystic ovary syndrome (PCOS) poly = many cyst/o = fluid filled sac -ic = pertaining to	polycystic ovary syndrome (PCOS) is a complex health problem that can affect a woman's menstrual cycle, fertility, heart, blood vessels, and appearance; a hormonal imbalance seems to be the main underlying problem; some ovarian follicles exhibit as fluid filled cysts and do not produce mature ovum; genetics may play a role in PCOS

(continues)

TABLE 13-5 FEMALE REPRODUCTIVE SYSTEM DISEASE
AND DISORDER TERMS (continued)

Term with Pronunciation	Definition
premenstrual syndrome (PMS) (pre-**MEN**-stroo-al) pre- = before men/o = menstruation -al = pertaining to	a group of symptoms such as irritability, anxiety, mood changes, headaches, breast swelling, and water retention that begin several days before the onset of menstruation and end a short time after the onset of menstruation; PMS
prolapse of the uterus	protrusion of the uterus into the vaginal opening (Figure 13-6)

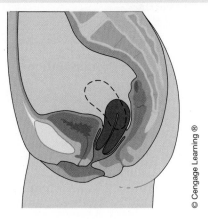

© Cengage Learning ®

Figure 13-6 Prolapse of the uterus.

retroversion of the uterus (**reh**-troh-**VER**-shun) retro- = backward; toward the back -version = to turn	backward displacement of the uterus
salpingitis (**sal**-pin-**JIGH**-tis) salping/o = fallopian tube -itis = inflammation	inflammation of the fallopian tube
toxic shock syndrome (TSS)	a rare and sometimes fatal disease caused by an infection of the female reproductive organs associated with certain strains of *Staphylococcus aureus*

(continues)

TABLE 13-5   FEMALE REPRODUCTIVE SYSTEM DISEASE AND DISORDER TERMS (continued)

Term with Pronunciation	Definition
vaginitis (vaj-in-**EYE**-tis) vagin/o = vagina -itis = inflammation	inflammation of the vagina
vulvovaginitis (**vull**-voh-**vaj**-in-**EYE**-tis vulv/o = vulva vagin/o = vagina -itis = inflammation	inflammation of the vulva (external genitalia) and vagina

© 2016 Cengage Learning®

EXERCISE 11

Analyze each term by writing the prefix, root, combining vowel, and suffix separated by vertical slashes. Based on the meaning of the word parts, write a definition for each term. Check the definition in a medical dictionary. Note that some terms might have more than one root.

1. oophoritis

   _____

   prefix   *root*   *combining vowel*   *suffix*

   DEFINITION: _____

2. retroversion

   _____

   prefix   *root*   *combining vowel*   *suffix*

   DEFINITION: _____

3. salpingitis

   _____

   prefix   *root*   *combining vowel*   *suffix*

   DEFINITION: _____

4. vaginitis

   _____

   prefix   *root*   *combining vowel*   *suffix*

   DEFINITION: _____

5. vulvovaginitis

   _____

   prefix   *root*   *combining vowel*   *suffix*

   DEFINITION: _____

EXERCISE 12

Write the medical term for each definition or abbreviation.

1. malignant tumor of the ovary   _____

2. fluid-filled sac in the ovary   _____

3. PID   _____

4. PMS   _____

5. TSS   _____

6. displacement of the uterus
   into the vagina   _____

Female Reproductive System Diagnostic and Treatment Terms

Review the pronunciation and definition of the diagnostic and treatment terms in Table 13-6. Complete the exercises for each set of terms.

TABLE 13-6   FEMALE REPRODUCTIVE SYSTEM DIAGNOSTIC
AND TREATMENT TERMS

Term with Pronunciation	Definition
colposcopy (kol-**POSS**-koh-pee) colp/o = vagina -scopy = examination with a scope	examination of vaginal and cervical tissue using a scope
conization (kon-ih-**ZAY**-shun)	surgical removal of a cone-shaped segment of the cervix for diagnosis or treatment; cone biopsy
cryosurgery (**krigh**-oh-**SER**-jer-ree) cry/o = cold	destruction and removal of tissue by rapid freezing
dilation and curettage (D&C) (digh-**LAY**-shun and koo-reh-**TAHZ**)	widening of the cervical canal followed by scraping of the uterine lining (Figure 13-7)
hysterectomy (**hiss**-ter-**EK**-toh-mee) hyster/o = uterus -ectomy = surgical removal	surgical removal of the uterus
hysterosalpingography (**hiss**-ter-oh-**sal**-pin-**GOG**-rah-fee) hyster/o = uterus salping/o = fallopian tubes -graphy = process of recording	process of recording an image or x-ray of the uterus and fallopian tubes using a contrast medium; a fertility test to examine the internal female genitalia in order to identify structural problems, such as stenosis or blockage that interfers with fertilization or implantation

(continues)

TABLE 13-6 FEMALE REPRODUCTIVE SYSTEM DIAGNOSTIC
AND TREATMENT TERMS (continued)

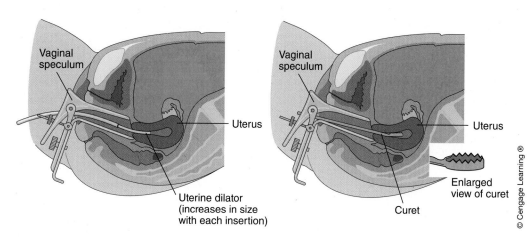

Figure 13-7 Dilation of the cervix and curettage of the uterus.

Term with Pronunciation	Definition
laparoscopy (lap-ar-**OSS**-koh-pee) lapar/o = abdominal wall -scopy = examination with a scope	examination of the contents of the abdominal and pelvic cavity using a scope
mammography (mam-**OG**-rah-fee) mamm/o = breast -graphy = process of recording	process of recording an image or x-ray examination of the soft tissue of the breast; screening mammography is used to establish a baseline record of a woman's breast tissue; diagnostic mammography is used to check for breast disease, including cancer, after a lump or other sign or symptom of a disease is found (Figure 13-8)
mastectomy (mass-**TEK**-toh-mee) mast/o = breast -ectomy = surgical removal	surgical removal of the breast and surrounding tissues
oophorectomy (oh-**off**-or-**EK**-toh-mee)	surgical removal of the ovary
oophoropexy (oh-**off**-or-oh-**PEK**-see) oophor/o = ovary -pexy = surgical fixation	surgical fixation of the ovary

(continues)

© Cengage Learning ®

TABLE 13-6 FEMALE REPRODUCTIVE SYSTEM DIAGNOSTIC
AND TREATMENT TERMS (continued)

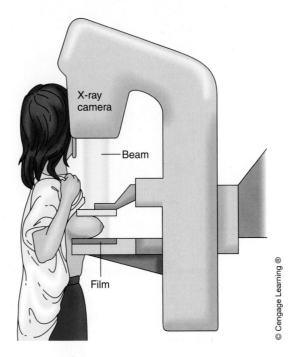

© Cengage Learning ®

Figure 13-8 Mammography.

Term with Pronunciation	Definition
ovariopexy (oh-**vay**-ree-oh-**PEK**-see) ovari/o = ovary -pexy = surgical fixation	surgical fixation of the ovary
Papanicolaou smear (pap-ah-**NIK**-oh-low)	microscopic examination of cervical cells; diagnostic test for cervical cancer; Pap smear, Pap test (Figure 13-9)
salpingo-oophorectomy (sal-ping-goh-oh-off-or-**EK**-toh-me) salping/o = fallopian tubes oophor/o = ovary -ectomy = surgical removal	surgical removal of the fallopian tubes and ovaries
total abdominal hysterectomy (TAH)	surgical removal of the uterus and cervix through an incision in the lower abdomen
tubal ligation (**TOO**-bal ligh-**GAY**-shun)	surgical cutting and tying of the fallopian tubes to prevent passage of the sperm and ova through the tube; female sterilization (Figure 13-10)

(continues)

**TABLE 13-6   FEMALE REPRODUCTIVE SYSTEM DIAGNOSTIC
AND TREATMENT TERMS** (continued)

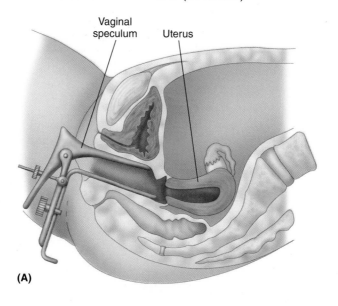

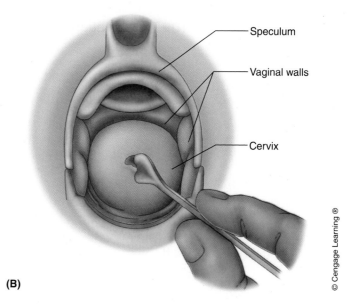

Figure 13-9   Pap smear: (A) speculum widens the vaginal opening;
(B) cervical cells are removed for microscopic evaluation.

Term with Pronunciation	Definition
uteropexy (**YOO**-ter-oh-**pek**-see) uter/o = uterus -pexy = surgical fixation	surgical fixation of the uterus to the abdominal wall

(continues)

TABLE 13-6 FEMALE REPRODUCTIVE SYSTEM DIAGNOSTIC AND TREATMENT TERMS (continued)

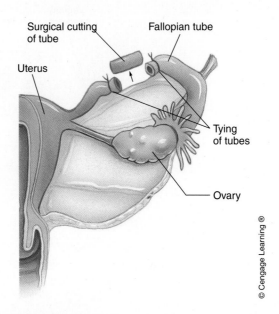

Figure 13-10 Tubal ligation.

© 2016 Cengage Learning®

EXERCISE 13

Analyze each term by writing the prefix, root, combining vowel, and suffix separated by vertical slashes. Based on the meaning of the word parts, write a definition for each term. Check the definition in a medical dictionary. Note that some terms might have more than one root.

1. colposcopy

prefix	*root*	*combining vowel*	*suffix*

   DEFINITION: _____

2. hysterectomy

prefix	*root*	*combining vowel*	*suffix*

   DEFINITION: _____

3. hysterosalpingography

prefix	*root*	*combining vowel*	*suffix*

   DEFINITION: _____

4. laparoscopy

prefix	*root*	*combining vowel*	*suffix*

   DEFINITION: _____

5. mammography

prefix	_root_	_combining vowel_	_suffix_

DEFINITION: _____

6. mastectomy

prefix	_root_	_combining vowel_	_suffix_

DEFINITION: _____

7. ovariopexy

prefix	_root_	_combining vowel_	_suffix_

DEFINITION: _____

8. oophoropexy

prefix	_root_	_combining vowel_	_suffix_

DEFINITION: _____

9. uteropexy

prefix	_root_	_combining vowel_	_suffix_

DEFINITION: _____

10. salpingo-oophorectomy

prefix	_root_	_combining vowel_	_suffix_

EXERCISE 14

Replace the italicized phrase with the correct medical term.

1. Carmen made every effort to have an annual _x-ray examination of her breasts._

   _____

2. Melinda's initial _microscopic examination of cervical cells_ was abnormal.

   _____

3. Helen chose _female sterilization_ to prevent future pregnancies.

   _____

4. Irregular menstrual periods sometimes necessitate a _widening of the cervical canal and scraping of the uterine lining._

   _____

5. After two abnormal cervical smears, the physician recommended a _surgical removal of cone-shaped segment of the cervix._

   _____

6. _Rapid freezing, destruction, and removal of tissue_ is a procedure for treating abnormal cervical tissue growth.

   _____

Abbreviations

Review the female reproductive system abbreviations in Table 13-7. Practice writing out the meaning of each abbreviation.

TABLE 13-7   ABBREVIATIONS

Abbreviation	Meaning
D&C	dilation and curettage
GYN	gynecology
Pap smear	Papanicolaou smear
PCOS	polycystic ovary syndrome
PID	pelvic inflammatory disease
PMS	premenstrual syndrome
TAH	total abdominal hysterectomy
TSS	toxic shock syndrome
TVH	total vaginal hysterectomy

© 2016 Cengage Learning®

Pregnancy

This section of the chapter covers medical terms related to pregnancy. The generic medical term for male and female sex cells (ovum and sperm) is **gamete** (**GAM**-eet). Pregnancy occurs when an ovum has been fertilized by a sperm and is implanted into the endometrium. Fertilization usually takes place in the fallopian tube. The fertilized ovum is called a **zygote** (**ZIGH**-goht). From the second through the eighth week of pregnancy, the fertilized ovum is called an **embryo** (**EM**-bree-oh). For the remainder of the pregnancy, the fertilized ovum is called a **fetus** (**FEE**-tus). Pregnancy lasts 40 weeks or 280 days, which is about 9 calendar months or 10 lunar months. A lunar month is 4 weeks or 28 days.

Pregnancy is divided into trimesters; each trimester is about three months long. The time between fertilization, also known as conception, and labor is called **gestation** (JESS-**TAY**-shun), or the gestational period.

Pregnancy Word Roots

Word roots with the combining vowel are listed in Table 13-8. Review the word roots and complete the exercises that follow.

TABLE 13-8   PREGNANCY WORD ROOTS

Word Root/Combining Form	Meaning
amni/o; amnion/o	amnion
chori/o	chorion

(continues)

TABLE 13-8   PREGNANCY WORD ROOTS (continued)

Word Root/Combining Form	Meaning
embry/o	embryo
episi/o; vulv/o	vulva
fet/o; fet/i	fetus
gravid/o	pregnancy
lact/o	milk
nat/o	birth
par/o; part/o	bear; give birth to; labor; childbirth
pelv/i	pelvis
perine/o	perineum
puerper/o	childbirth
salping/o	fallopian tube
vagin/o	vagina

© 2016 Cengage Learning®

EXERCISE 15

Write the definitions of the following word roots.

1. fet/o   _____

2. nat/o   _____

3. par/o   _____

4. amni/o   _____

5. episi/o   _____

6. salping/o   _____

7. perine/o   _____

8. pueper/o   _____

9. pelv/i   _____

10. lact/o   _____

EXERCISE 16

Write the word root and its meanings on the spaces provided.

1. gravidarum

   ROOT: _____   MEANING: _____

2. perinatal

   ROOT: _____   MEANING: _____

3. salpingectomy

   ROOT: _____   MEANING: _____

4. fetoscope

   ROOT: _____   MEANING: _____

5. amniocentesis

ROOT: _____   MEANING: _____

6. puerperium

ROOT: _____   MEANING: _____

7. vaginal

ROOT: _____   MEANING: _____

8. chorionitis

ROOT: _____   MEANING: _____

9. lactorrhea

ROOT: _____   MEANING: _____

10. episiotomy

ROOT: _____   MEANING: _____

Structures Related to Pregnancy

In addition to the female reproductive organs already presented, Figure 13-11 illustrates specific structures related to pregnancy. Refer to the figure as you read about the structures. The (1) **amniotic sac** (**am**-nee-**OT**-IK sac), also called the **fetal membrane** or **amnion**, houses the developing fetus. The outer layer of the amniotic sac is the (2) **chorion** (**KOR**-ee-on). The sac is filled with (3) **amniotic fluid** that cushions and protects the fetus. The (4) **placenta** (plah-**SEN**-tah) is a temporary organ embedded in the wall of the uterus. Nutrients, oxygen, and waste are exchanged between the mother and fetus via the (5) **umbilical cord**, also called the **umbilicus** (um-**BILL**-ih-kus), which is connected to the placenta. The placenta also produces other hormones necessary for a normal pregnancy.

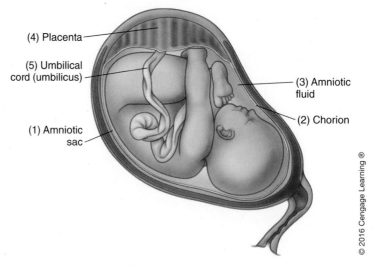

© 2016 Cengage Learning ®

Figure 13-11 Amniotic sac.

EXERCISE 17

Write the medical term for each definition.

1. fertilized ovum _____

2. fertilized ovum, 9th to 40th
   week of pregnancy _____

3. fertilized ovum, second to eighth
   week of pregnancy _____

4. male and female sex cell _____

5. period between fertilization and labor _____

6. temporary organ embedded in the
   uterine wall _____

7. structure that houses the developing fetus _____

8. connects the fetus to the placenta _____

9. inner layer of the structure that houses
   the developing fetus _____

10. outer layer of the structure that houses
    the developing fetus _____

Medical Terms Related to Pregnancy

Pregnancy medical terms are organized as: (1) general medical terms; (2) complications and disorders of pregnancy; and (3) diagnostic, surgical, and laboratory test terms. Prefixes and suffixes used in pregnancy terms are listed in Table 13-9. Review these word parts and complete the exercises that follow.

TABLE 13-9 PREFIXES AND SUFFIXES FOR PREGNANCY TERMS

Prefix	Meaning	Suffix	Meaning
ante-	before	-centesis	surgical puncture
micro-	small	-graphy	process of recording
multi-	many	-(o)logy	study of
nulli-	none	-metry	to measure
post-	after	-(o)tomy	incision into
primi-	first; one	-(r)rhexis	rupture
		-scopy	visualization with a scope
		-tocia	labor; birth

EXERCISE 18

Write the prefixes, suffixes, and their meanings in the spaces provided. Note that some terms have both a prefix and suffix, and some terms have only one or the other.

1. dystocia

   PREFIX: _____ MEANING: _____

   SUFFIX: _____ MEANING: _____

2. nullipara

   PREFIX: _____ MEANING: _____

   SUFFIX: _____ MEANING: _____

3. postpartum

   PREFIX: _____ MEANING: _____

   SUFFIX: _____ MEANING: _____

4. fetoscopy

   PREFIX: _____ MEANING: _____

   SUFFIX: _____ MEANING: _____

5. antepartum

   PREFIX: _____ MEANING: _____

   SUFFIX: _____ MEANING: _____

6. amniocentesis

   PREFIX: _____ MEANING: _____

   SUFFIX: _____ MEANING: _____

7. primigravida

   PREFIX: _____ MEANING: _____

   SUFFIX: _____ MEANING: _____

8. hysterorrhexis

   PREFIX: _____ MEANING: _____

   SUFFIX: _____ MEANING: _____

9. multigravida

   PREFIX: _____ MEANING: _____

   SUFFIX: _____ MEANING: _____

10. microscope

    PREFIX: _____ MEANING: _____

    SUFFIX: _____ MEANING: _____

EXERCISE 19

Write the prefix or suffix for each definition.

1. after _____

2. before _____

3. first _____

4. labor; birth _____

5. many _____

6. none _____

7. process of recording _____

8. rupture _____

9. surgical puncture _____

10. visualization with a scope _____

Pregnancy General Medical Terms

Review the pronunciation and meaning for each term in Table 13-10. Note that some terms are built from word parts and some are not. Complete the exercises for these terms.

TABLE 13-10 PREGNANCY GENERAL MEDICAL TERMS

Term with Pronunciation	Definition
antepartum (an-tee-**PAR**-tum) ante- = before part/o = giving birth; labor -um = noun ending	before the onset of labor; before giving birth
Braxton Hicks contraction	irregular and nonproductive contractions of the uterus that might occur throughout pregnancy
effacement (eh-**FACE**-ment)	normal thinning and shortening of the cervix during the birth process
embryologist (em-bree-**ALL**-oh-jist) embry/o = embryo -(o)logist = specialist in the study of	physician who specializes in the study and treatment of the growth and development of the human organism
embryology (em-bree-**ALL**-oh-jist) embry/o = embryo -(o)logy = study of	study and treatment of the growth and development of the human organism
lochia (**LOH**-kee-ah)	vaginal discharge from the uterus that occurs for the first week or two after childbirth

(continues)

TABLE 13-10 PREGNANCY GENERAL MEDICAL TERMS (continued)

Term with Pronunciation	Definition
meconium (meh-**KOH**-nee-um)	first feces of a newborn
multigravida (mull-tee-**GRAV**-ih-dah) multi- = many gravid/o = pregnancy	having been pregnant more than two times
multipara (mull-**TIP**-ah-rah) multi- = many par/o = giving birth to -a = noun ending	having given birth to a viable fetus more than two times
nulligravida (null-ee-**GRAV**-ih-dah) nulli- = none gravid/o = pregnancy -a = noun ending	never having been pregnant
nullipara (null-**IP**-ah-rah) nulli- = none par/o = giving birth to -a = noun ending	never having given birth to a viable fetus
obstetrician (**ob**-steh-**TRISH**-an)	physician who specializes in the study and treatment of pregnancy and delivery
obstetrics (ob-**STEH**-triks)	medical specialty related to pregnancy and delivery
parturition (par-too-**RISH**-un)	act of giving birth; childbirth; delivery
postpartum (post-**PAR**-tum) post- = after part/o = giving birth to -um = noun ending	occurring after childbirth
primigravida (prigh-mih-**GRAV**-ih-dah) primi- = first gravid/o = pregnancy -a = noun ending	first pregnancy
primipara (prigh-**MIP**-ah-rah) primi- = first par/o = giving birth to -a = noun ending	giving birth for the first time following 20 or more weeks of gestation

(continues)

TABLE 13-10   PREGNANCY GENERAL MEDICAL TERMS (continued)

Term with Pronunciation	Definition
puerperium (pyoo-er-**PEER**-ee-um) puerper/o = childbirth -um = noun ending	three- to six-week time period following childbirth

© 2016 Cengage Learning®

EXERCISE 20

Analyze each term by writing the prefix, root, combining vowel, and suffix separated by vertical slashes. Based on the meaning of the word parts, write a definition for each term. Check the definition in a medical dictionary. Note that some terms might have more than one root

EXAMPLE: gynecologist

	/gynec	/o	/logist
prefix	*root*	*combining vowel*	*suffix*

DEFINITION: specialist in the female reproductive system

1. antepartum

prefix	*root*	*combining vowel*	*suffix*

DEFINITION: _____

2. embryologist

prefix	*root*	*combining vowel*	*suffix*

DEFINITION: _____

3. embryology

prefix	*root*	*combining vowel*	*suffix*

DEFINITION: _____

4. multigravida

prefix	*root*	*combining vowel*	*suffix*

DEFINITION: _____

5. multipara

prefix	*root*	*combining vowel*	*suffix*

DEFINITION: _____

6. nulligravida

prefix	*root*	*combining vowel*	*suffix*

DEFINITION: _____

7. nullipara

prefix	root	combining vowel	suffix

DEFINITION: _____

8. postpartum

prefix	root	combining vowel	suffix

DEFINITION: _____

9. primigravida

prefix	root	combining vowel	suffix

DEFINITION: _____

10. primipara

prefix	root	combining vowel	suffix

DEFINITION:_____

EXERCISE 21

Write the medical term for each definition.

1. childbirth _____

2. first childbirth after 20 weeks of gestation _____

3. first feces of a newborn _____

4. irregular, nonproductive contractions at any
   time during pregnancy _____

5. medical specialty related to pregnancy and delivery _____

6. more than one pregnancy _____

7. thinning and shortening of the cervix during the
   birth process _____

8. physician who specializes in pregnancy and delivery _____

9. specialty related to the growth and development
   of humans _____

10. three to six weeks following childbirth _____

11. vaginal discharge lasting a few weeks after childbirth _____

Pregnancy Complication and Disorder Terms

Complications and disorders associated with pregnancy and delivery include familiar problems such as ectopic, or tubal, pregnancy as well as more serious complications such as abruptio placentae (ah-**BRUP**-shee-oh plah-**SEN**-tee). Review the medical terms, pronunciations, and definitions in Table 13-11 and complete the exercises.

TABLE 13-11   PREGNANCY COMPLICATION AND DISORDER TERMS

Term with Pronunciation	Definition
abortion (ah-**BOR**-shun)	spontaneous or induced termination of a pregnancy; a spontaneous abortion is commonly called a *miscarriage*
abruptio placentae (ah-**BRUP**-shee-oh plah-**SEN**-tee)	premature separation of the placenta from the uterine wall
amnionitis (**am**-nee-oh-**NIGH-** tis) amni/o = amnion -itis = inflammation	inflammation of the amnion
amniorrhea (**am**-nee-oh-**REE**-ah) amni/o = amnion -(r)rhea = flow; discharge	discharge of amniotic fluid from the amniotic sac; leaking of amniotic fluid
breech birth	delivery presentation with the buttocks appearing first
dystocia (diss-**TOH**-see-ah) dys- = abnormal; painful; difficult -tocia = labor; birth	difficult or painful labor
eclampsia (ee-**KLAMP-** see-ah)	most severe form of gestational hypertension characterized by seizures
ectopic pregnancy (ek-**TOP**-ik)	abnormal implantation of a fertilized ovum outside the uterus; also called a *tubal pregnancy* when implantation occurs in the fallopian tube (Figure 13-12)

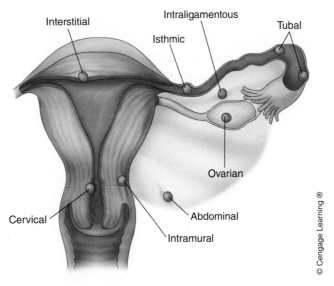

© Cengage Learning ®

Figure 13-12   Potential sites of an ectopic pregnancy.

(continues)

**TABLE 13-11   PREGNANCY COMPLICATION
AND DISORDER TERMS** (continued)

Term with Pronunciation	Definition
gestational diabetes (jess-**TAY**-shun-al digh-ah-**BEE**-teez)	diabetes that develops during pregnancy and that usually resolves after pregnancy
gestational hypertension (jess-**TAY**-shun-al high-per-**TEN**-shun)	hypertension that develops during pregnancy and usually resolves after pregnancy; also called pregnancy-induced hypertension (PIH)
hydatidiform mole (**high**-dah-**TID**-ih-form)	a cystic mass resembling a cluster of grapes that develops in place of a placenta and fetus; also called a *molar pregnancy*
hyperemesis gravidarum (**high**-per-**EM**-eh-sis **grav**-ih-**DAR**-um) hyper- = excessive -emesis = vomiting gravid/o = pregnancy -um = noun ending	condition characterized by excessive and severe vomiting that results in maternal dehydration and weight loss
hysterorrhexis (**hiss**-ter-oh-**REKS**-iss) hyster/o = uterus -(r)rhexis = rupture	rupture of the uterus
incompetent cervix	inability of the cervix to retain the contents of the pregnant uterus that results in a spontaneous abortion
placenta previa (plah-**SEN**-tah **PREE**-vee-ah)	condition in which the placenta is implanted in a lower part of the uterus and precedes the fetus during delivery (Figure 13-13)
pre-eclampsia (**pre**-ee-**KLAMP**-see-ah)	gestational hypertension characterized by edema and proteinuria, the presence of protein in the urine
Rh incompatibility	reaction between maternal Rh negative (Rh–) blood and fetal Rh positive (Rh+) during a first pregnancy that causes the immune system of the mother to develop antibodies against Rh+ blood cells; in subsequent pregnancies, the antibodies will attack Rh+ fetal blood cells
tubal pregnancy	implantation of a fertilized ovum in the wall of a fallopian tube; also called *ectopic pregnancy*

(continues)

**TABLE 13-11   PREGNANCY COMPLICATION
AND DISORDER TERMS** (continued)

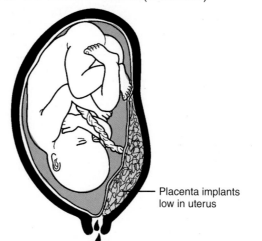

Placenta implants
low in uterus

© Cengage Learning ®

Figure 13-13 Placenta previa.

© 2016 Cengage Learning®

EXERCISE 22

Analyze each term by writing the prefix, root, combining vowel, and suffix separated by vertical slashes. Based on the meaning of the word parts, write a definition for each term. Check the definitions in a medical dictionary. Note that some terms might have more than one root.

1. amnionitis

prefix	*root*	*combining vowel*	*suffix*

DEFINITION: _____

2. amniorrhea

prefix	*root*	*combining vowel*	*suffix*

DEFINITION: _____

3. dystocia

prefix	*root*	*combining vowel*	*suffix*

DEFINITION: _____

4. hyperemesis gravidarum

prefix	*root*	*combining vowel*	*suffix*

prefix	*root*	*combining vowel*	*suffix*

DEFINITION: _____

5. hysterorrhexis

prefix	*root*	*combining vowel*	*suffix*

DEFINITION: _____

EXERCISE 23

Replace the italicized phrase with the correct medical term.

1. At 12 weeks gestation, Marcia had a spontaneous *termination of pregnancy*.

   _____

2. *Premature separation of the placenta* is a life-threatening condition for both mother and child.

   _____

3. Cheryl experienced *diabetes during pregnancy* for each of her pregnancies.

   _____

4. Due to an *implantation of a fertilized ovum outside the uterus*, Sara underwent removal of a fallopian tube.

   _____

5. Melinda's labor was prolonged due to a *delivery presentation with buttocks appearing first*.

   _____

EXERCISE 24

Match the condition in Column 1 with the correct definition in Column 2.

COLUMN 1

_____ 1. abruptio placentae
_____ 2. breech birth
_____ 3. dystocia
_____ 4. eclampsia
_____ 5. hydatidiform mole
_____ 6. hysterorrhexis
_____ 7. incompetent cervix
_____ 8. PIH
_____ 9. placenta previa
_____ 10. pre-eclampsia
_____ 11. Rh incompatibility
_____ 12. tubal pregnancy

COLUMN 2

a. rupture of the uterus
b. reaction between maternal and fetal blood
c. premature separation of the placenta
d. placenta precedes the fetus during delivery
e. most severe form of gestational hypertension
f. inability of the cervix to retain contents of pregnant uterus
g. gestational hypertension with edema and proteinuria
h. ectopic pregnancy
i. development of hypertension during pregnancy
j. difficult or painful labor
k. delivery presentation with buttocks appearing first
l. cystic mass that develops in place of a placenta and fetus

Pregnancy Diagnostic, Treatment, and Surgical Terms

Review the pronunciation and definition for the terms listed in Table 13-12 and complete the exercises.

TABLE 13-12 PREGNANCY DIAGNOSTIC, TREATMENT, AND SURGICAL TERMS

Term with Pronunciation	Definition
amniocentesis (**am**-nee-oh-sen-**TEE**-sis) amni/o = amnion -centesis = surgical puncture to remove fluid	surgical puncture into the amniotic sac to remove fluid for analysis to identify genetic disorders of the fetus; usually performed during the 15th week of pregnancy or later (Figure 13-14)

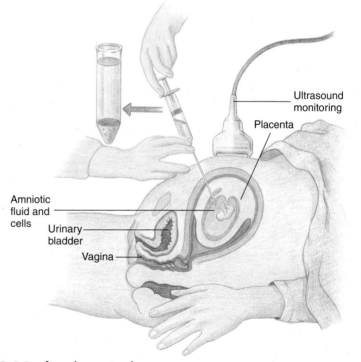

Amniotic fluid and cells

Urinary bladder

Vagina

Ultrasound monitoring

Placenta

© Cengage Learning ®

Figure 13-14 Amniocentesis.

amnioscopy (**am**-nee-**OSS**-koh-pee) amni/o = amnion -scopy = visualization with a scope	visualization of the fetus with a scope that enters the amniotic cavity through the abdominal wall
amniotomy (**am**-nee-**OT**-oh-mee) amni/o = amnion -(o)tomy = incision into	incision into or rupture of the amniotic membranes to induce labor; also called "breaking the water"

(continues)

TABLE 13-12   PREGNANCY DIAGNOSTIC, TREATMENT, AND SURGICAL
TERMS (continued)

Term with Pronunciation	Definition
cerclage (ser-**KLOZH**)	suturing the cervical opening to prevent spontaneous abortion; treatment for a history of incompetent cervix
cesarean section (see-**SAYR**-ee-an) (C-section)	incision into the abdominal wall and uterus to deliver a baby
chorionic villus sampling (**kor**-ee-**ON**-ik **VILL**-us) (CVS) chori/o = chorion -ic = pertaining to	removal of a small sample of the placenta by inserting a catheter or needle through the cervix and withdrawing placental tissue for analysis to identify genetic disorders of the fetus; usually performed between the 10th and 12th weeks of pregnancy
contraction stress test (CST)	introduction of a diluted intravenous (IV) solution containing the hormone oxytocin to stimulate uterine contractions to evaluate whether the fetus can tolerate the stress of labor and delivery; also called the *oxytocin challenge test*
electronic fetal monitoring	application and use of an internal or external electronic device to monitor fetal heart rate and maternal uterine contractions; such monitoring can assess the quality of the uterine contractions and the effects of labor on the fetus
episiotomy (eh-**pihz**-ee-**OT**-oh-mee) episi/o = vulva -(o)tomy = incision into	incision into the perineum to facilitate delivery and prevent perineal laceration or tearing
fetal ultrasonography (**ull**-trah-soh-**NOG**-rah-fee)	noninvasive examination of the fetus in utero using high-frequency sound waves (Figure 13-15)
fetometry (fee-**TOM**-eh-tree) fet/o = fetus -metry = process of measuring	measuring or estimating the size of the fetus or the fetal head before delivery

(continues)

TABLE 13-12   PREGNANCY DIAGNOSTIC, TREATMENT, AND SURGICAL TERMS (continued)

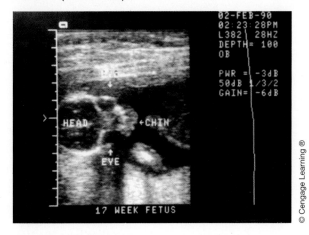

© Cengage Learning®

Figure 13-15   Fetal ultrasound.

Term with Pronunciation	Definition
pelvimetry (pell-**VIM**-eh-tree) pelv/i = pelvis -metry = process of measuring	measuring the pelvic outlet to determine if its size is adequate for childbirth
pregnancy test	laboratory blood and urine tests to determine pregnancy

© 2016 Cengage Learning®

EXERCISE 25

Analyze each term by writing the root, combining vowel, and suffix separated by vertical slashes. Based on the meaning of the word parts, write a definition for each term. Check the definition in a medical dictionary.

1. amniocentesis

prefix	*root*	*combining vowel*	*suffix*

DEFINITION: _____

2. amnioscopy

prefix	*root*	*combining vowel*	*suffix*

DEFINITION: _____

3. amniotomy

prefix	*root*	*combining vowel*	*suffix*

DEFINITION: _____

4. episiotomy

prefix	*root*	*combining vowel*	*suffix*

DEFINITION: _____

5. fetography

prefix	root	combining vowel	suffix

DEFINITION: _____

6. fetometry

prefix	root	combining vowel	suffix

DEFINITION: _____

7. pelvimetry

prefix	root	combining vowel	suffix

DEFINITION: _____

EXERCISE 26

Circle the medical term that best fits the description.

DESCRIPTION	CIRCLE ONE ITEM
1. surgical puncture to remove fluid	*amniotomy* OR *amniocentesis*
2. estimating fetal size before delivery	*fetometry* OR *fetography*
3. x-ray examination of the fetus	*fetography* OR *fetoscopy*
4. incision into the perineum	*cerclage* OR *episiotomy*
5. endoscopic visualization of the fetus	*fetal ultrasound* OR *amnioscopy*
6. measuring the pelvic outlet	*pelvimetry* OR *CST*
7. rupture of the amniotic membranes	*amniotomy* OR *C-section*
8. suturing the cervical opening	*CVS* OR *cerclage*
9. labor and delivery fetal stress test	*electronic fetal monitoring* OR *CST*
10. incision to deliver a baby	*cesarean section* OR *amniotomy*

Abbreviations

Review the abbreviations in Table 13-13. Practice writing out the meaning of each abbreviation.

TABLE 13-13 ABBREVIATIONS

Abbreviation	Meaning
C-section	cesarean section
CST	contraction stimulation test
CVS	chorionic villus sampling
EDB	expected date of birth
EDC	expected or estimated date of confinement
EDD	expected date of delivery

(continues)

TABLE 13-13   ABBREVIATIONS (continued)

Abbreviation	Meaning
FHR	fetal heart rate
L&D	labor and delivery
LMP	last menstrual period
NSD	normal spontaneous delivery
OB	obstetrics
PIH	pregnancy-induced hypertension
SVD	spontaneous vaginal delivery

© 2016 Cengage Learning®

CHAPTER REVIEW

The Chapter Review can be used as a self-test. Go through each exercise and answer as many questions as you can without referring to previous exercises or earlier discussions within this chapter. Check your answers and fill in any blanks. Practice writing any terms you might have misspelled.

EXERCISE 27

Write the medical term for each definition.

1. physician who specializes in the female reproductive system _____

2. study of the female reproductive system _____

3. absence or lack of menstrual flow _____

4. painful or difficult menstrual flow _____

5. excessive bleeding during the menstrual period _____

6. excessive uterine bleeding at times other than the menstrual period _____

7. excessive uterine bleeding during and between the regular menstrual period _____

8. diminished menstrual flow _____

9. inflammation of the ovaries _____

10. inflammation of the fallopian tubes _____

11. examination of the vagina with a scope _____

12. process of recording an x-ray of the uterus and fallopian tubes _____

13. process of recording an x-ray of the breasts _____

14. surgical removal of the breast _____

15. surgical fixation of the ovaries _____

16. surgical removal of the uterus _____

17. surgical removal of the fallopian tubes
    and ovaries _____

18. surgical fixation of the uterus to the
    abdominal wall _____

19. inflammation of the vagina _____

20. inflammation of the vulva and vagina _____

EXERCISE 28

Read the following operative report and write a brief definition for each italicized medical term on the spaces provided.

OPERATIVE REPORT
PREOPERATIVE DIAGNOSIS: (1) *Menometrorrhagia* and (2) *cervical* stenosis.
POSTOPERATIVE DIAGNOSIS: Menometrorrhagia and cervical stenosis.
OPERATION: Diagnostic (3) *hysteroscopy* and (4) *dilation and curettage* of the uterus.
DESCRIPTION OF PROCEDURE: Under adequate general anesthesia, the patient was prepped and draped in the low lithotomy position. Bimanual examination revealed the (5) *uterus* to be 6-weeks' size and midline. A speculum was placed in the (6) *vagina*, and the (7) *cervix* was grasped with a single-toothed tenaculum. It was very stenotic, and we started with the smallest dilator available and dilated up to a No. 9 Pratt. An Olympus fiberoptic (8) *hysteroscope* was then inserted, and inspection was carried out. There was extensive glandular- and abnormal-appearing tissue along the entire posterior wall of the uterus that appeared to be hyperplastic. The hysteroscope was removed from the uterus, and the cervix was then dilated. (9) *Endometrial* curettage was performed, with removal of a very large amount of glandular-appearing tissue. The patient tolerated the procedure well and left the operating room in good condition.

1. _____

2. _____

3. _____

4. _____

5. _____

6. _____

7. _____

8. _____

9. _____

EXERCISE 29

Write out the abbreviations and provide a brief description of the disease or procedure.

1. D&C _____

   DEFINITION: _____

2. PID _____

   DEFINITION: _____

3. PMS _____

   DEFINITION: _____

4. TAH _____

   DEFINITION: _____

5. TSS _____

   DEFINITION: _____

EXERCISE 30

Select the best answer for each statement or question.

1. Which structures coax the ovum into the fallopian tubes?
   a. villi
   b. fimbriae
   c. vulva
   d. adnexa

2. Which term means the outer layer of the uterus?
   a. endometrium
   b. epimetrium
   c. perimetrium
   d. myometrium

3. Select the medical term for the external genitalia.
   a. fimbriae
   b. vulva
   c. adnexa
   d. villi

4. Which term is used to describe the fallopian tubes and ovaries?
   a. fimbriae
   b. vulva
   c. adnexa
   d. villi

5. Select the term for the ovarian structures where ova mature.
   a. graafian follicles
   b. ovarian cyst
   c. adnexa
   d. ovarial follicles

6. Select the medical term for the muscle layer of the uterus.
   a. endometrium
   b. perimetrium
   c. myometrium
   d. musculometrium

7. Which female reproductive structure is commonly called the womb?
   a. vulva
   b. uterus
   c. adnexa
   d. vagina

8. Select the medical term for the onset of menstruation.
   a. menarche
   b. menses
   c. menopause
   d. menstrual period

9. Which term means the inner layer of the uterus?
   a. perimetrium
   b. endometrium
   c. myometrium
   d. endometriosis

10. Select the term for the periodic release of ovum.
    a. menstruation
    b. menses
    c. menarche
    d. ovulation

EXERCISE 31

Write the medical term for each definition.

1. physician who specializes in the growth and development of the human organism _____

2. has been pregnant many times _____

3. occurring after childbirth _____

4. first pregnancy _____

5. discharge or leaking of amniotic fluid _____

6. never has been pregnant _____

7. difficult or painful labor _____

8. inflammation of the amnion _____

9. excessive and severe vomiting during pregnancy _____

10. uterine rupture _____

11. incision into the amniotic membranes   _____

12. surgical puncture into the amniotic sac to remove fluid   _____

13. incision into the perineum to facilitate delivery   _____

14. measuring the size of the fetus before delivery   _____

15. study of the growth and development of the human organism   _____

16. physician who specializes in pregnancy and delivery   _____

17. act of giving birth   _____

18. three- to six-week time period following childbirth   _____

19. delivery presentation with buttocks appearing first   _____

20. most severe form of gestational hypertension characterized by seizures   _____

EXERCISE 32

Match the medical terms in Column 1 with the correct definition in Column 2.

COLUMN 1

_____ 1. abruptio placentae
_____ 2. Braxton Hicks contractions
_____ 3. cerclage
_____ 4. effacement
_____ 5. hydatidiform mole
_____ 6. lochia
_____ 7. meconium
_____ 8. nullipara
_____ 9. obstetrics
_____ 10. placenta previa
_____ 11. pre-eclampsia
_____ 12. Rh incompatibility
_____ 13. tubal pregnancy
_____ 14. eclampsia

COLUMN 2

a. cystic grapelike mass in the uterus
b. severe gestational hypertension
c. ectopic pregnancy
d. first feces of a newborn
e. gestational hypertension with proteinuria
f. implantation of the placenta toward the cervix
g. reaction between maternal and fetal blood
h. irregular, nonproductive contractions
i. medical specialty related to pregnancy
j. normal thinning of the cervix during childbirth
k. never having given birth to a viable fetus
l. premature separation of the placenta
m. suturing of the cervical opening
n. vaginal discharge from the uterus

EXERCISE 33

Read the following progress note and write the meaning of the italicized terms.

PROGRESS NOTE

The patient was admitted to the (1) *obstetrical* unit with contractions 5 minutes apart. According to her history, she is (2) *multigravida* and (3) *nullipara*. She has had two miscarriages and (4) *cerclage* was done at 8 weeks gestation, due to (5) *incompetent cervix*. She presents at 39 weeks gestation with (6) *amniorrhea* that is negative for (7) *meconium*. (8) *Effacement* was noted during her (9) *prenatal* visit last Friday. The patient states that she is comfortable with her current pain level. Prenatal (10) *pelvimetry* supported her decision for (11) *SVD*. However, given her history (12) *electronic fetal monitoring* is appropriate and the patient has signed a consent for a (13) *C-section*, should that be necessary.

1. _____
2. _____
3. _____
4. _____
5. _____
6. _____
7. _____
8. _____
9. _____
10. _____
11. _____
12. _____
13. _____

CHALLENGE EXERCISE

1. *Endometriosis is a painful, chronic disease that affects 5.5 million females in the United States and Canada alone. Access the Endometriosis Association's (EA) website at www.endometriosisassn.org to learn more about this condition. Prepare a handout that answers these questions: What are the symptoms, causes, and treatments for endometriosis? What languages are available for EA brochures? Does the site provide links for additional information about endometriosis? What startling discovery was made regarding toxic chemicals such as dioxin?*

2. *Amniocentesis and chorionic villus sampling (CVS) are tests that help identify fetal genetic disorders before birth. Access the American Academy of Family Physician's (AAFP) website at www.familydoctor.org to learn more about these tests. After reviewing the information, answer the following questions; What is the difference between amniocentesis and CVS? Who should consider having these tests? What are the risks involved with these tests?*

Pronunciation Review

Review the terms in the chapter. Pronounce each term using the following phonetic pronunciations. Check off the term when you are comfortable saying it.

TERM	PRONUNCIATION
☐ abortion	ah-**BOR**-shun
☐ abruptio placentae	ah-**BRUP**-shee-oh plah-**SEN**-tee
☐ amenorrhea	**ah**-men-oh-**REE**-ah
☐ amniocentesis	**am**-nee-oh-sen-**TEE**-sis
☐ amniography	**am**-nee-**OG**-rah-fee
☐ amnionitis	**am**-nee-oh-**NIGH**-tis
☐ amniorrhea	**am**-nee-oh-**REE**-ah
☐ amnioscopy	**am**-nee-**OSS**-koh-pee
☐ amniotic sac	**am**-nee-**OT**-ik sac
☐ anteflexion	an-tee-**FLEX**-shun
☐ antepartum	an-tee-**PAR**-tum
☐ Braxton Hicks contraction	**BRACKS**-ton Hicks contraction
☐ carcinoma of the breast	**kar**-sin-**OH**-mah of the breast
☐ cerclage	sar-**KLOZH**
☐ cervical carcinoma	**SER**-vih-kal **kar**-sin-**OH**-mah
☐ cervicitis	serv-vih-**SIGH**-tis
☐ cesarean section (C-section)	see-**SAYR**-ee-an section
☐ colposcopy	kol-**POSS**-koh-pee
☐ cone biopsy	cone **BIGH**-op-see
☐ conization	kon-ih-**ZAY**-shun
☐ cryosurgery	**krigh**-oh-**SER**-jer-ree
☐ cystocele	**SISS**-toh-seel
☐ dilatation and curettage	dill-ah-**TAY**-shun and koo-reh-**TAHZ**
☐ dysmenorrhea	**diss**-men-oh-**REE**-ah
☐ dystocia	diss-**TOH**-see-ah
☐ eclampsia	ee-**KLAMP**-see-ah
☐ ectopic pregnancy	ek-**TOP**-ik pregnancy
☐ effacement	eh-**FACE**-ment
☐ embryo	**EM**-bree-oh
☐ embryologist	em-bree-**ALL**-oh-jist
☐ embryology	em-bree-**ALL**-oh-jee
☐ endometriosis	**en**-doh-**mee**-tree-**OH**-sis
☐ episiotomy	eh-**pihz**-ee-**OT**-oh-mee
☐ fetal ultrasonography	**FEE**-tal **ull**-trah-soh-**NOG**-rah-fee
☐ fetometry	fee-**TOM**-eh-tree
☐ fetus	**FEE**-tus
☐ fibrocystic breast disease	**figh**-broh-**SIS**- tik breast disease
☐ gamete	**GAM**-eet
☐ gestation	jess-**TAY**-shun
☐ gestational diabetes	jess-**TAY**-shun-al digh-ah-**BEE**- teez
☐ gestational hypertension	jess-**TAY**-shun-al high-per-**TEN**-shun
☐ gynecologist	gigh-neh-**KALL**-oh-jist OR jin-eh-**KALL**-oh-jist
☐ gynecology	gigh-neh-**KALL**-oh-jee OR jin-eh-**KALL**-oh-jee

☐ hydatidiform mole	**high**-dah-**TID**-ih-form mole
☐ hyperemesis gravidarum	**high**-per-**EM**-eh-sis **grav**-ih-**DAR**-um
☐ hysterectomy	**hiss-** ter-**EK**-toh-mee
☐ hysterorrhexis	**hiss**-teh-roh-**EK**-sis
☐ hysterosalpingography	**hiss**-ter-oh-**sal**-pin-**GOG**-rah-fee
☐ laparoscopy	lap-ah-**ROSS**-koh-pee
☐ lochia	**LOH**-kee-ah
☐ mammography	mam-**OG**-rah-fee
☐ mastectomy	mass-**TEK**-toh-mee
☐ meconium	meh-**KOH**-nee-um
☐ menometrorrhagia	**men**-oh-**met**-roh-**RAY**-jee-ah
☐ menopause	**MEN**-oh-pawz
☐ menorrhagia	men-oh-**RAY**-jee-ah
☐ menorrhea	men-oh-**REE**-ah
☐ metrorrhagia	meh-troh-**RAY**-jee-ah
☐ multigravida	mull-tee-**GRAV**-ih-dah
☐ multipara	mull-**TIP**-ah-rah
☐ nulligravida	null-ee-**GRAV**-ih-dah
☐ nullipara	null-**IP**-ah-rah
☐ obstetrician	**ob**-steh-**TRISH**-an
☐ obstetrics	ob-**STEH**-triks
☐ oligomenorrhea	**oh**-lig-oh-**men**-oh-**REE**-ah
☐ oophorectomy	oh-**off**-or-**EK**-toh-mee
☐ oophoritis	oh-**off**-or-**EYE**-tis
☐ oophoropexy	oh-**off**-or-**PEK**-see
☐ ovarian carcinoma	oh-**VAY**-ree-an **kar**-sin-**OH**-mah
☐ ovarian cyst	oh-**VAY**-ree-an **SIST**
☐ ovariopexy	oh-**vay**-ree-oh-**PEK**-see
☐ ovary	**OH**-vah-ree
☐ Papanicolaou smear	pap-ah-**NIK**-oh-loh smear
☐ parturition	par-too-**RISH**-un
☐ pelvimetry	pell-**VIM**-eh-tree
☐ placenta	plah-**SEN**-tah
☐ placenta previa	plah-**SEN**-tah **PREE**-vee-ah
☐ postpartum	post-**PAR**-tum
☐ pre-eclampsia	**pree-** ee-**KLAM**-see-ah
☐ premenstrual syndrome	pree-**MEN**-strool syndrome
☐ primigravida	prigh-mih-**GRAV**-ih-dah
☐ primipara	prigh-**MIP**-ah-rah
☐ puerperium	pyoo-er-**PEE**-ree-um
☐ retroversion of the uterus	**reh-** troh-**VER**-shun of the uterus
☐ salpingitis	**sal**-pin-**JIGH**-tis
☐ salpingo-oophorectomy	sal-**ping**-oh-**oh**-off-or-**EK**-toh-mee
☐ tubal ligation	**TOO**-bal ligh-**GAY**-shun
☐ tubal pregnancy	**TOO**-bal pregnancy
☐ umbilicus	um-**BILL**-ih-kus
☐ vaginitis	vaj-in-**EYE**-tis
☐ vulvovaginitis	**vull**-voh-**vaj**-in-**EYE**-tis
☐ zygote	**ZIGH**-goht

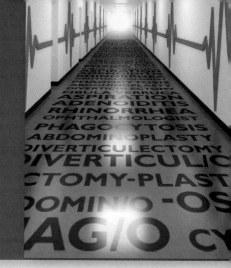

CHAPTER 14

Nervous System

OBJECTIVES

At the completion of this chapter, the student should be able to:

1. Identify, define, and spell word roots associated with the nervous system.
2. Label the basic structures of the nervous system.
3. Discuss the functions of the nervous system.
4. Provide the correct spelling of nervous system terms, given the definition of the terms.
5. Analyze nervous system terms by defining the roots, prefixes, and suffixes of these terms.
6. Identify, define, and spell disease, disorder, and procedure terms related to the nervous system.

OVERVIEW

The nervous system includes nerve cells, the brain, the spinal cord, 12 pairs of cranial nerves, and 31 pairs of spinal nerves. The brain and spinal cord are known as the **central nervous system (CNS)**. The cranial and spinal nerves are known as the **peripheral** (peh-**RIF**-er-al) **nervous system (PNS)**. Spinal nerves are also called the peripheral nerves. Figure 14-1 illustrates the divisions of the nervous system.

The structures of the nervous system function together to (1) regulate all activities of the body, (2) control consciousness, (3) detect environmental stimuli, (4) respond to environmental stimuli, (5) process and store sensory and motor information, and (6) transmit sensory and motor impulses between the brain and all parts of the body.

Nervous System Word Roots

To understand and use nervous system medical terms, it is necessary to acquire a thorough knowledge of the associated word roots. These word roots are listed with the combining vowel in Table 14-1. Review the word roots and complete the exercises that follow.

TABLE 14-1 NERVOUS SYSTEM WORD ROOTS

Word Root/Combining Form	Meaning
cephal/o	head
cerebell/o	cerebellum
cerebr/o	cerebrum
crani/o	cranium; skull

(continues)

TABLE 14-1 NERVOUS SYSTEM WORD ROOTS (continued)

Word Root/Combining Form	Meaning
dendr/o	branching
encephal/o	brain
gli/o	neuroglia; nerve cell
mening/o	meninges
myel/o	spinal cord (also bone marrow)
neur/o	nerve
olig/o	few; diminished amount
thec/o	sheath
ventricul/o	ventricle

© 2016 Cengage Learning®

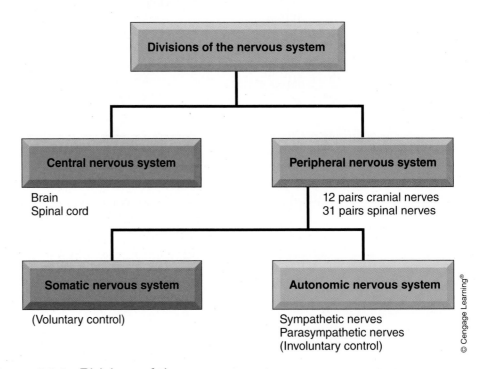

Figure 14-1 Divisions of the nervous system.

EXERCISE 1

Write the definitions of the following word roots.

1. encephal/o _____

2. crani/o _____

3. cerebell/o _____

4. neur/o _____

5. mening/o _____

6. cerebr/o   _____

7. gli/o   _____

8. olig/o   _____

9. dendr/o   _____

10. myel/o   _____

EXERCISE 2

Write the nervous system word root(s) and meanings for each term.

1. craniotomy

   ROOT: _____ MEANING: _____

2. neuropathy

   ROOT: _____ MEANING: _____

3. intrathecal

   ROOT: _____ MEANING: _____

4. cephalalgia

   ROOT: _____ MEANING: _____

5. cerebrovascular

   ROOT: _____ MEANING: _____

6. meningitis

   ROOT: _____ MEANING: _____

7. glioma

   ROOT: _____ MEANING: _____

8. myeloma

   ROOT: _____ MEANING: _____

9. oligodendroglia

   ROOT: _____ MEANING: _____

   ROOT: _____ MEANING: _____

10. ventriculitis

   ROOT: _____ MEANING: _____

EXERCISE 3

Write the correct word root(s) for the following definitions.

1. brain   _____

2. cerebellum   _____

3. cerebrum   _____

4. cranium   _____

5. head _____

6. meninges _____

7. nerve _____

8. nerve cell _____

9. sheath _____

10. spinal cord _____

11. ventricle _____

Cells of the Nervous System

Nerve cells are the basic structure or unit of the nervous system. There are two general categories of nerve cells: **neurons** (**NOO**-ronz), which transmit nerve impulses from the body to the brain and back to the body, and **neuroglia** (noo-**ROG**-lee-ah), the nerve cells that support the nervous system.

Neurons consist of a (1) **cell body** that contains the cell nucleus; (2) **dendrites** (**DEN**-drights), which are branchlike structures that receive impulses and send them to the cell body; an (3) **axon** (**ACKS**-on), which sends impulses away from the cell body; (4) **myelin** (**MIGH**-eh-lin), a white fatty tissue that covers the axon; and (5) **terminal end fibers**, branching fibers that lead the impulse away from the axon. The space between neurons or a neuron and an organ is called a (6) **synapse** (**SIN**-apps). Figure 14-2 illustrates a neuron.

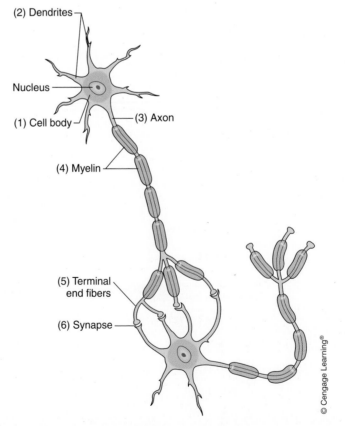

© Cengage Learning®

Figure 14-2 Structures of a neuron.

Neuroglia are the supportive and connective cells of the nervous system and do not conduct impulses. There are three types of neuroglial cells: (1) **astrocytes** (**ASS**-troh-sights), (2) **microglia** (my-**KROG**-lee-ah), and (3) **oligodendroglia** (**all**-ih-goh-den-**DROG**-lee-ah). Figure 14-3 illustrates the neuroglia.

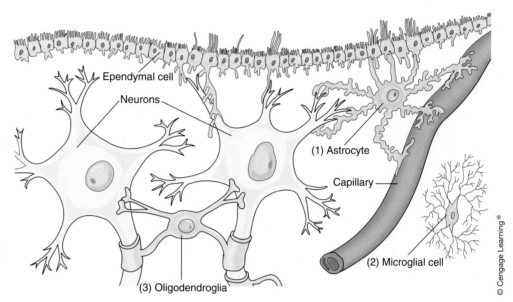

Figure 14-3   Neuroglial cells.

EXERCISE 4

Label the parts of the neuron shown in Figure 14-4. Write your answers in the spaces provided.

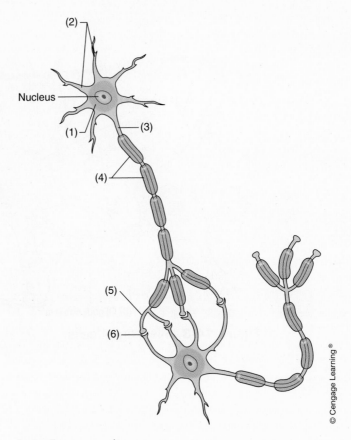

Nucleus

Figure 14-4   Labeling exercise.

1. _____

2. _____

3. _____

4. _____

5. _____

6. _____

Brain and Spinal Cord

As previously stated, the brain and spinal cord are known as the *central nervous system*. The brain weighs about three pounds and controls almost every physical and mental activity of the body. The spinal cord is a tubelike structure that begins at the end of the brainstem and continues almost to the bottom of the spinal column. The spinal cord is protected by the vertebral column, **meninges** (meh-**NIN**-jeez), and **cerbrospinal fluid**. Meninges are layers of tissue that surround the brain and spinal cord. Cerbrospinal fluid flows in and around the brain and spinal cord. These components of the nervous system are described later in this chapter. The parts of the brain are illustrated in Figure 14-5. Refer to this figure as you learn about these structures.

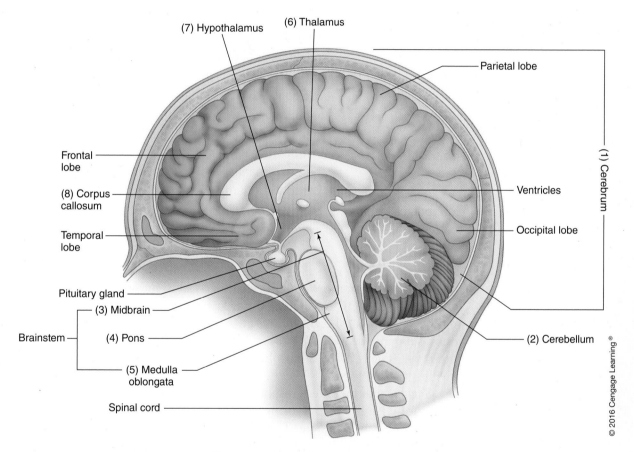

Figure 14-5   Structures of the brain.

Major structures of the brain include the (1) **cerebrum** (seh-**REE**-brum), (2) **cerebellum** (ser-eh-**BELL**-um), (3) **midbrain**, (4) **pons** (PONZ), (5) **medulla oblongata** (meh-**DULL**-ah ob-long-**AH**-tah), (6) **thalamus** (**THAL**-ah-mus), (7) **hypothalamus** (**high**-poh-**THAL**-ah-mus), and (8) **corpus callosum** (**KOR**-pus kal-**OH**-sum). The midbrain, pons, and medulla oblongata are collectively known as the **brainstem**. Table 14-2 lists the parts of the brain and describes their functions.

TABLE 14-2   PARTS OF THE BRAIN WITH DESCRIPTIONS

Parts of the Brain	Description
cerebrum	largest section of the brain; controls consciousness, memory, sensations, emotions, and voluntary movement
cerebellum	attaches the brain to the brainstem; maintains muscle tone, movement, and balance; sometimes called the "tree of life"
midbrain	area of the brain that provides nerve-conduction pathways to and from the brain
pons	literally means "bridge"; nerve cells cross from one side of the brain to control the opposite side of the body
medulla oblongata	lowest section of the brainstem; controls the muscles of respiration, heart rate, and blood pressure
thalamus	relays nerve impulses to and from the cerebral cortex and the sense organs of the body
hypothalamus	regulates heart rate, blood pressure, respiratory rate, digestive activities, emotional responses, behavior, body temperature, water balance and thirst, sleep-wake cycles, hunger sensations, and endocrine system activities; often called the "thermostat" of the body
corpus callosum	structure that connects the two hemispheres of the brain

© 2016 Cengage Learning®

The cerebrum is divided into right and left hemispheres. The **cerebral cortex** (seh-**REE**-bral **KOR**-teks) is the outer layer of the cerebrum; it is characterized by folds and grooves. The cerebral cortex folds are called **gyri** (**JIGH**-righ), and the grooves are called **sulci** (**SULL**-kigh), or fissures. A single fold is a gyrus, and a single groove is a sulcus. Each hemisphere of the cerebrum has four distinct lobes, which are illustrated in Figure 14-6.

The (1) **frontal lobe** is responsible for motor function. The (2) **temporal** (**TEM**-por-al) **lobe** is responsible for hearing and smell. The (3) **occipital** (ok-**SIP**-ih-tal) **lobe** is responsible for sight. The (4) **parietal** (pah-**RIGH**-eh-tal) **lobe** receives and interprets nerve impulses from the sensory receptors located throughout the body.

Nerve fibers in the brainstem cross over each other so that the brain hemispheres control the side of the body opposite to the name of the hemisphere. Figure 14-7 illustrates the hemispheres of the brain. The (1) **right hemisphere** controls most of the function on the *left* side of the body. An injury to the right hemisphere may result in sensory or motor deficits on the left side of the body. The (2) **left hemisphere** controls most of the functions on the *right* side of the body. An injury to the left hemisphere may result in sensory or motor deficits on the right side of the body.

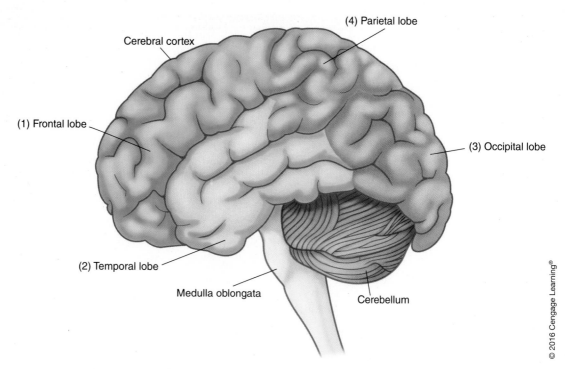

Figure 14-6   Lobes of the cerebrum.

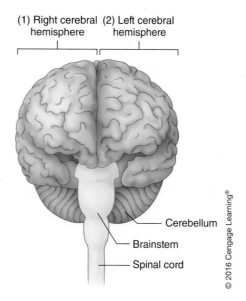

Figure 14-7   Right and left hemispheres of the brain.

Label the structures of the brain shown in Figure 14-8. Write your answers on the spaces provided.

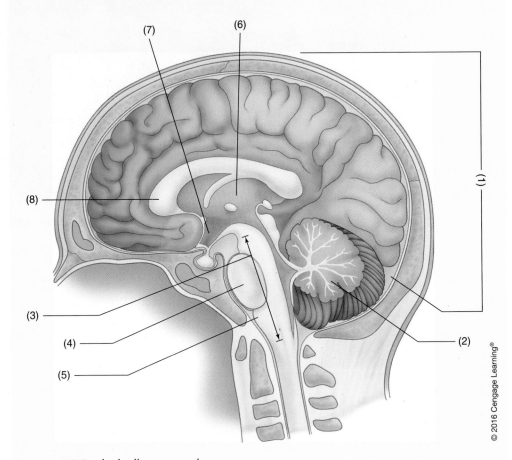

Figure 14-8 Labeling exercise.

1. _____
2. _____
3. _____
4. _____
5. _____
6. _____
7. _____
8. _____

EXERCISE 6

Match the medical term in Column 1 with the correct definition in Column 2.

COLUMN 1

_____ 1. cerebellum

_____ 2. cerebral cortex

_____ 3. cerebrum

_____ 4. corpus callosum

_____ 5. frontal lobe

_____ 6. gyri

_____ 7. hypothalamus

_____ 8. medulla oblongata

_____ 9. occipital lobe

_____ 10. pons

_____ 11. sulci

_____ 12. temporal lobe

_____ 13. thalamus

COLUMN 2

a. attaches the brain to the brainstem

b. connects the two hemispheres of the brain

c. folds of the cerebral cortex

d. grooves of the cerebral cortex

e. largest section of the brain

f. literally means "bridge"

g. lowest section of the brainstem

h. outer layer of the cerebrum

i. relays impulses between the cerebral cortex and sense organs

j. responsible for hearing and smell

k. responsible for motor function

l. responsible for sight

m. "thermostat" of the body

Meninges and Cerebrospinal Fluid

The **meninges** (men-**IN**-jeez) are three layers of membranes that surround and protect the brain and spinal cord. The meninges are illustrated in Figure 14-9. The outer membrane layer is the (1) **dura mater** (**DOO**-rah **MAY**-ter), which is a tough, white connective tissue just beneath the skull. The middle layer is the (2) **arachnoid** (ah-**RAK**-noyd) **membrane**, a weblike tissue with several strands that attach to the inner membrane layer. The inner membrane layer is the (3) **pia mater** (**PEE**-ah **MAY**-ter), which is attached directly to the surface of the brain and spinal cord.

(4) **Cerebrospinal** (seh-**ree**-broh-**SPIGH**-nal) **fluid (CSF)** flows in and around the brain and spinal cord. CSF is produced by specialized capillaries within the **ventricles**, open spaces located in the middle region of the cerebrum. Cerebrospinal fluid cushions the brain and spinal cord and also provides some nutrition to those structures.

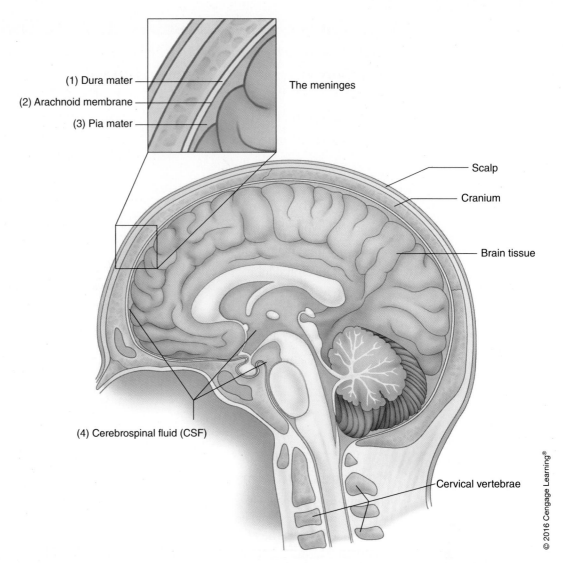

(1) Dura mater
(2) Arachnoid membrane
(3) Pia mater

The meninges

Scalp

Cranium

Brain tissue

(4) Cerebrospinal fluid (CSF)

Cervical vertebrae

© 2016 Cengage Learning®

Figure 14-9 Meninges and cerebrospinal fluid.

Cranial and Spinal Nerves

As stated previously, the 12 pairs of cranial nerves and 31 pairs of spinal nerve are known as the *peripheral nervous system* (PNS). The peripheral nervous system transmits information from all parts of the body to the brain and back to the body. **Afferent**, or **sensory**, nerves carry impulses from the body to the brain, and **efferent**, or **motor**, nerves carry impulses from the brain to the appropriate body structure.

The peripheral nervous system is further classified as the **somatic** (soh-**MAT**-ik) **nervous system** (**SNS**) and the **autonomic** (ot-oh-**NOM**-ik) **nervous system** (**ANS**). The somatic nervous system is responsible for voluntary movements and also for responses such as walking, talking, and swimming. The autonomic nervous system is responsible for involuntary movement and responses such as hormone secretion, heart rate, blood flow, and digestive system functions. Figure 14-10 illustrates the body areas and functions that are controlled by the autonomic nervous system.

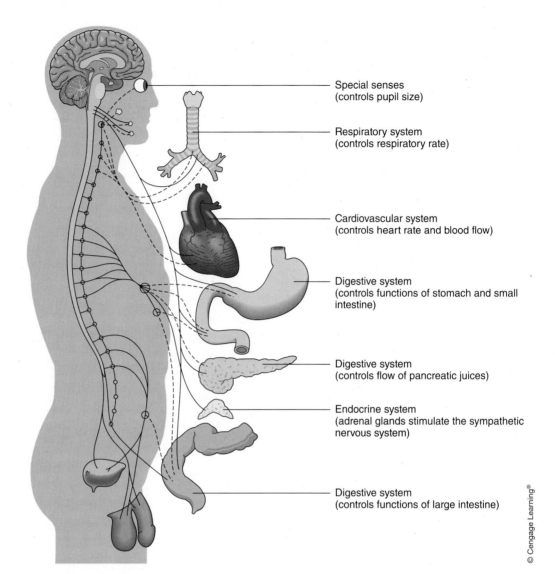

Special senses
(controls pupil size)

Respiratory system
(controls respiratory rate)

Cardiovascular system
(controls heart rate and blood flow)

Digestive system
(controls functions of stomach and small
intestine)

Digestive system
(controls flow of pancreatic juices)

Endocrine system
(adrenal glands stimulate the sympathetic
nervous system)

Digestive system
(controls functions of large intestine)

© Cengage Learning®

Figure 14-10   Body areas affected by the autonomic nervous system.

The cranial nerves are numbered from 1 to 12, using Roman numerals. Table 14-3 lists the cranial nerves and provides a brief description of their functions. Figure 14-11 illustrates the body areas affected by the 12 pairs of cranial nerves.

TABLE 14-3 CRANIAL NERVES

Cranial Nerves	Description
I olfactory nerve (ohl-**FAK**-tor-ee)	transmits sensory impulses necessary for the sense of smell
II optic nerve (**OP**-tik)	transmits sensory impulses necessary for sight
III oculomotor nerve (**ok**-yoo-loh-**MOH**-tor)	transmits impulses necessary for eye movement
IV trochlear nerve (**TROK**-lee-ar)	transmits impulses necessary for eye movement and eye muscle sensations
V trigeminal nerve (trigh-**JEM**-ih-nal)	transmits impulses necessary for chewing and facial sensations
VI abducens nerve (ab-**DOO**-senz)	transmits impulses necessary to turn the eyeball outward or away from the midline
VII facial nerve (**FAY**-shee-al)	transmits impulses to the scalp, forehead, eyelids, cheek, jaw, and other facial muscles
VIII acoustic nerve (ah-**KOO**-stik)	transmits impulses necessary for hearing and balance; also called the *auditory nerve*
IX glossopharyngeal nerve (**gloss**-oh-fair-in-**JEE**-al)	transmits impulses necessary for taste, some sensations from the viscera, and secretions from some glands
X vagus nerve (**VAY**-gus)	transmits impulses necessary for speech, swallowing, as well as the activity of cardiac muscle, smooth muscle, and glands and ducts of the endocrine system
XI accessory nerve	transmits impulses necessary for speech, swallowing, and some head and shoulder movements
XII hypoglossal nerve (**high**-poh-**GLOSS**-al)	transmits impulses necessary for swallowing and moving the tongue

© 2016 Cengage Learning®

The 31 pairs of spinal or peripheral nerves transmit impulses to all parts of the body. The spinal nerves are attached to the spinal cord and exit the vertebral column through openings between the vertebrae. These nerves have many branches that eventually reach every part of the body.

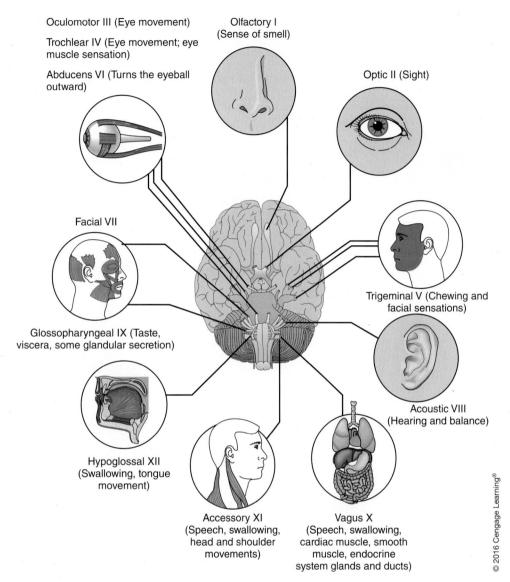

Oculomotor III (Eye movement)

Trochlear IV (Eye movement; eye muscle sensation)

Abducens VI (Turns the eyeball outward)

Olfactory I (Sense of smell)

Optic II (Sight)

Facial VII

Trigeminal V (Chewing and facial sensations)

Glossopharyngeal IX (Taste, viscera, some glandular secretion)

Acoustic VIII (Hearing and balance)

Hypoglossal XII (Swallowing, tongue movement)

Accessory XI (Speech, swallowing, head and shoulder movements)

Vagus X (Speech, swallowing, cardiac muscle, smooth muscle, endocrine system glands and ducts)

© 2016 Cengage Learning®

Figure 14-11 Body areas and functions affected by the cranial nerves.

Write the medical term for each definition.

1. membranes that surround and protect the brain and spinal cord

   _____

2. weblike membrane located between the outer and inner membrane

   _____

3. outer membrane just beneath the skull

   _____

4. inner membrane attached directly to the surface of the brain

   _____

5. fluid that flows around the brain and spinal cord

   _____

6. nerves that carry impulses from the body to the brain

   _____

7. nerves that carry impulses from the brain to the body structures

   _____

8. 12 pairs of nerves that are identified by name and number

   _____

9. 31 pairs of nerves that are also called peripheral nerves

   _____

Write out the following abbreviations.

1. ANS _____

2. CSF _____

3. PNS _____

4. SNS _____

Nervous System Medical Terminology

Nervous system medical terms are organized into three main categories: (1) general medical terms; (2) disease and condition terms; and (3) diagnostic procedure, surgery, and laboratory test terms. The roots, prefixes, and suffixes associated with the nervous system are listed in Table 14-4. Review these word parts and complete the related exercises.

TABLE 14-4   ROOTS, PREFIXES, AND SUFFIXES FOR NERVOUS SYSTEM TERMS

Root	Meaning	Prefix	Meaning	Suffix	Meaning
arachn/o	spider	an-; a-	lack of; without	-algia	pain
electr/o	electricity	dura-	hard	-cele	hernia; protrusion
hemat/o	blood	echo-	sound	-gram	picture; record
hydr/o	water; fluid	epi-	above; upon	-graphy	process of recording
quadr/i	four	hemi-	half	-itis	inflammation
thromb/o	clot	poly-	many	-malacia	softening
		sub-	beneath; below	-oma	tumor
				-osis	condition
				-(o)tomy	incision into
				-paresis	partial paralysis
				-pathy	disease
				-plegia	paralysis

EXERCISE 8

Write and define the root(s), prefix, and suffix for each medical term. Note: *Anencephaly has the noun ending -y as a suffix. Based on the meaning of the word parts, write a definition for each term. Check the definition in a medical dictionary.*

1. anencephaly

    ROOT: _____ MEANING: _____

    PREFIX: _____MEANING:_____

    SUFFIX: _____MEANING:_____

    DEFINITION: _____

2. cephalalgia

    ROOT: _____ MEANING: _____

    PREFIX:_____ MEANING: _____

    SUFFIX:_____ MEANING: _____

    DEFINITION: _____

3. cerebromalacia

    ROOT: _____ MEANING: _____

    PREFIX: _____ MEANING: _____

    SUFFIX: _____ MEANING: _____

    DEFINITION: _____

4. electromyelography

ROOT: _____ MEANING: _____

PREFIX: _____ MEANING: _____

SUFFIX: _____ MEANING: _____

DEFINITION: _____

5. epidural

ROOT: _____ MEANING: _____

PREFIX: _____ MEANING: _____

SUFFIX: _____ MEANING: _____

DEFINITION: _____

6. hematoma

ROOT: _____ MEANING: _____

PREFIX: _____ MEANING: _____

SUFFIX: _____ MEANING: _____

DEFINITION: _____

7. hydrocephalus

ROOT: _____ MEANING: _____

PREFIX: _____ MEANING: _____

SUFFIX: _____ MEANING: _____

DEFINITION: _____

8. meningocele

ROOT: _____ MEANING: _____

PREFIX: _____ MEANING: _____

SUFFIX: _____ MEANING: _____

DEFINITION: _____

9. neuritis

ROOT: _____ MEANING: _____

PREFIX: _____ MEANING: _____

SUFFIX: _____ MEANING: _____

DEFINITION: _____

10. thrombosis

ROOT: _____ MEANING: _____

PREFIX: _____ MEANING: _____

SUFFIX: _____ MEANING: _____

DEFINITION: _____

Nervous System General Medical Terms

Review the pronunciation and meaning of each term in Table 14-5. Note that some terms are built from word parts and some are not. Complete the exercises for these terms.

TABLE 14-5 NERVOUS SYSTEM GENERAL MEDICAL TERMS

Term with Pronunciation	Definition
afferent nerves (**AFF**-er-ent)	nerves that carry impulses toward the brain
cauda equina (**KAW**-dah ee-**KWIGH**-nah)	lower end of the spinal cord and spinal nerve roots; resembles a horse's tail
cerebral (seh-**REE**-bral) cerebr/o = cerebrum -al = pertaining to	pertaining to the cerebrum
craniocerebral (**kray**-nee-oh-seh-**REE**-bral) crani/o = skull; cranium cerebr/o = cerebrum -al = pertaining to	pertaining to the cranium or skull and cerebrum
efferent nerves (**EE**-fair-ent)	nerves that carry impulses away from the brain
epidural (ep-ih-**DOO**-ral) epi- = above; over dura- = hard -al = pertaining to	above or over the dura mater
neurologist (noo-**RALL**-oh-jist) neur/o = nerve -(o)logist = specialist	physician who specializes in nervous system diseases
neurology (noo-**RALL**-oh-jee) neur/o = nerve -(o)logy = study of	medical specialty related to diseases and disorders of the nervous system
neurosurgeon (**noo**-roh-**SER**-jun) neur/o = nerve	surgeon who specializes in surgical techniques related to the nervous system

(continues)

TABLE 14-5 NERVOUS SYSTEM GENERAL MEDICAL TERMS (continued)

Term with Pronunciation	Definition
neurosurgery (**noo**-roh-**SER**-jer-ree) neur/o = nerve	surgical specialty related to diseases and disorders of the nervous system; any nervous system surgery
plexus (**PLECKS**-us)	network of interwoven nerves
subarachnoid (sub-ah-**RAK**-noyd) sub- = beneath; below arachn/o = spider -oid = like; resembling	beneath or below the arachnoid membrane
subdural (sub-**DOO**-ral) sub- = beneath; below dura- = hard -al = pertaining to	beneath or below the dura mater
ventricle (**VEN**-trih-kal)	small hollow or space within the brain that is filled with cerebrospinal fluid

© 2016 Cengage Learning®

EXERCISE 9

Analyze each term by writing the prefix, root, combining vowel, and suffix separated by vertical slashes. Based on the meaning of the word parts, write a definition for each term. Check the definition in a medical dictionary. Note that some terms might have more than one root.

EXAMPLE: cerebromalacia

	/ cerebr	/ o	/ malacia
prefix	*root*	*combining vowel*	*suffix*

DEFINITION: softening of the cerebrum

1. craniocerebral

prefix	*root*	*combining vowel*	*suffix*

DEFINITION: _____

2. epidural

prefix	*root*	*combining vowel*	*suffix*

DEFINITION: _____

3. neurologist

prefix	root	combining vowel	suffix
DEFINITION: _____

4. neurology

prefix	root	combining vowel	suffix
DEFINITION: _____

5. subarachnoid

prefix	root	combining vowel	suffix
DEFINITION: _____

6. subdural

prefix	root	combining vowel	suffix
DEFINITION: _____

7. cerebral

prefix	root	combining vowel	suffix
DEFINITION: _____

EXERCISE 10

Write the medical term for each definition.

1. carrying impulses away from the brain   _____
2. carrying impulses toward the brain   _____
3. lower end of the spinal cord   _____
4. network of interwoven nerves   _____
5. any nervous system surgery   _____
6. space or hollow within the brain   _____
7. specialist in nervous system surgery   _____

Nervous System Disease and Disorder Terms

Nervous system diseases and disorders include familiar problems such as headaches as well as more complex and less familiar diagnoses such as encephalomalacia. The medical terms are presented in alphabetical order in Table 14-6. Review the pronunciation and definition for each term and complete the exercises.

TABLE 14-6 NERVOUS SYSTEM DISEASE AND DISORDER TERMS

Term with Pronunciation	Definition
Alzheimer's disease (**ALTS**-high-merz)	progressive, extremely debilitating deterioration of an individual's intellectual functioning
amyotrophic lateral sclerosis (ALS) (ah-migh-oh-**TROFF**-ik **LAT**-er-al skleh-**ROH**-sis)	severe weakening and wasting of various muscle groups due to loss of motor neuron function in the brainstem and spinal cord
anencephaly (an-en-**SEFF**-ah-lee) an- = lack of; absence encephal/o = brain -y = noun ending	congenital absence of the brain and, in some cases, the spinal cord
ataxia (ah-**TAK**-see-ah)	lacking muscular coordination, especially voluntary muscle movement
Bell's palsy (Bell's **PALL**-zee)	weakness or paralysis of the muscles of one side of the face
cephalalgia (seff-al-**AL**-jee-ah) cephal/o = head -algia = pain	pain in the head; headache
cerebral aneurysm (seh-**REE**-bral **AN**-yoo-rizm)	dilatation of a cerebral artery that might put pressure on cerebral tissue and interfere with cerebral function
cerebral hemorrhage (seh-**REE**-bral **HEM**-oh-rij) hem/o = blood -(r)rhage = bursting forth	bursting forth of blood into cerebral tissue due to rupture of a cerebral vessel (Figure14-12)
cerebral palsy (CP) (seh-**REE**-bral **PALL**-zee)	lack of voluntary muscle control and/or coordination caused by a lack of oxygen to the brain at or near the time of birth

(continues)

TABLE 14-6   NERVOUS SYSTEM DISEASE AND DISORDER TERMS (continued)

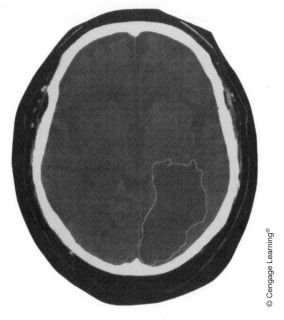

© Cengage Learning®

Figure 14-12   Cerebral hemorrhage, lower-right area.

Term with Pronunciation	Definition
cerebral thrombosis (seh-**REE**-bral throm-**BOH**-sis) thromb/o = clot -osis = condition	presence of an atherosclerotic clot in a cerebral blood vessel that causes death of a specific portion of brain tissue
cerebrovascular accident (CVA) (seh-**REE**-broh-**VASS**-kyoo-lar) cerebr/o = brain vascul/o = vessel -al = pertaining to	occlusion or rupture of a cerebral blood vessel resulting in decreased blood flow to the affected area and death of a specific portion of brain tissue; a *stroke*
concussion (kon-**KUSH**-on)	violent jarring, shaking, or other blunt nonpenetrating injury to the brain; may or may not involve loss of consciousness
contusion (kon-**TOO**-zhun)	small venous hemorrhages in the brain caused by the brain striking the cranium; also called a bruise
dementia (deh-**MEN**-shee-ah)	progressive, irreversible deterioration of memory, judgment, and other thought processes

(continues)

TABLE 14-6   NERVOUS SYSTEM DISEASE AND DISORDER TERMS (continued)

Term with Pronunciation	Definition
encephalitis (**en**-seff-ah-**LIGH**-tis) encephal/o = brain -itis = inflammation	inflammation of the brain
encephalomalacia (**en**-seff-ah-loh-mah-**LAY**-shee-ah) encephal/o = brain -malacia = softening	softening of brain tissue
encephalopathy (**en**-seff-ah-**LOP**-ah-thee) encephal/o = brain -pathy = disease	any disease of the brain
epidural hematoma (ep-ih-**DOO**-ral **hee**-mah-**TOH**-ah) epi- = above dura- = dura mater -al = pertaining to hemat/o = blood -oma = tumor	a swelling or mass of blood between the cranium and dura mater that applies pressure on the brain tissue in the affected area (Figure 14-13)

© 2016 Cengage Learning®

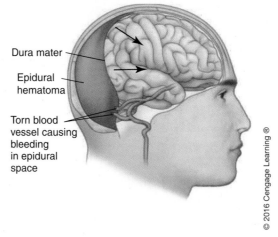

Dura mater

Epidural
hematoma

Torn blood
vessel causing
bleeding
in epidural
space

© 2016 Cengage Learning ®

Figure 14-13   Epidural hematoma.

EXERCISE 11

Analyze each term by writing the prefix, root, combining vowel, and suffix separated by vertical slashes. Based on the meaning of the word parts, write a definition for each term. Check the definition in a medical dictionary.

1. anencephaly

   _____

   prefix   *root*   *combining vowel*   *suffix*

   DEFINITION: _____

2. cephalalgia

   _____

   prefix   .   *root*   *combining vowel*   *suffix*

   DEFINITION: _____

3. encephalitis

   _____

   prefix   *root*   *combining vowel*   *suffix*

   DEFINITION: _____

4. encephalomalacia

   _____

   prefix   *root*   *combining vowel*   *suffix*

   DEFINITION: _____

5. encephalopathy

   _____

   prefix   *root*   *combining vowel*   *suffix*

   DEFINITION: _____

EXERCISE 12

Replace the italicized phrase or abbreviation with the correct medical term.

1. The computed tomography (CT) scan revealed a *dilation of a cerebral artery.*

   _____

2. Erik sustained a *blunt nonpenetrating injury to the brain* as a result of being struck with a baseball.

   _____

3. Shayna's diagnosis of *facial muscle paralysis* was established by her family physician.

   _____

4. After a *stroke,* Victoria was paralyzed on her left side.

   _____

5. An *atherosclerotic clot* resulted in temporal lobe brain tissue death.

   _____

6. *ALS* is also called Lou Gehrig's disease, after the famous baseball player who had this condition.

_____

7. Bridget was diagnosed with *CP* as a result of a lack of oxygen during delivery.

_____

Review the pronunciation and definition for each term in Table 14-7 and complete the exercises.

TABLE 14-7   NERVOUS SYSTEM DISEASE AND DISORDER TERMS

Term with Pronunciation	Definition
epilepsy (**EP**-ih-lep-see)	recurring episodes of excessive or irregular electrical activity of the central nervous system; commonly called *seizures*
glioma (gligh-**OH**-mah) gli/o = neuroglia; nerve cell -oma = tumor	malignant tumor of neuroglial cells
Guillain-Barré syndrome (**GEE**-yon bah-**RAY SIN**-drohm)	disorder in which the body's immune system attacks part of the peripheral nervous system, causing tingling and weakness in both legs; the weakness and abnormal sensations can travel to the arms and other areas of the body resulting in partial or total paralysis; in severe cases, the inflammation can affect respiration, heart rate, and blood pressure
hemiparesis (**hem**-ee-pah-**REE**-sis) hemi- = half -paresis = partial paralysis	partial paralysis of one side of the body
hemiplegia (**hem**-ee-**PLEE**-jee-ah) hemi- = half -plegia = paralysis	paralysis of one side of the body

(continues)

TABLE 14-7   NERVOUS SYSTEM DISEASE AND DISORDER TERMS (continued)

Term with Pronunciation	Definition
Huntington's disease (HD)	genetic disorder characterized by progressive, irreversible degeneration of cerebral neurons that results in uncontrolled movements, loss of intellectual capabilities, and emotional disturbances; also called *Huntington's chorea*
hydrocephalus (**high**-droh-**SEFF**-ah-lus) hydr/o = water; fluid cephal/o = head -us = noun ending	abnormal accumulation of cerebrospinal fluid around the brain, often causing swelling of the head; commonly called "water on the brain"
meningioma (men-**in**-jee-**OH**-mah) mening/o = meninges -oma = tumor	slow-growth tumor of the meninges of the brain, primarily from the arachnoid membrane
meningitis (**men**-in-**JIGH**-tis) mening/o = meninges; -itis = inflammation	infection or inflammation of the membranes covering the brain or spinal cord (meninges); may be bacterial or viral and is characterized by severe headache, vomiting, and pain and stiffness in the neck (Figure 14-14)
meningocele (men-**IN**-goh-seel) mening/o = meninges -cele = hernia; protrusion	herniation of the meninges through a hole in the skull or vertebral column
meningomyelocele (men-**in**-goh-my-**ELL**-oh-seel) mening/o = meninges myel/o = spinal cord -cele = hernia; protrusion	herniation of the spinal cord and meninges through a defect in the vertebral column
multiple sclerosis (MS) (sklair-**OH**-sis)	degenerative inflammatory disease of the central nervous system that attacks the myelin sheath of the spinal cord and brain, resulting in hardening and scarring
myelomalacia (**migh**-eh-loh-mah-**LAY**-shee-ah) myel/o = spinal cord -malacia = softening	abnormal softening of the spinal cord

(continues)

TABLE 14-7 NERVOUS SYSTEM DISEASE AND DISORDER TERMS (continued)

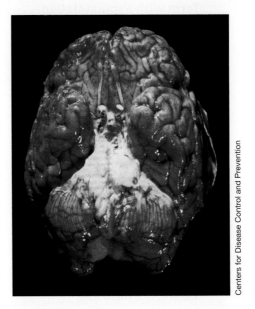

Centers for Disease Control and Prevention

Figure 14-14 Meningitis cerebral tissue damage (Centers for Disease Control and Prevention).

Term with Pronunciation	Definition
neuralgia (noo-**RAL**-jee-ah) neur/o = nerve -algia = pain	severe sharp pain of a nerve or along the course of a nerve
neuritis (noo-**RIGH**-tis) neur/o = nerve -itis = inflammation	inflammation of nerve or nerves

EXERCISE 13

Analyze each term by writing the prefix, root, combining vowel, and suffix separated by vertical slashes. Based on the meaning of the word parts, write a definition for each term. Check the definition in a medical dictionary.

1. glioma

prefix	*root*	*combining vowel*	*suffix*

DEFINITION: _____

2. hemiplegia

prefix	*root*	*combining vowel*	*suffix*

DEFINITION: _____

3. hydrocephalus

prefix	root	combining vowel	suffix
DEFINITION: _____

4. meningioma

prefix	root	combining vowel	suffix
DEFINITION: _____

5. meningitis

prefix	root	combining vowel	suffix
DEFINITION: _____

6. meningocele

prefix	root	combining vowel	suffix
DEFINITION: _____

7. meningomyelocele

prefix	root	combining vowel	suffix
DEFINITION: _____

8. neuralgia

prefix	root	combining vowel	suffix
DEFINITION: _____

9. neuritis

prefix	root	combining vowel	suffix
DEFINITION: _____

EXERCISE 14

Replace the italicized phrase or abbreviation with the correct medical term.

1. Lillian's diagnosis was a _malignant tumor of neuroglial cells._

   _____

2. _MS_ is a debilitating disease that often strikes young adults.

   _____

3. Armando's _seizure disorder_ was successfully treated with medication.

   _____

4. _Inflammation of the meninges_ can result in severe brain damage.

   _____

5. The cause of _an acute inflammation of many nerves of the peripheral nervous system_ is unknown.

   _____

6. *Paralysis of one side of the body* can be the result of a stroke.

_____

7. Belinda's *abnormal accumulation of cerebrospinal fluid around the brain* was relieved by the placement of a shunt.

_____

Review the pronunciation and definition for each term in Table 14-8 and complete the exercises.

TABLE 14-8 NERVOUS SYSTEM DISEASE AND DISORDER TERMS

Term with Pronunciation	Definition
neuroblastoma (**noo**-roh-blast-**OH**-mah) neur/o = nerve blast/o = embryonic state of development -oma = tumor	highly malignant tumor composed of cells derived from embryonic neural tissue; usually occurs in young children
neuropathy (noo-**ROP**-ah-thee) neur/o = nerve -pathy = disease	any disease of the nerves
paraplegia (**pair**-ah-**PLEE**-jee-ah) para- = around -plegia = paralysis	paralysis of the lower half of the body, including the legs
Parkinson's disease	chronic, progressive nervous disease characterized by tremor, muscular weakness, and rigidity
poliomyelitis (**poh**-lee-oh-**migh**-eh-**LIGH**-tis)	infectious viral disease that affects the motor (efferent) neurons of the brain and spinal cord, resulting in muscle paralysis and wasting
polyneuritis (**pall**-ee-noo-**RIGH**-tis) poly- = many neur/o = nerve -itis = inflammation	inflammation of many nerves or nerve fibers
postpolio syndrome (**post-POH**-lee-oh **SIN**-drom)	slow, progressive weakening of muscles that occurs in approximately 25% of poliomyelitis survivors 20–30 years after the initial illness

(continues)

TABLE 14-8 NERVOUS SYSTEM DISEASE AND DISORDER TERMS (continued)

Term with Pronunciation	Definition
quadriplegia (**kwad**-rih-**PLEE**-jee-ah) quadr/i = four -plegia = paralysis	paralysis of all four limbs, usually resulting from a spinal cord injury
Reye's syndrome (**RIGH's SIN**-drohm)	acute encephalopathy following an acute viral infection
sciatica (sigh-**AT**-ih-kah)	severe pain along the course of the sciatic nerve, from the back of the thigh and down the inside of the leg
seizure (**SEE**-zhoor)	excessive irregular electrical activity of the central nervous system associated with epilepsy
shingles; herpes zoster (**HER**-peez **ZOSS**-ter)	acute viral infection characterized by an inflammation of a spinal or cranial nerve pathway that produces painful vesicular eruptions on the skin (Figure 14-15)

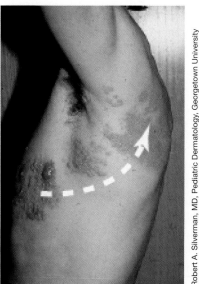

Robert A. Silverman, MD, Pediatric Dermatology, Georgetown University

Figure 14-15 Shingles (Robert A. Silverman, MD, pediatric dermatology, Georgetown University).

(continues)

TABLE 14-8 NERVOUS SYSTEM DISEASE AND DISORDER TERMS (continued)

Term with Pronunciation	Definition
subdural hematoma (sub-**DOO**-ral **hee**-mah-**TOH**-mah) sub- = beneath; below dura- = hard -al = pertaining to hemat/o = blood -oma = tumor	collection of blood below the dura mater and above the arachnoid membrane, usually the result of a closed head injury (Figure 14-16)

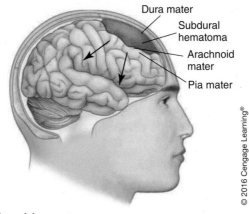

Dura mater
Subdural hematoma
Arachnoid mater
Pia mater

© 2016 Cengage Learning®

Figure 14-16 Subdural hematoma.

syncope (**SIN**-koh-pee)	loss of consciousness due to a lack of blood supply to the brain; fainting
transient ischemic attack (TIA) (iss-**KEE**-mik)	temporary interference or interruption of the blood supply to a portion of the brain
trigeminal neuralgia; tic douloureaux (trigh-**JEM**-ih-nal noo-**RAL**-jee-ah; **TIK DOO**-loh-roo)	severe pain that radiates along the fifth cranial nerve (trigeminal nerve) and usually affects one side of the head and face

© 2016 Cengage Learning®

EXERCISE 15

Write the medical term for each definition.

1. any disease of the nerves   _____

2. paralysis of the lower half of the body   _____

3. inflammation of many nerves   _____

4. paralysis of all four limbs   _____

5. severe pain along the sciatic nerve   _____

6. fainting   _____

EXERCISE 16

Match the medical term in Column 1 with the definition in Column 2.

COLUMN 1

_____ 1. neuropathy

_____ 2. paraplegia

_____ 3. Parkinson's disease

_____ 4. poliomyelitis

_____ 5. polyneuritis

_____ 6. quadriplegia

_____ 7. Reye's syndrome

_____ 8. shingles

_____ 9. syncope

_____ 10. transient ischemic attack

_____ 11. trigeminal neuralgia

COLUMN 2

a. acute encephalopathy following an acute viral infection

b. any disease of the nerves

c. chronic progressive nerve disease with tremors

d. fainting

e. infectious viral disease of the motor neurons

f. inflammation of many nerves

g. inflammation of a nerve pathway with skin eruptions

h. paralysis of all four limbs

i. paralysis of the lower half of the body, including the legs

j. severe pain along the fifth cranial nerve

k. temporary interruption of the blood supply to the brain

Nervous System Diagnostic and Treatment Terms

Review the pronunciation and definition of the diagnostic and treatment terms in Table 14-9. Complete the exercises for each set of terms.

TABLE 14-9   NERVOUS SYSTEM DIAGNOSTIC AND TREATMENT TERMS

Term with Pronunciation	Definition
cerebrospinal fluid analysis (seh-**ree**-broh-**SPIGH**-nal) cerebr/o = cerebrum spin/o = spine -al = pertaining to	laboratory analysis of cerebrospinal fluid (CSF) to detect the presence of bacteria, blood, and malignant cells, and to measure glucose and protein content
craniotomy (**kray**-nee-**OT**-oh-me) crani/o = skull -(o)tomy = incision into	incision into the skull to provide access to the brain
echoencephalography (EEG) (**ek**-oh-en-**seff**-ah-**LOG**-rah-fee) echo- = sound encephal/o = brain -graphy = process of recording	process of recording a picture of the structures of the brain using sound waves

(continues)

TABLE 14-9   NERVOUS SYSTEM DIAGNOSTIC AND TREATMENT TERMS
(continued)

Term with Pronunciation	Definition
electroencephalogram (ee-**lek**-troh-en-**SEFF**-ah-loh-gram) electr/o = electricity encephal/o = brain -gram = record of	graphic record of the electrical activity of the brain
electroencephalography (ee-**lek**-troh-en-**seff**-ah-**LOG**-rah-fee) electr/o = electricity encephal/o = brain -graphy = process of recording	process of recording the electrical activity of the brain
evoked potential studies (ee-**VOHKT**)	electroencephalographic test that measures the brain activity in response to various types of electrical stimulation
lumbar puncture (LP) (**LUM**-bar)	insertion of a needle into the subarachnoid space, usually between the third and fourth lumbar vertebrae, to withdraw cerebrospinal fluid; also called *spinal tap* (Figure 14-17).

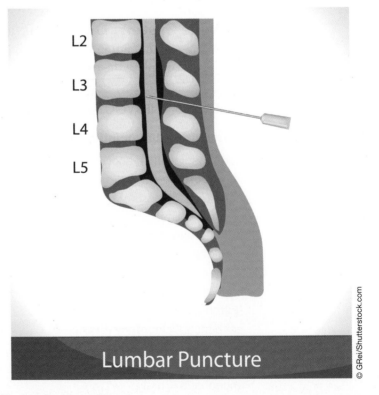

© GRei/Shutterstock.com

Figure 14-17   Lumbar puncture.

(continues)

TABLE 14-9 NERVOUS SYSTEM DIAGNOSTIC AND TREATMENT TERMS
(continued)

Term with Pronunciation	Definition
myelography (**migh**-eh-**LOG**-rah-fee) myel/o = spinal cord -graphy = process of recording	process of recording an x-ray picture of the spinal cord and spinal cavity after the injection of a contrast medium via a lumbar puncture; used to diagnose and evaluate abnormalities of the spinal canal, spinal cord, nerve roots, and surrounding tissues and structures
myelogram (**MIGH**-eh-loh-gram) myel/o = spinal cord -gram = record of	record or image of the spinal cord, subarachnoid space, and surrounding structures accomplished by x-rays or scans enhanced with a contrast medium
neurectomy (noo-**REK**-toh-me) neur/o = nerve -ectomy = surgical removal	surgical excision of a nerve or nerve fibers
neurorrhaphy (new-**ROR**-ah-fee) neur/o = nerve -rrhaphy = suture of	suturing together the ends of a severed nerve
pneumoencephalography (noo-moh-en-s**eff**-ah-**LOG**-rah-fee) pneum/o = air encephal/o = brain -graph = process of recording	process of recording an x-ray picture of the ventricles and other fluid-filled cavities of the central nervous system; air or another type of gas is used as the contrast medium
Romberg test (**ROM**-berg)	technique used to assess and evaluate cerebellar function and balance
transcutaneous electrical nerve stimulation (TENS) (**tranz**-kyoo-**TAY**-nee-us) trans- = across, through cutane/o = skin -ous = pertaining to	pain-relief treatment during which electrical impulses are delivered through the skin to nerve endings near the pain site; the impulses prevent the transmission of pain signals to the brain

© 2016 Cengage Learning®

EXERCISE 17

Analyze each term by writing the prefix, root, combining vowel, and suffix separated by vertical slashes. Based on the meaning of the word parts, write a definition for each term. Check the definition in a medical dictionary. Note that some terms have more than one root.

1. craniotomy

_____

prefix   *root*   *combining vowel*   *suffix*

DEFINITION: _____

2. electroencephalogram

| prefix | root | combining vowel | suffix |

DEFINITION: _____

3. electroencephalography

| prefix | root | combining vowel | suffix |

DEFINITION: _____

4. myelogram

| prefix | root | combining vowel | suffix |

DEFINITION: _____

5. neurectomy

| prefix | root | combining vowel | suffix |

DEFINITION: _____

EXERCISE 18

Match the medical term in Column 1 with the definition in Column 2.

COLUMN 1

_____ 1. cerebrospinal fluid analysis

_____ 2. craniotomy

_____ 3. echoencephalography

_____ 4. electroencephalogram

_____ 5. electroencephalography

_____ 6. evoked potential studies

_____ 7. lumbar puncture

_____ 8. myelogram

_____ 9. neurectomy

_____ 10. Romberg test

COLUMN 2

a. excision of a nerve or nerve fibers

b. graphic record of the electrical activity of the brain

c. incision into the skull

d. laboratory test of CSF

e. recording the electrical activity of the brain

f. spinal tap

g. technique for assessing cerebellar function and balance

h. ultrasound analysis of the structures of the brain

i. x-ray record of the spinal cord and spinal cavity

j. measure the brain's response to electrical stimulation

Abbreviations Review the nervous system abbreviations in Table 14-10. Practice writing out the meaning of each abbreviation.

TABLE 14-10   ABBREVIATIONS

Abbreviation	Meaning
ALS	amyotrophic lateral sclerosis
ANS	autonomic nervous system
CNS	central nervous system
CP	cerebral palsy
CSF	cerebrospinal fluid
CVA	cerebrovascular accident
EEG	electroencephalography
HD	Huntington's disease
ICP	intracranial pressure
LP	lumbar puncture
MS	multiple sclerosis
PEG	pneumoencephalogram
PNS	peripheral nervous system
PPS	postpolio syndrome
SNS	somatic nervous system
TENS	transcutaneous electrical nerve stimulation
TIA	transient ischemic attack

© 2016 Cengage Learning®

CHAPTER REVIEW

The Chapter Review can be used as a self-test. Go through each exercise and answer as many questions as you can without referring to previous exercises or earlier discussions within this chapter. Check your answers and fill in any blanks. Practice writing any terms you might have misspelled.

EXERCISE 19

Write the medical term for each definition.

1. pertaining to the cranium and cerebrum _____

2. above the dura mater _____

3. physician who specializes in the nervous system _____

4. study of the nervous system _____

5. below the arachnoid membrane _____

6. congenital absence of the brain _____

7. pain in the head; headache _____

8. inflammation of the brain _____

9. malignant tumor of the neuroglial cells _____

10. inflammation of the meninges _____

11. herniation of the meninges through a hole in the skull or vertebral column _____

12. sharp pain along the course of a nerve _____

13. paralysis of the lower half of the body, including the legs _____

14. inflammation of many nerves or nerve fibers _____

15. paralysis of all four limbs _____

16. incision into the skull _____

17. recording the electrical activity of the brain _____

18. excision of a nerve or nerve fibers _____

19. partial paralysis of one side of the body _____

20. any disease of the brain _____

EXERCISE 20

Replace the italicized phrase or abbreviation with the correct medical term.

1. Vaneesha was accepted into a residency program for *surgery related to the nervous system.*

   _____

2. After receiving a blow to the head, Patrick had *below the dura mater* bleeding.

   _____

3. A *blunt, nonpenetrating injury to the brain* can be caused by violent jarring or shaking.

   _____

4. A closed head injury can result in a *collection of blood below the dura mater.*

   _____

5. Marko underwent *an incision into the skull* to relieve the pressure on his brain.

   _____

6. Dr. Rodriguez ordered an *LP* to obtain a sample of cerebrospinal fluid.

   _____

7. The *ANS* is responsible for involuntary movements, including hormone secretion.

   _____

8. *Lack of muscular coordination* is associated with several neuromuscular diseases.

   _____

9. A *dilatation of a cerebral artery* puts the patient at risk for a stroke.

   _____

10. *Irregular electrical activity of the central nervous system* can be congenital or caused by trauma.

    _____

EXERCISE 21

Read the discharge summary and write a brief definition for each italicized medical term or phrase.

DISCHARGE SUMMARY
FINAL DIAGNOSIS: (1) *Subarachnoid* hemorrhage. (2) *Hydrocephalus.* Anterior communicating artery aneurysm and (3) *cerebral* failure.
PROCEDURES: CT head scans. (4) *Cerebral angiography.*
HOSPITAL COURSE: The patient was admitted in a comatose condition and was intubated. CT head scans revealed blood in the subarachnoid space and demyelination patterns consistent with (5) *MS.* There was excessive blood in the (6) *ventricular* space. Due to the extensive nature of the subarachnoid hemorrhage, the patient's comatose state, and the fact that surgery was not an option, the patient's comfort was maintained. The (7) *EEG* done on the third day of hospitalization showed no brain wave activity. Mechanical life support was discontinued, per the patient's advance directive.

1. _____
2. _____
3. _____
4. _____
5. _____
6. _____
7. _____

EXERCISE 22

Write out the abbreviation and provide a brief definition for the abbreviation.

EXAMPLE: EEG = electroencephalogram
DEFINITION: record of the electrical activity of the brain

1. ALS _____
   DEFINITION: _____
2. ANS _____
   DEFINITION: _____
3. CNS _____
   DEFINITION: _____
4. CVA _____
   DEFINITION: _____
5. ICP _____
   DEFINITION: _____
6. LP _____
   DEFINITION: _____

7. MS _____

   DEFINITION: _____

8. PNS _____

   DEFINITION: _____

9. SNS _____

   DEFINITION: _____

10. TIA _____

   DEFINITION: _____

EXERCISE 23

Match the cranial nerve in Column 1 with the description in Column 2. Note: Each cranial nerve is also identified by its Roman numeral, which is the number in the parentheses.

COLUMN 1

_____ 1. olfactory nerve (I)

_____ 2. optic nerve (II)

_____ 3. oculomotor nerve (III)

_____ 4. trochlear nerve (IV)

_____ 5. trigeminal nerve (V)

_____ 6. abducens nerve (VI)

_____ 7. facial nerve (VII)

_____ 8. acoustic nerve (VIII)

_____ 9. glossopharyngeal nerve (IX)

_____ 10. vagus nerve (X)

_____ 11. accessory nerve (XI)

_____ 12. hypoglossal nerve (XII)

COLUMN 2

a. chewing and facial sensations

b. eye movement

c. eye movement and eye muscle sensations

d. hearing and balance

e. innervates the scalp, forehead, eyelids, cheek, and jaw

f. sense of smell

g. speech and swallowing

h. speech, swallowing, and head and shoulder movements

i. swallowing and moving the tongue

j. taste, visceral sensations, and glandular secretions

k. transmits impulses necessary for sight

l. turning the eyeball outward

EXERCISE 24

Select the best answer for each question or statement.

1. Which part of the brain is often called the thermostat?
   a. thalamus
   b. pons
   c. midbrain
   d. hypothalamus

2. Select the correct term for the part of the brain that literally means bridge.
   a. thalamus
   b. pons
   c. midbrain
   d. hypothalamus

3. Which part of the brain is responsible for maintaining muscle tone, movement, and balance?
   a. cerebrum
   b. midbrain
   c. cerebellum
   d. medulla oblongata

4. Select the type of nerves that carry impulses toward the brain.
   a. efferent
   b. cauda equina
   c. afferent
   d. neuroglia

5. Which type of nerves carry impulses away from the brain?
   a. efferent
   b. cauda equina
   c. afferent
   d. neuroglia

6. Select the term that means a network of interwoven nerves.
   a. cauda equina
   b. plexus
   c. nerve fiber
   d. neuroglia

7. Which term describes a progressive and debilitating deterioration of intellectual functioning?
   a. amyotrophic lateral sclerosis
   b. multiple sclerosis
   c. cerebral palsy
   d. Alzheimer's disease

8. Select the term that describes a weakness or paralysis of the muscles of one side of the face.
   a. cerebrovascular accident
   b. Bell's palsy
   c. cerebral palsy
   d. multiple sclerosis

9. Which term best describes a swelling or mass of blood between the cranium and dura mater?
   a. epidural hematoma
   b. subdural hematoma
   c. subarachnoid hematoma
   d. concussion

10. Select the term for an acute polyneuritis of the peripheral nervous system.
   a. amyotrophic lateral sclerosis
   b. multiple sclerosis
   c. Guillain-Barré syndrome
   d. Bell's palsy

11. Which term best describes a hardening and scarring of the myelin sheath of the brain and spinal cord?
   a. cerebral palsy
   b. multiple sclerosis
   c. amyotrophic lateral sclerosis
   d. Guillain-Barré syndrome

12. Select the term for a chronic and progressive condition of tremors, muscular rigidity, and weakness.
   a. Bell's palsy
   b. Guillain-Barré syndrome
   c. Reye's syndrome
   d. Parkinson's disease

13. Which term best describes an acute encephalopathy that follows an acute viral infection?
   a. Bell's palsy
   b. Guillain-Barré syndrome
   c. Reye's syndrome
   d. Parkinson's disease

14. Select the term that means the process of recording the electrical activity of the brain.
   a. electroencephalography
   b. electroencephalogram
   c. evoked potential studies
   d. echoencephalography

15. Which test or procedure is used to assess and evaluate cerebellar function?
   a. electroencephalography
   b. evoked potential studies
   c. cerebrospinal fluid analysis
   d. Romberg test

CHALLENGE EXERCISE

Alzheimer's disease is a debilitating disease for the patient and presents many challenges to family and friends. Using current medical references, research the effects this disease has on the brain and the behaviors of the affected individual.

Pronunciation Review

Review the terms in the chapter. Pronounce each term using the following phonetic pronunciations. Check off the term when you are comfortable saying it.

MEDICAL TERM	PRONUNCIATION
☐ afferent nerves	**AFF**-er-ent nerves
☐ Alzheimer's disease	**ALTS**-high-merz disease
☐ amyotrophic lateral sclerosis (ALS)	ah-**migh**-oh-**TROFF**-ik **LAT**-er-al skleh-**ROH**-sis
☐ anencephaly	an-en-**SEFF**-ah-lee
☐ arachnoid membrane	ah-**RAK**-noyd membrane
☐ astrocyte	**ASS**-troh-sight
☐ ataxia	ah-**TAK**-see-ah
☐ autonomic nervous system	ot-oh-**NOM**-ik nervous system
☐ axon	**ACKS**-on
☐ Bell's palsy	Bell's **PALL**-zee
☐ cauda equina	**KAW**-dah ee-**KWIGH**-nah
☐ cephalalgia	seff-al-**AL**-jee-ah
☐ cerebellum	ser-eh-**BELL**-um
☐ cerebral	seh-**REE**-bral
☐ cerebral aneurysm	seh-**REE**-bral **AN**-yoo-rizm
☐ cerebral cortex	seh-**REE**-bral **KOR**-teks
☐ cerebral palsy (CP)	seh-**REE**-bral **PALL**-zee
☐ cerebral thrombosis	seh-**REE**-bral throm-**BOH**-sis
☐ cerebrospinal fluid (CSF)	seh-**ree**-broh-**SPIGH**-nal fluid
☐ cerebrospinal fluid analysis	seh-**ree**-broh-**SPIGH**-nal fluid analysis
☐ cerebrovascular accident (CVA)	seh-**REE**-broh-**VASS**-kyoo-lar accident
☐ cerebrum	seh-**REE**-brum
☐ contusion	kon-**TOO**-zhun
☐ concussion	kon-**KUSH**-on
☐ corpus callosum	**KOR**-pus kal-**OH**-sum
☐ craniocerebral	**kray**-nee-oh-seh-**REE**-bral
☐ craniotomy	**kray**-nee-**OT**-oh-me
☐ dementia	deh-**MEN**-shee-ah
☐ dendrite	**DEN**-dright
☐ dura mater	**DOO**-rah **MAY**-ter
☐ echoencephalography	**ek**-oh-en-**seff**-ah-**LOG**-rah-fee
☐ efferent nerves	**EE**-fair-ent nerves
☐ electroencephalogram	ee-**lek**-troh-en-**SEFF**-ah-loh-gram
☐ electroencephalography	ee-**lek**-troh-en-**seff**-ah-**LOG**-rah-fee
☐ encephalitis	**en**-seff-ah-**LIGH**-tis

MEDICAL TERM	PRONUNCIATION
☐ encephalopathy	**en**-seff-ah-**LOP**-ah-thee
☐ epidural	ep-ih-**DOO**-ral
☐ epidural hematoma	ep-ih-**DOO**-ral **hee**-mah-**TOH**-mah
☐ epilepsy	**EP**-ih-lep-see
☐ evoked potential studies	ee-**VOHKT** potential studies
☐ glioma	gligh-**OH**-mah
☐ Guillain-Barré syndrome	**GEE**-yon bah-**RAYSIN**-drohm
☐ gyrus; gyri (pl.)	**JIGH**-rus; **JIGH**-righ
☐ hemiparesis	**hem**-ee-pah-**REE**-sis
☐ hemiplegia	**hem**-ee-**PLEE**-jee-ah
☐ hydrocephalus	**high**-droh-**SEFF**-ah-lus
☐ hypothalamus	high-poh-**THAL**-ah-mus
☐ lumbar puncture (LP)	**LUM**-bar puncture
☐ medulla oblongata	meh-**DULL**-ah ob-long-**AH**-tah
☐ meninges	men-**IN**-jeez
☐ meningitis	**men**-in-**JIGH**-tis
☐ meningioma	men-**in**-jee-**OH**-mah
☐ meningitis	**men**-in-**JIGH**-tis
☐ meningocele	men-**IN**-goh-seel
☐ meningomyelocele	men-**in**-goh-my-**ELL**-oh-seel
☐ microglia	my-**KROG**-lee-ah
☐ multiple sclerosis (MS)	multiple sklair-**OH**-sis
☐ myelin	**MIGH**-eh-lin
☐ myelogram	**MIGH**-eh-loh-gram
☐ myelography	**migh**-eh-**LOG**-rah-fee
☐ myelomalacia	**migh**-eh-loh-mah-**LAY**-shee-ah
☐ neuralgia	noo-**RAL**-jee-ah
☐ neurectomy	noo-**REK**-toh-me
☐ neuritis	noo-**RIGH**-tis
☐ neuroblastoma	**noo**-roh-blast-**OH**-mah
☐ neuroglia	noo-**ROG**-lee-ah
☐ neurologist	noo-**RALL**-oh-jist
☐ neurology	noo-**RALL**-oh-jee
☐ neurons	**NOO**-ronz
☐ neuropathy	noo-**ROP**-ah-thee
☐ neurosurgeon	**noo**-roh-**SER**-jun
☐ neurosurgery	**noo**-roh-**SER**-jer-ree
☐ occipital lobe	ok-**SIP**-ih-tal lobe
☐ oligodendroglia	**all**-ih-goh-den-**DROG**-lee-ah
☐ paraplegia	**pair**-ah-**PLEE**-jee-ah
☐ parietal lobe	pah-**RIGH**-eh-tal lobe
☐ peripheral nervous system (PNS)	peh-**RIF**-er-al nervous system
☐ pia mater	**PEE**-ah **MAY**-ter
☐ plexus	**PLECKS**-us
☐ pneumoencephalography	noo-moh-en-**seff**-ah-**LOG**-rah-fee
☐ poliomyelitis	**poh**-lee-oh-**migh**-eh-**LIGH**-tis
☐ polyneuritis	**pall**-ee-noo-**RIGH**-tis

MEDICAL TERM	**PRONUNCIATION**
☐ pons	PONZ
☐ postpolio syndrome	**post**-**POH**-lee-oh **SIN**-drom
☐ quadriplegia	**kwad**-rih-**PLEE**-jee-ah
☐ Reye's syndrome	**RIGH's SIN**-drohm
☐ Romberg test	**ROM**-berg test
☐ sciatica	sigh-**AT**-ih-kah
☐ seizure	**SEE**-zhoor
☐ shingles; herpes zoster	shingles; **HER**-peez **ZOSS**-ter
☐ somatic nervous system	soh-**MAT**-ik nervous system
☐ subarachnoid	sub-ah-**RAK**-noyd
☐ subdural	sub-**DOO**-ral
☐ subdural hematoma	sub-**DOO**-ral **hee**-mah-**TOH**-mah
☐ sulcus; sulci (pl.)	**SULL**-kus; **SULL**-kigh
☐ syncope	**SIN**-koh-pee
☐ temporal lobe	**TEM**-por-al lobe
☐ thalamus	**THAL**-ah-mus
☐ transcutaneous electrical nerve stimulation	**tranz**-kyoo-**TAY**-nee-us electrical nerve stimulation
☐ trigeminal neuralgia; tic douloureux	trigh-**JEM**-ih-nal noo-**RAL**-jee-ah; **TIKDOO**-loh-roo
☐ ventricle	**VEN**-trih-kal

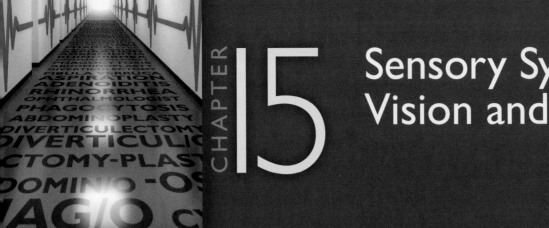

CHAPTER 15

Sensory System: Vision and Hearing

OBJECTIVES

At the completion of this chapter, the student should be able to:

1. Identify, define, and spell word roots associated with the eyes and ears.
2. Label the basic structures of the eyes and ears.
3. Discuss the functions of the eyes and ears.
4. Provide the correct spelling of eye and ear terms, given the definition of the terms.
5. Analyze the eye and ear terms by defining the roots, prefixes, and suffixes of these terms.
6. Identify, define, and spell disease, disorder, and procedure terms related to the eyes and ears.

OVERVIEW

The eyes and ears are primary sense organs that capture information through sight and sound. The information is transmitted via the nervous system to areas of the brain responsible for vision and hearing. This chapter presents information about the structures, functions, diseases, procedures, and tests related to these important organs.

The Eye

The eyes are located in the bony orbits at the front of the skull. The structures of the eyes are arranged in three layers, also called tunics. The eyes receive light rays; bend, or **refract**, those rays; and transmit the nerve impulses generated by the light rays to the occipital lobe of the brain. After the impulses reach the occipital lobe, they are interpreted as images and we are able to "see." Our vision is dependent on the health of our eyes, our sight-related nerves, and our brain.

Word Roots Related to the Eyes

To understand and use the medical terms related to the eyes, it is necessary to acquire a thorough knowledge of the associated word roots and combining forms. Review the word roots in Table 15-1 and complete the exercises that follow.

TABLE 15-1   WORD ROOTS RELATED TO THE EYES

Word Root/Combining Form	Meaning
aque/o	watery
blephar/o	eyelid
conjunctiv/o	conjunctiva

(continues)

TABLE 15-1 WORD ROOTS RELATED TO THE EYES (continued)

Word Root/Combining Form	Meaning
corne/o	cornea
dacry/o	tears
dacryocyst/o	tear sac
glauc/o	silver; gray
ir/o; irid/o	iris
kerat/o	cornea
lacrim/o	tears
ocul/o	eye
ophthalm/o	eye
opt/o	eye; vision
palpebr/o	eyelid
phac/o; phak/o	lens
phot/o	light
pupill/o	pupil
retin/o	retina
scler/o	sclera; hard
uve/o	uvea
vitre/o	glassy; jellylike

© 2016 Cengage Learning®

EXERCISE 1

Write the definitions of the following word roots.

1. corne/o _____

2. dacry/o _____

3. retin/o _____

4. scler/o _____

5. ocul/o _____

6. irid/o _____

7. glauc/o _____

8. ir/o _____

9. aque/o _____

10. conjunctiv/o _____

11. dacryocyst/o _____

12. vitre/o _____

13. opt/o _____

14. phac/o _____

15. lacrim/o _____

16. ophthalm/o _____

17. kerat/o _____

18. blephar/o   _____

19. phak/o   _____

20. pupill/o   _____

Write the combining form of the word root and its meaning for each of the listed terms.

1. aqueous

   ROOT: _____   MEANING: _____

2. blepharoptosis

   ROOT: _____   MEANING: _____

3. conjunctivitis

   ROOT: _____   MEANING: _____

4. corneitis

   ROOT: _____   MEANING: _____

5. glaucoma

   ROOT: _____   MEANING: _____

6. keratotomy

   ROOT: _____   MEANING: _____

7. lacrimal

   ROOT: _____   MEANING: _____

8. oculomotor

   ROOT: _____   MEANING: _____

9. ophthalmoscope

   ROOT: _____   MEANING: _____

10. optic

    ROOT: _____   MEANING: _____

11. palpebral

    ROOT: _____   MEANING: _____

12. photophobia

    ROOT: _____   MEANING: _____

13. pupillary

    ROOT: _____   MEANING: _____

14. retinitis

    ROOT: _____   MEANING: _____

15. vitreous

    ROOT: _____   MEANING: _____

EXERCISE 3

Write the correct word root(s) with the combining form for the following definitions.

1. cornea   _____

2. eye   _____

3. eyelid   _____

4. tears   _____

5. glassy   _____

6. sclera   _____

7. lens   _____

8. light   _____

9. pupil   _____

10. retina   _____

11. silver   _____

12. tear sac   _____

13. watery   _____

Structures of the Eye

As stated previously, the structures of the eye are arranged in three layers, or tunics. The outer layer is the **sclera** (**SKLAIR**-ah), the middle layer is the **choroid** (**KOH**-royd), and the inner layer is the **retina** (**RET**-ih-nah). Each layer consists of additional structures and provides specific functions related to sight. Figure 15-1 illustrates the structures of the eye. Refer to this figure as you learn about each layer and its structures.

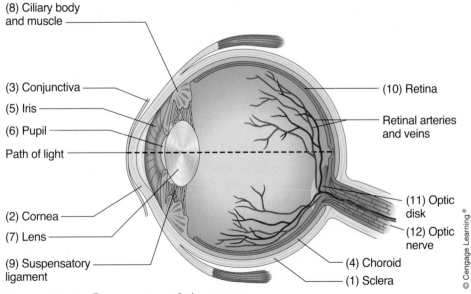

(8) Ciliary body and muscle

(3) Conjunctiva

(5) Iris

(6) Pupil

Path of light

(2) Cornea

(7) Lens

(9) Suspensatory ligament

(10) Retina

Retinal arteries and veins

(11) Optic disk

(12) Optic nerve

(4) Choroid

(1) Sclera

© Cengage Learning ®

Figure 15-1   Structures of the eye.

Outer Layer

The outer layer of the eye consists of the sclera, cornea, and conjunctiva. The (1) **sclera** is a tough or fibrous tissue that maintains the shape of the eyeball and serves as its protective covering. The sclera is commonly called the "white of the eyes." The (2) **cornea** (**KOR**-nee-ah) is the transparent anterior portion of the sclera that covers the iris. The (3) **conjunctiva** (kon-junk- **TIGH**-vah) is a mucous membrane that lines the outer surface of the eye and the inside of the eyelid.

Middle Layer

The middle layer of the eye includes the choroid, iris, pupil, lens, and ciliary body. The (4) **choroid** is a layer of tissue beneath the sclera that contains blood vessels that supply oxygen and nutrients to the eye. The (5) **iris**, which gives our eyes their unique color, is a muscular ring that surrounds the (6) **pupil**. The iris adjusts the opening of the pupil to control the amount of light that enters the eye. The (7) **lens**, also called the **crystalline** (**KRIS**-tah-lin) **lens**, is connected to the choroid by the (8) **ciliary** (**SILL**-ee-air-ee) **body** and the (9) **suspensatory** (suh- **SPEN**-sah-tor-ee) **ligaments**. The choroid, iris, and ciliary body are collectively known as the **uvea** (**YOO**-vee-ah).

The ciliary body and suspensatory ligaments adjust the shape of the lens to help focus light rays on the retina. When an object is near, the lens is shortened and becomes thicker; when an object is distant, the lens is lengthened and becomes thinner.

Inner Layer

The inner layer of the eye includes the retina, nerve cells, and optic disk. The (10) **retina** is the sensory nerve tissue that coats the inside of the eye. It contains nerve cells called **rods** and **cones**, which convert light rays into nerve impulses. Rods are responsible for vision in dim light and also peripheral vision. Cones are responsible for the vision in bright light, central vision, and color vision. The (11) **optic disk**, located at the back of the eye, is the area where the nerve endings of the retina come together to form the (12) **optic nerve**. The optic nerve transmits impulses to the occipital lobe of the brain.

Cavities of the Eye

The interior of the eye has two cavities: the anterior cavity and the posterior cavity. Figure 15-2 illustrates the cavities of the eyeball. Refer to Figure 15-2 as you learn about the cavities. The anterior cavity makes up the front one-third of the eyeball. The anterior cavity consists of the (1) **anterior chamber**, the area in the front of the iris; and the (2) **posterior chamber**, the area behind the iris and in front of the ligaments that hold the lens in place. These chambers are filled with a watery fluid called (3) **aqueous** (**AY**-kwee-us) **humor**. Aqueous humor helps the eyeball maintain its shape; maintains the proper pressure within the eye; and nourishes structures in the eyeball. **Intraocular** (in-trah-**OCK**-yoo-lar) pressure is a measurement of the fluid pressure inside the eyeball.

The posterior cavity makes up the remaining two-thirds of the eyeball. The (4) **retina** (**REH**-tin-ah) lines the posterior cavity. (5) **Vitreous** (**VIH**-ree-us) **humor**, also called vitreous gel, is a soft, clear, jellylike substance that contains millions of fine fibers. These fibers are attached to the retina and also help the eyeball retain its shape.

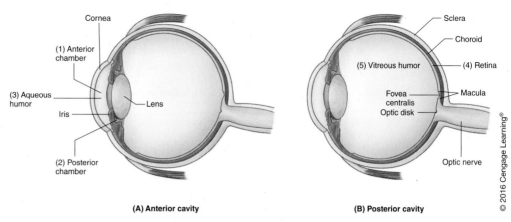

Figure 15-2   Anterior and posterior cavities and chambers of the eye.

Vitreous humor is necessary for sight. If the eyeball is injured and vitreous humor escapes, blindness can result. Both aqueous and vitreous humor help bend light rays as they pass through the eye and focus on the retina.

EXERCISE 4

Write the name of the labeled structures in Figure 15-3 on the spaces provided.

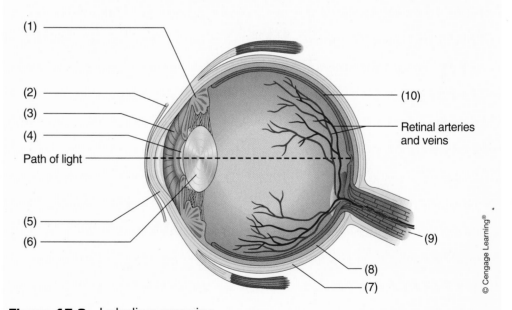

Figure 15-3   Labeling exercise.

1. _____

2. _____

3. _____

4. _____

5. _____

6. _____

7. _____

8. _____

9. _____

10. _____

EXERCISE 5

Match the medical term in Column 1 with the definition in Column 2.

COLUMN 1	COLUMN 2
_____ 1. choroid	a. adjusts to focus light rays on the retina
_____ 2. ciliary body	b. area where retinal nerve endings come together
_____ 3. conjunctiva	c. clear jelly like substance necessary for sight
_____ 4. cornea	d. colorful muscular ring that adjusts the pupil
_____ 5. iris	e. fibrous outer layer of the eye; white of the eye
_____ 6. lens	f. helps adjust the shape of the lens
_____ 7. optic disk	g. membrane that lines the outer surface of the eye
_____ 8. optic nerve	h. opening or hole in the eye
_____ 9. pupil	i. sensory nerve tissue; inner layer of the eye
_____ 10. retina	j. tissue containing the blood vessels of the eye
_____ 11. sclera	k. transmits impulses to the brain
_____ 12. vitreous humor	l. transparent, anterior portion of the sclera

---

Accessory Structures of the Eye

Accessory structures of the eye include the orbit; eyebrows; eyelashes; oil glands; and lacrimal glands, fluid, sacs, and ducts. The purpose of the accessory structures is to protect the eye from disease and injury. Refer to Figure 15-4 as you learn about these structures.

The **orbit**, also called the **eye socket**, is the bony cavity of the skull that houses and protects the eyeball. The (1) **upper** and (2) **lower eyelids** and (3) **eyelashes**, along with the (4) **eyebrows**, prevent foreign matter from reaching the eyes. The **meibomian** (migh-**BOH**-mee-an) **glands**, located between the conjunctiva and

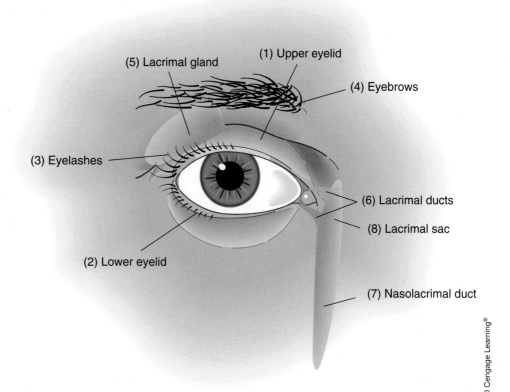

(5) Lacrimal gland   (1) Upper eyelid

(4) Eyebrows

(3) Eyelashes

(6) Lacrimal ducts

(8) Lacrimal sac

(2) Lower eyelid

(7) Nasolacrimal duct

© Cengage Learning®

Figure 15-4 Accessory structures of the eye.

the tissue of the upper and lower eyelids, are small oil glands that lubricate the eyes. These glands are not visible unless they become obstructed. The (5) **lacrimal** (**LAK**-rih-mal) **glands**, located above the outer corner of each eye, produce **lacrimal fluid** (tears) that moisten the anterior surface of the eyeball. The (6) **lacrimal ducts** drain lacrimal fluid away from the eye and into the nose via the (7) **nasolacrimal duct**. The upper expanded portion of the nasolacrimal duct is called the (8) **lacrimal sac**.

In addition to the accessory structures, there are three pairs of major eye muscles. The six muscles, illustrated in Figure 15-5, allow the eyes to execute a wide range of very precise movements. *Rectus* means straight and therefore a rectus muscle appears straight. *Oblique* means slanted and therefore an oblique muscle appears slanted.

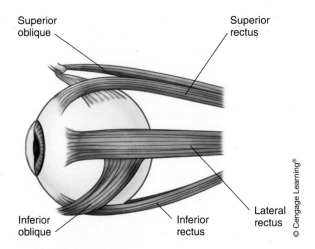

Figure 15-5 Major muscles related to eye movement.

© Cengage Learning®

EXERCISE 6

Write the name of the accessory structure of the eye.

1. bony cavity of the skull; houses the eyes   _____

2. oil glands; lubricate the eye   _____

3. drain tears away from the eye   _____

4. tears   _____

5. produce tears   _____

Medical Terms Related to the Eye

Medical terms related to the eye are organized into three main categories: (1) general medical terms; (2) disease and condition terms; and (3) diagnostic procedure, surgery, and laboratory test terms. The roots, prefixes, and suffixes associated with the eye are listed in Table 15-2. Review these word parts and complete the exercises.

TABLE 15-2   ROOTS, PREFIXES, AND SUFFIXES FOR THE EYE

Root	Meaning	Prefix	Meaning	Suffix	Meaning
blast/o	immature	ect-	outside; out	-ectomy	surgical removal
dipl/o	two; double	en-; eso-	in; inward	-ist	specialist
fund/o	fundus; base	ex-	out; outward	-itis	inflammation
nas/o	nose	intra-	within	-metry	to measure
		presby-	old	-opia	vision
				-(o)tomy	incision into
				-pathy	disease
				-plasty	surgical repair
				-ptosis	drooping

(continues)

TABLE 15-2   ROOTS, PREFIXES, AND SUFFIXES FOR THE EYE (continued)

-scope	instrument for viewing
-tropia; -tropio	to turn; turning

EXERCISE 7

Write the root, prefix, suffix, and their meanings on the spaces provided. Based on these meanings, write a brief definition for each term.

1. blepharoplasty

   ROOT: _____   MEANING: _____

   PREFIX: _____   MEANING: _____

   SUFFIX: _____   MEANING: _____

   DEFINITION: _____

2. blepharoptosis

   ROOT: _____   MEANING: _____

   PREFIX: _____   MEANING: _____

   SUFFIX: _____   MEANING: _____

   DEFINITION: _____

3. conjunctivitis

   ROOT: _____   MEANING: _____

   PREFIX: _____   MEANING: _____

   SUFFIX: _____   MEANING: _____

   DEFINITION: _____

4. diplopia

   ROOT: _____   MEANING: _____

   PREFIX: _____   MEANING: _____

   SUFFIX: _____   MEANING: _____

   DEFINITION: _____

5. exophthalmia

   ROOT: _____   MEANING: _____

   PREFIX: _____   MEANING: _____

   SUFFIX: _____   MEANING: _____

   DEFINITION: _____

6. exotropia

ROOT: _____ MEANING: _____

PREFIX: _____ MEANING: _____

SUFFIX: _____ MEANING: _____

DEFINITION: _____

7. intraocular

ROOT: _____ MEANING: _____

PREFIX: _____ MEANING: _____

SUFFIX: _____ MEANING: _____

DEFINITION: _____

8. iridectomy

ROOT: _____ MEANING: _____

PREFIX: _____ MEANING: _____

SUFFIX: _____ MEANING: _____

DEFINITION: _____

9. keratotomy

ROOT: _____ MEANING: _____

PREFIX: _____ MEANING: _____

SUFFIX: _____ MEANING: _____

DEFINITION: _____

10. nasolacrimal

ROOT: _____ MEANING: _____

PREFIX: _____ MEANING: _____

SUFFIX: _____ MEANING: _____

DEFINITION: _____

11. ophthalmoscope

ROOT: _____ MEANING: _____

PREFIX: _____ MEANING: _____

SUFFIX: _____ MEANING: _____

DEFINITION: _____

12. presbyopia

ROOT: _____ MEANING: _____

PREFIX: _____ MEANING: _____

SUFFIX: _____ MEANING: _____

DEFINITION: _____

13. retinopathy

ROOT: _____ MEANING: _____

PREFIX: _____ MEANING: _____

SUFFIX: _____ MEANING: _____

DEFINITION: _____

General Medical Terms of the Eye

Review the pronunciation and meaning of each term in Table 15-3. Note that some terms are built from word parts and some are not. Complete the exercises for these terms.

TABLE 15-3 GENERAL MEDICAL TERMS OF THE EYE

Term with Pronunciation	Definition
intraocular (**in**-trah-**OK**-yoo-lar) intra- = within ocul/o = eye -ar = pertaining to	pertaining to within the eye
lacrimal (**LAK**-rih-mal) lacrim/o = tears -al = pertaining to	pertaining to tears
miotic (my-**OT**-ik)	pertaining to constricting the pupil; agent that constricts the pupil
mydriatic (mid-ree-**AT**-ik)	pertaining to dilating the pupil; agent that dilates the pupil
nasolacrimal (**nay**-zoh-**LAK**-rih-mal) nas/o = nose lacrim/o = tears -al = pertaining to	pertaining to the nose and tear duct
ophthalmologist (**off**-thall-**MALL**-oh-jist) ophthalm/o = eye -(o)logist = specialist	physician who specializes in diseases, disorders, and treatments of the eye
ophthalmology (**off**-thall-**MALL**-oh-jee) ophthalm/o = eye -(o)logy = study of	medical specialty related to the study of diseases, disorders, and treatments of the eye
optician (op-**TIH**-shun)	individual who measures and fits eyeglasses

(continues)

TABLE 15-3 GENERAL MEDICAL TERMS OF THE EYE (continued)

Term with Pronunciation	Definition
optometrist (op-**TOM**-eh-trist) opt/o = eye -metr = to measure; measurement -ist = specialist	doctor of optometry; health care provider who measures visual acuity, prescribes corrective lenses, and may diagnose and treat some eye problems
optometry (op-**TOM**-eh-tree) opt/o = eye -metr = to measure; measurement -y = noun ending	measuring and testing the eyes for visual acuity and corrective lenses
visual acuity (**VIZH**-yoo-al ah-**KYOO**-ih-tee)	sharpness or clearness of vision in one or both eyes

© 2016 Cengage Learning ®

EXERCISE 8

Analyze each term by writing the prefix, root, combining vowel, and suffix separated by vertical slashes. Based on the meaning of the word parts, write a definition for each term. Check the definition in a medical dictionary. Note that some terms might have more than one root.

EXAMPLE: retinopathy

	/retin	/ o	/ pathy
prefix	*root*	*combining vowel*	*suffix*

DEFINITION: <u>disease of the retina</u>

1. intraocular

prefix	*root*	*combining vowel*	*suffix*

DEFINITION: _____

2. nasolacrimal

prefix	*root*	*combining vowel*	*suffix*

DEFINITION: _____

3. ophthalmologist

prefix	*root*	*combining vowel*	*suffix*

DEFINITION: _____

4. ophthalmology

prefix	*root*	*combining vowel*	*suffix*

DEFINITION: _____

5. optometrist

_____

| _prefix_ | _root_ | _combining vowel_ | _suffix_ |

DEFINITION:_____

6. optometry

_____

| _prefix_ | _root_ | _combining vowel_ | _suffix_ |

DEFINITION: _____

EXERCISE 9

Write the medical term for each definition.

1. agent that constricts the pupil   _____

2. agent that dilates the pupil   _____

3. sharpness or clearness of vision   _____

4. pertaining to tears   _____

5. individual who measures and fits eyeglasses   _____

Disease and Disorder Terms of the Eye

Eye diseases and disorders include familiar problems such as cataract as well as more complex and less familiar diagnoses such as retinitis pigmentosa. The medical terms are presented in alphabetic order in Table 15-4. Review the pronunciation and definition for each term and complete the exercises.

TABLE 15-4   DISEASE AND DISORDER TERMS OF THE EYE

Term with Pronunciation	Definition
astigmatism (ah-**STIG**-mah-tizm)	a refractive error causing light rays to be focused irregularly on the retina due to an abnormally shaped cornea
blepharitis (**bleh**-fah-**RIGH**-tis) blephar/o = eyelids -itis = inflammation	inflammation of the eyelids
blepharoptosis (**bleh**-fah-roh-**TOH**-sis) blephar/o = eyelid -ptosis = drooping	drooping of an eyelid
cataract (**KAT**-ah-rakt)	progressive cloudiness of the crystalline lens (Figure 15-6)

(continues)

TABLE 15-4 DISEASE AND DISORDER TERMS OF THE EYE (continued)

Term with Pronunciation	Definition

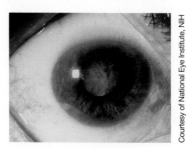

Figure 15-6 Cataract (National Eye Institute, NIH).

chalazion (kah-**LAY**-zee-on)	cyst or nodule on the eyelid as a result of an obstructed meibomian gland (Figure 15-7)

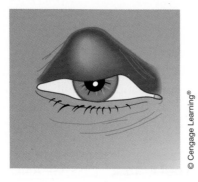

Figure 15-7 Chalazion.

conjunctivitis (kon-**junk**-tih-**VIGH**-tis) conjunctiv/o = conjunctiva -itis = inflammation	inflammation of the conjunctiva; commonly called pinkeye
dacryocystitis (**dak**-ree-oh-sis-**TIGH**-tis) dacryocyst/o = tear sac -itis = inflammation	inflammation of the tear sac or lacrimal sac
detached retina	separation of the retina from the choroid layer of the eye

(continues)

TABLE 15-4   DISEASE AND DISORDER TERMS OF THE EYE (continued)

Term with Pronunciation	Definition
diabetic retinopathy (**digh**-ah-**BEH**-tik **reh**-tin-**OP**-ah-thee) retin/o = retina -pathy = disease	disease of the retina and its capillaries caused by long-standing and usually poorly controlled diabetes mellitus (Figure 15-8)

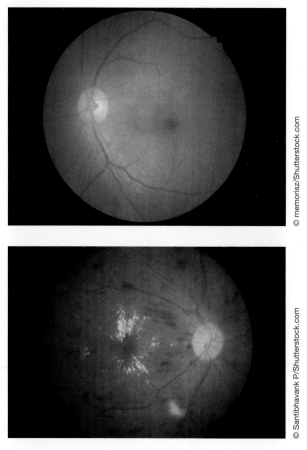

Figure 15-8 (A) Normal retina; (B) Diabetic retinopathy, proliferative (National Eye Institute, NIH).

diplopia (dih-**PLOH**-pee-ah) dipl/o = two; double -opia = vision	double vision; may be in one or both eyes
ectropion (ek-**TROH**-pee-on) ect- = outside; out -tropion = turning	turning outward of the eyelash margins, usually affects the lower eyelid (Figure 15-9)

(continues)

TABLE 15-4 DISEASE AND DISORDER TERMS OF THE EYE (continued)

Term with Pronunciation	Definition

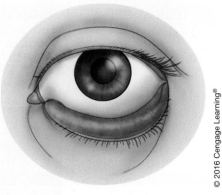

Figure 15-9 Ectropion.

Term with Pronunciation	Definition
entropion (en-**TROH**-pee-on) en- = in; inward -tropion = turning	turning inward of the eyelash margins, usually affects the lower eyelid
esotropia (ess-oh-**TROH**-pee-ah) eso- = in; inward -tropia = turning	inward turning of the eyes; also known as *convergent strabismus*; commonly called *cross-eyed*
exophthalmia (**ecks**-off-**THAL**-mee-ah) ex- = out; outward ophthalm/o = eye -ia = noun ending	abnormal protrusion of the eyeball(s)
exotropia (**ecks**-oh-**TROH**-pee-ah) ex- = out; outward -tropia = turning	outward turning of the eyes; also known as *divergent strabismus*; commonly called *walleyed*
glaucoma (glaw-**KOH**-mah)	increased intraocular pressure

EXERCISE 10

Analyze each term by writing the prefix, root, combining vowel, and suffix separated by vertical slashes. Based on the meaning of the word parts, write a definition for each term. Check the definition in a medical dictionary. Note that some terms might have more than one root.

1. blepharitis

prefix	*root*	*combining vowel*	*suffix*

DEFINITION: _____

2. blepharoptosis

prefix	root	combining vowel	suffix

DEFINITION: _____

3. conjunctivitis

prefix	root	combining vowel	suffix

DEFINITION: _____

4. dacryocystitis

prefix	root	combining vowel	suffix

DEFINITION: _____

5. exophthalmia

prefix	root	combining vowel	suffix

DEFINITION: _____

6. diplopia

prefix	root	combining vowel	suffix

DEFINITION: _____

7. entropion

prefix	root	combining vowel	suffix

DEFINITION: _____

8. esotropia

prefix	root	combining vowel	suffix

DEFINITION: _____

9. exotropia

prefix	root	combining vowel	suffix

DEFINITION: _____

EXERCISE 11

Replace the italicized phrase with the correct medical term.

1. *Cloudiness of the crystalline lens* is a common problem associated with aging.

   _____

2. *A refractive error of irregularly focused light rays* can be corrected with glasses.

   _____

3. Trauma to the eye can result in *double vision*.

   _____

4. Surgical intervention might be needed to correct *convergent strabismus*.

   _____

5. A thorough eye examination includes an assessment for *increased intraocular pressure*.

   _____

6. *Walleye* is often caused by a problem with the muscles of the eye.

   _____

7. An obstructed meibomian gland is a common cause of a *cyst on the eyelid*.

   _____

8. *Abnormal protrusion of the eyeballs* is often seen in severe hyperthyroidism.

   _____

9. *Turning outward of the eyelash margin* usually affects the lower eyelid.

   _____

10. *Turning inward of the eyelash margin* might cause irritation of the eye.

    _____

Review the pronunciation and definition for each term in Table 15-5 and complete the exercises.

TABLE 15-5 DISEASE AND DISORDER TERMS OF THE EYE

Term with Pronunciation	Definition
hordeolum (hor-**DEE**-oh-lum)	bacterial infection of an eyelash follicle or sebaceous gland; commonly called a *sty*
hyperopia (**high**-per-**OH**-pee-ah) hyper- = increased; excessive -opia = vision	impaired vision of close objects; light rays focus beyond the retina; commonly called *farsightedness* (Figure 15-10)

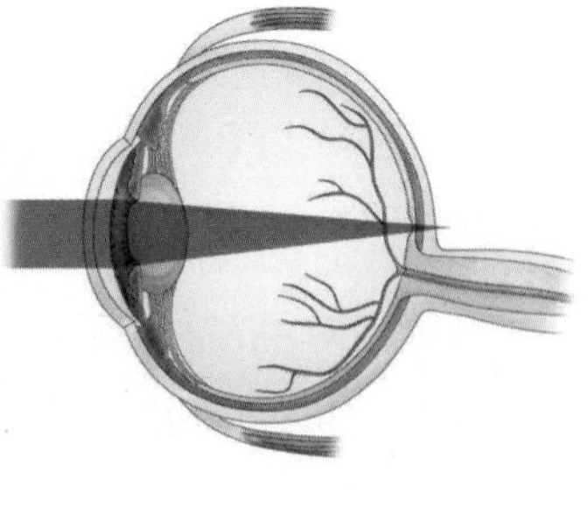

© 2016 Cengage Learning®

Figure 15-10 Hyperopia.

iritis (ir-**RIGH**-tis) ir/o = iris -itis = inflammation	inflammation of the iris
keratitis (**kair**-ah-**TIGH**-tis) kerat/o = cornea -itis = inflammation	inflammation of the cornea

(continues)

TABLE 15-5   DISEASE AND DISORDER TERMS OF THE EYE (continued)

Term with Pronunciation	Definition
monochromatism (mon-oh-**KROH**-mah-tizm) mono- = one, single chromat/o = color -ism = condition	impaired ability to differentiate colors; in some cases only certain colors are affected; in other cases all colors appear as shades of one color; layman's term *color blindness*
myopia (my-**OH**-pee-ah)	impaired vision of distant objects; light rays focus in front of the retina; commonly called *nearsightedness* (Figure 15-11)

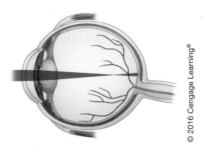

© 2016 Cengage Learning®

Figure 15-11   Myopia.

nyctalopia (**nik**-tah-**LOH**-pee-ah)	impaired or inadequate vision at night; commonly called *night blindness*
nystagmus (niss-**TAG**-mus)	involuntary movements of the eye(s), which may or may not be apparent to the individual
ophthalmia neonatorum (off-**THAL**-mee-ah nee-oh-nay-**TOR**-um) ophthalm/o = eye -ia = condition neo- = new nat/o = birth	inflammation of the conjunctiva of a newborn caused by irritation, a blocked tear duct, or a bacterial or viral infection contracted as the infant passes through the birth canal; bacterial infections include chlamydia and viral infections include genital herpes; also called *newborn* or *neonatal conjunctivitis* (Figure15-12)
photophobia (foh-toh-**FOH**-bee-ah) phot/o = light -phobia = fear	abnormal sensitivity to light
photoretinitis (**foh**-toh-reh-tih-**NIGH**-tis) phot/o = light retin/o = retina -itis = inflammation	damage or inflammation of the retina due to excessive exposure to light

TABLE 15-5 DISEASE AND DISORDER TERMS OF THE EYE (continued)

Term with Pronunciation	Definition

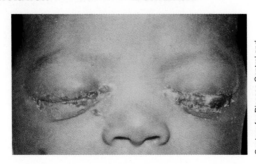

Figure 15-12 Bacterial ophthalmia neonatorum (Centers for Disease Control and Prevention/J. Pledger).

Term with Pronunciation	Definition
presbyopia (prez-bee-**OH**-pee-ah) presby- = old -opia = vision	impaired vision due to aging
pterygium (ter-**IJ**-ee-um)	irregular growth and thickening of the conjunctiva on the nasal side of the cornea
retinitis pigmentosa (**reh**-tih-**NIGH**-tis **pig**-men-**TOH**-sah) retin/o = retina -itis = inflammation	degenerative disease of the retina without inflammation that results in defective night vision and a decreased field of vision
retinoblastoma (**reh**-tih-noh-blass-**TOH**-mah) retin/o = retina blast/o = immature cell -oma = tumor	malignant tumor of the retina
retinopathy (**reh**-tih-**NOP**-ah-thee) retin/o = retina -pathy = disease	any disease or disorder of the retina
sclerokeratitis (**sklair**-oh-**kair**-ah-**TIGH**-tis) scler/o = sclera kerat/o = cornea -itis = inflammation	inflammation of the sclera and cornea
strabismus (strah-**BIZ**-mus)	inability of the eyes to gaze in the same direction because of weakness of the eye muscles
trachoma (tray-**KOH**-mah)	chronic, contagious form of conjunctivitis characterized by hypertrophy of the conjunctiva
uveitis (yoo-vee-**EYE**-tis) uve/o = uvea -itis = inflammation	inflammation of the iris, ciliary body, and choroid

EXERCISE 12

Analyze each term by writing the prefix, root, combining vowel, and suffix separated by vertical slashes. Based on the meaning of the word parts, write a definition for each term. Check the definition in a medical dictionary. Note that some terms might have more than one root.

1. hyperopia

prefix	root	combining vowel	suffix

DEFINITION: _____

2. iritis

prefix	root	combining vowel	suffix

DEFINITION: _____

3. keratitis

prefix	root	combining vowel	suffix

DEFINITION: _____

4. photophobia

prefix	root	combining vowel	suffix

DEFINITION: _____

5. photoretinitis

prefix	root	combining vowel	suffix

DEFINITION: _____

6. presbyopia

prefix	root	combining vowel	suffix

DEFINITION: _____

7. retinoblastoma

prefix	root	combining vowel	suffix

DEFINITION: _____

8. retinopathy

prefix	root	combining vowel	suffix

DEFINITION: _____

9. sclerokeratitis

prefix	root	combining vowel	suffix

DEFINITION: _____

EXERCISE 13

Replace the italicized phrase with the correct medical term.

1. *Involuntary eye movements* might not be apparent to the patient.

   _____

2. Excessive ultraviolet light exposure can cause *irregular growth of the conjunctiva.*

   _____

3. During Shawna's well-baby visit, the pediatrician noted *an inability of the eyes to gaze in the same direction.*

   _____

4. *Conjunctivitis with hypertrophy of the conjunctiva* is prevalent in third-world countries.

   _____

5. Linda's *sty* was resolved without medical intervention.

   _____

6. *Nearsightedness* is a vision problem that requires corrective lenses.

   _____

7. Because of his *night blindness,* Wade seldom drove his car after dusk.

   _____

8. A decreased field of vision is often the result of *a degenerative disease of the retina.*

   _____

Diagnostic and Treatment Terms Related to the Eye

Review the pronunciation and definition of the diagnostic and treatment terms in Table 15-6. Complete the exercises for each set of terms.

TABLE 15-6 DIAGNOSTIC AND TREATMENT TERMS RELATED TO THE EYE

Term with Pronunciation	Definition
blepharoplasty (**BLEFF**-ah-roh-**plass**-tee) blephar/o = eyelid -plasty = surgical repair	surgical repair or plastic surgery of the eyelid
corneal transplant (**KOR**-nee-al) corne/o = cornea -al = pertaining to	surgical transplantation of a donor cornea into the eye of a recipient

(continues)

TABLE 15-6 DIAGNOSTIC AND TREATMENT TERMS RELATED TO THE EYE (continued)

Term with Pronunciation	Definition
cryoextraction of the lens (**krigh**-oh-ecks-**TRAK**-shun)	removal of the crystalline lens with a cooling probe
enucleation of the eye (ee-**noo**-klee-**AY**-shun)	removal of the eye from the orbit
extracapsular cataract extraction (ECCE) (**eks**-trah-**KAP**-syoo-lar **KAT**-ah-rakt)	removal of the crystalline lens and the anterior segment of the lens capsule
fundoscopy (fun-**DOSS**-koh-pee) fund/o = fundus; base -scopy = examination with a scope	examination of the posterior inner part of the eye, known as the *fundus*, using an ophthalmoscope
intraocular lens implant (**in**-trah-**OK**-yoo-lar) intra- = within ocul/o = eye -ar = pertaining to	surgical implantation of a crystalline lens; usually done at the same time as cataract extraction
iridectomy (ir-id-**EK**-toh-mee) irid/o = iris -ectomy = surgical removal	excision of a section of the iris
keratoplasty (**KAIR**-ah-toh-**plass**-tee) kerat/o = cornea -plasty = surgical repair	surgical repair of the cornea characterized by the excision of an opaque section of the cornea
laser in situ keratomileusis (LASIK) (**kair**-ah-toh-mill-**YOO**-sis)	procedure to correct vision problems, especially myopia, by removing corneal tissue and permanently changing the shape of the cornea
ophthalmoscope (off-**THAL**-moh-skohp) ophthalm/o = eye -scope = instrument for viewing	instrument for viewing the interior of the eye
ophthalmoscopy (**off**-thal-**MOSS**-koh-pee) ophthalm/o = eye -scopy = visualization with a scope	examination of the interior of the eye
phacoemulsification (**fak**-oh-ee-**MULL**-sih-fih-**kay**-shun)	breaking the crystalline lens or its cataract into tiny particles that can be removed by suction or aspiration

(continues)

TABLE 15-6 DIAGNOSTIC AND TREATMENT TERMS RELATED
TO THE EYE (continued)

Term with Pronunciation	Definition
photo-refractive keratectomy (PRK) (**FOH**-toh ree-**FRAK**-tiv kair-ah-**TEK**-toh-mee) kerat/o = cornea -ectomy = surgical removal	surgical removal of corneal surface cells to correct or reduce myopia
radial keratotomy (RK) (**RAY**-dee-al **kair**-ah-**TOT**-oh-mee) kerat/o = cornea -(o)tomy = incision into	spoke-like incisions into the cornea to correct nearsightedness
retinal photocoagulation (**REH**-tin-al **foh**-toh-koh-**ag**-yoo-**LAY**-shun) retin/o = retina -al = pertaining to	laser surgery of the retina to correct retinal detachment and prevent hemorrhage of retinal blood vessels
scleral buckling (**SKLAIR**-al **BUK**-ling) scler/o = sclera -al = pertaining to	repair of retinal detachment by resecting or folding in the sclera
trabeculectomy (trah-**bek**-yoo-**LEK**-toh-mee)	surgical excision of a portion of corneal and scleral tissue to decrease intraocular pressure
trabeculoplasty (trah-**BEK**-yoo-loh-**plass**-tee)	surgical creation of a permanent fistula to drain excess aqueous humor from the anterior chamber of the eye in order to relieve the intraocular pressure associated with glaucoma
vitrectomy (vih-**TREK**-toh-mee) vitre/o = glassy; jelly-like -ectomy = surgical removal	surgical removal of all or part of the vitreous humor

© 2016 Cengage Learning®

EXERCISE 14

Analyze each term by writing the prefix, root, combining vowel, and suffix separated by vertical slashes. Based on the meaning of the word parts, write a definition for each term. Check the definition in a medical dictionary.

1. blepharoplasty

_____

prefix   root   combining vowel   suffix

DEFINITION: _____

2. funduscopy

prefix	root	combining vowel	suffix

DEFINITION: _____

3. iridectomy

prefix	root	combining vowel	suffix

DEFINITION: _____

4. keratoplasty

prefix	root	combining vowel	suffix

DEFINITION: _____

5. ophthalmoscope

prefix	root	combining vowel	suffix

DEFINITION: _____

6. ophthalmoscopy

prefix	root	combining vowel	suffix

DEFINITION: _____

7. vitrectomy

prefix	root	combining vowel	suffix

DEFINITION: _____

EXERCISE 15

Match each medical term in Column 1 with the correct definition in Column 2.

COLUMN 1

_____ 1. corneal transplant

_____ 2. cryoextraction of the lens

_____ 3. ECCE

_____ 4. enucleation of the eye

_____ 5. intraocular lens implant

_____ 6. phacoemulsification

_____ 7. photo-refractive keratectomy

_____ 8. radial keratotomy

_____ 9. retinal photocoagulation

_____ 10. scleral buckling

_____ 11. trabeculectomy

_____ 12. vitrectomy

COLUMN 2

a. breaking the lens into tiny particles

b. extracapsular cataract extraction

c. excision of corneal and scleral tissue

d. folding in of the sclera to repair a detached retina

e. laser surgery of the retina

f. removal of corneal surface cells

g. removal of the eye from the orbit

h. removal of the lens with a cooling probe

i. spoke-like incisions into the cornea

j. surgical implantation of a lens

k. surgical removal of vitreous humor

l. surgical transplantation of a donor cornea

Abbreviations

Review the abbreviations related to the eye in Table 15-7. Practice writing out the meaning of each abbreviation.

TABLE 15-7 ABBREVIATIONS

Abbreviation	Meaning
ECCE	extracapsular cataract extraction
EOM	extraocular movement
ICCE	intracapsular cataract extraction
IOL	intraocular lens
IOP	intraocular pressure
LASIK	laser in situ keratomileusis
OD	right eye (oculus dexter)
OS	left eye (oculus sinister)
OU	each eye (oculus uterque)
PERRLA	pupils equal, round, reactive to light and accommodation
PRK	photo-refractive keratectomy
REM	rapid eye movement
RK	radial keratotomy
VA	visual acuity
VF	visual field

© 2016 Cengage Learning®

The Ear

The visible parts of our ears, located on either side of the head, are called the *external ear*. The internal ear structures, called the *middle* and *inner* ear, are buried in the bony framework of the cranium. The structures of the ear function to provide our sense of hearing, balance, and equilibrium. Sound waves enter the ear, travel through the structures of the middle and inner ear, and are converted to electrical impulses that are transmitted to the cerebral cortex. In the cerebral cortex, the impulses are interpreted into the sounds that we hear. Our sense of hearing is dependent on the health of our ears, our hearing-related nerves, and our brain.

Word Roots Related to Hearing

To understand and use medical terms related to hearing, it is necessary to acquire a thorough knowledge of the associated word roots. Review the word roots in Table 15-8 and complete the exercises.

TABLE 15-8   WORD ROOTS: EAR

Word Root/Combining Form	Meaning
acoust/o	hearing
audi/o	hearing; sound
cochle/o	cochlea
labyrinth/o	inner ear; labyrinth
myring/o	eardrum
ot/o	ear
staped/o	stapes; middle ear bone
tympan/o	eardrum

© 2016 Cengage Learning®

EXERCISE 16

Write the word root and its meaning on the spaces provided.

1. audiologist

   ROOT: _____   MEANING: _____

2. labyrinthitis

   ROOT: _____   MEANING: _____

3. myringotomy

   ROOT: _____   MEANING: _____

4. tympanoplasty

   ROOT: _____   MEANING: _____

5. otitis media

   ROOT: _____   MEANING: _____

6. stapedectomy

   ROOT: _____   MEANING: _____

7. cochleoma

   ROOT: _____   MEANING: _____

8. acoustic nerve

   ROOT: _____   MEANING: _____

EXERCISE 17

Write the correct word root(s) for the following definitions.

1. ear   _____

2. eardrum   _____

3. hearing   _____

4. inner ear   _____

5. middle ear bone _____

Structures of the Ear

The major structures of the ear are organized as the external, middle, and internal ear. Figure 15-13 illustrates these structures. Refer to the figure as you learn about the parts of the ear.

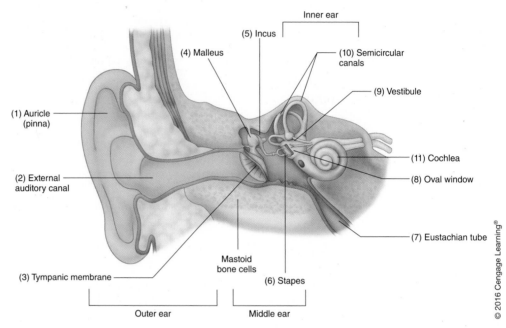

Figure 15-13 Structures of the ear shown in cross section.

The external ear includes the (1) **auricle** (**OR**-ih-kal), or **pinna** (**PIN**-ah), which is a cartilaginous flap that directs sound waves into the (2) **external auditory canal.** The auditory canal is lined with hairs called **cilia** (**SILL**-ee-ah) and **ceruminous** (seh- **ROOM**-ih-nus) **glands**. Cilia help direct sound waves through the canal, and the ceruminous glands produce **cerumen** (seh- **ROO**-men), a substance commonly called *earwax* that protects and lubricates the ear. The external ear is separated from the middle ear by the (3) **tympanic** (tim- **PAN**-ik) **membrane**, or eardrum. The tympanic membrane transmits sound waves to the middle ear.

The middle ear includes three small bones called the **ossicles** (**OSS**-ih-kuhlz). The bone closest to the tympanic membrane is the (4) **malleus** (**MAL**-ee-us), commonly known as the *hammer*; the next bone is the (5) **incus** (**INK**-us), commonly known as the *anvil*; and the third bone is the (6) **stapes** (**STAY**-peez), commonly known as the *stirrup*. The middle ear also includes the (7) **eustachian** (yoo- **STAY**-shun) **tube** that connects the middle ear to the pharynx. Yawning and swallowing cause the eustachian tube to open and equalize the pressure between the middle ear and the outside atmosphere.

Vibrations of the tympanic membrane, which are caused by sound waves, set the ossicles in motion. The malleus transmits sound waves to the incus, which in turn transmits sound waves to the stapes. The stapes vibrate against the (8) **oval window**, which separates the middle ear from the inner ear.

The inner ear, called the **labyrinth** (**LAB**-ih-rinth), includes the (9) **vestibule** (**VESS**-tih-byool), the (10) **semicircular canals**, and the (11) **cochlea** (**KOK**-lee-ah). The cochlea is a spiral or snail-shaped structure that contains auditory fluids and the **organ of Corti**. The organ of Corti receives sound wave vibrations and converts them into nerve impulses. The impulses are carried to the brain by the **acoustic** (ah- **KOO**-stik) **nerve** and are then recognized as specific sounds. The semicircular canals are continuous with the vestibule and are filled with fluid necessary for balance and equilibrium. The process of converting sound waves into hearing is illustrated in Figure 15-14.

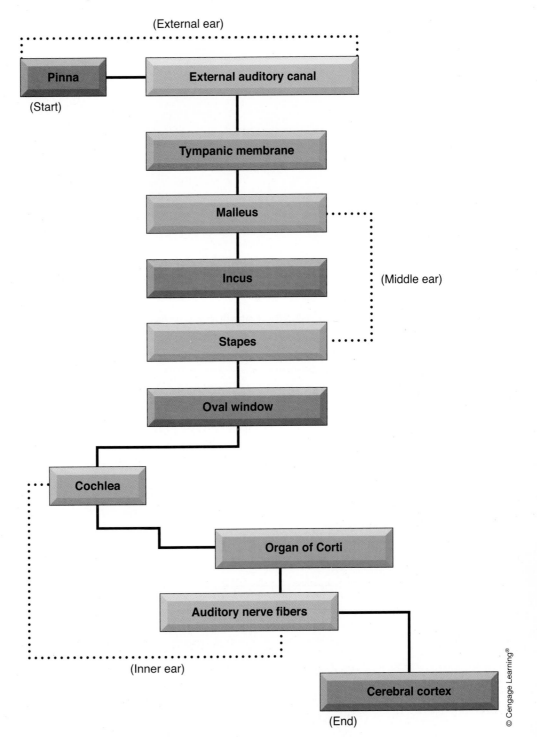

Figure 15-14 Converting sound waves to hearing.

Identify the names of the structures shown in Figure 15-15. Write your answers on the spaces provided.

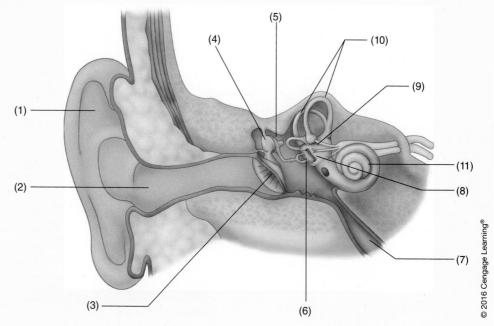

Figure 15-15 Labeling exercise.

1. _____

2. _____

3. _____

4. _____

5. _____

6. _____

7. _____

8. _____

9. _____

10. _____

11. _____

Write the name of each defined structure of the ear.

1. anvil   _____

2. converts sound waves into nerve impulses _____

3. eardrum   _____

4. flap of the outer ear   _____

5. hammer _____

6. inner ear _____

7. middle ear bones (one word) _____

8. secretes earwax _____

9. snail-shaped structure _____

10. stirrup _____

Medical Terminology Related to the Ear

Medical terms related to the ear are organized into three main categories: (1) general medical terms; (2) disease and condition terms; and (3) diagnostic procedure, surgery, and laboratory test terms. Table 15-9 lists roots, prefixes, and suffixes associated with these terms. Review the word parts in the table and complete the exercises.

TABLE 15-9   ROOTS, PREFIXES, AND SUFFIXES

Root	Meaning	Suffix	Meaning	Prefix	Meaning
laryng/o	larynx	-algia	pain	presby-	old
myc/o	fungus	-cusis; cusia	hearing		
rhin/o	nose	-gram	graphic record		
		-metry	to measure		
		-oma	tumor; mass		
		-plasty	surgical repair		
		-(r)rhea	flow; discharge		
		-(o)tomy	incision into		

© 2016 Cengage Learning®

EXERCISE 20

Write the root(s), suffix, and their meanings on the spaces provided. Based on the meaning of the word parts, write a definition for each term. Check the definition in a medical dictionary. Note that some terms might have more than one root.

1. otomycosis

   ROOT: _____ MEANING: _____

   ROOT: _____ MEANING: _____

   PREFIX: _____ MEANING: _____

   SUFFIX: _____ MEANING: _____

   DEFINITION: _____

2. otalgia

   ROOT: _____ MEANING: _____

   PREFIX: _____ MEANING: _____

   SUFFIX: _____ MEANING: _____

   DEFINITION: _____

3. otorrhea

ROOT: _____ MEANING: _____

PREFIX: _____ MEANING: _____

SUFFIX: _____ MEANING: _____

DEFINITION: _____

4. audiogram

ROOT: _____ MEANING: _____

PREFIX: _____ MEANING: _____

SUFFIX: _____ MEANING: _____

DEFINITION: _____

5. myringoplasty

ROOT: _____ MEANING: _____

PREFIX: _____ MEANING: _____

SUFFIX: _____ MEANING: _____

DEFINITION: _____

6. myringotomy

ROOT: _____ MEANING: _____

PREFIX: _____ MEANING: _____

SUFFIX: _____ MEANING: _____

DEFINITION: _____

7. presbycusis

ROOT: _____ MEANING: _____

PREFIX: _____ MEANING: _____

SUFFIX: _____ MEANING: _____

DEFINITION: _____

8. audiometry

ROOT: _____ MEANING: _____

PREFIX: _____ MEANING: _____

SUFFIX: _____ MEANING: _____

DEFINITION: _____

9. audiologist

ROOT: _____ MEANING: _____

PREFIX: _____ MEANING: _____

SUFFIX: _____ MEANING: _____

DEFINITION: _____

10. otorhinolaryngologist

ROOT: _____   MEANING: _____

ROOT: _____   MEANING: _____

ROOT: _____   MEANING: _____

PREFIX: _____   MEANING: _____

SUFFIX: _____   MEANING: _____

DEFINITION: _____

General Medical Terms Related to the Ear

Review the pronunciation and meaning of each term in Table 15-10 and complete the exercises.

TABLE 15-10 GENERAL MEDICAL TERMS RELATED TO THE EAR

Term with Pronunciation	Definition
acoustic (ah-**KOO**-stik) acoust/o = hearing -ic = pertaining to	pertaining to hearing
audiologist (**aw**-dee-**ALL**-oh-jist) audi/o = hearing -(o)logist = specialist	health professional who specializes in evaluating hearing potential and loss
audiology (**aw**-dee-**ALL**-oh-jee) audi/o = hearing -(o)logy = study of	health profession related to the study, evaluation, and measurement of hearing potential and loss
auditory (**AW**-dih-tor-ee) audi/o = hearing -tory = pertaining to	pertaining to hearing
cochlear (**KOK**-lee-ar) cochle/o = cochlea -ar = pertaining to	pertaining to the cochlea
otologist (oh-**TALL**-oh-jist) ot/o = ear -(o)logist = specialist	physician who specializes in the study and treatment of diseases of the ear
otology (oh-**TALL**-oh-jee) ot/o = ear -(o)logy = study of	medical specialty related to the study of the diseases and treatments of the ear

(continues)

TABLE 15-10 GENERAL MEDICAL TERMS RELATED TO THE EAR (continued)

Term with Pronunciation	Definition
otorhinolaryngologist (**oh**-toh-**righ**-noh-**lair**-in-**GALL**-oh-jist) ot/o = ear rhin/o = nose laryng/o = larynx; throat -(o)logist = specialist	physician who specializes in the study and treatment of diseases of the ear, nose, and throat
otorhinolaryngology (**oh**-toh-**righ**-noh-**lair**-in-**GALL**-oh-jee) ot/o = ear rhin/o = nose laryng/o = larynx; throat -(o)logy = study of	medical specialty related to the study and treatment of diseases of the ear, nose, and throat
otoscope (**OH**-toh-skohp) ot/o = ear -scope = instrument for visualization	instrument for visualizing the tympanic membrane and other structures of the ear

© 2016 Cengage Learning®

EXERCISE 21

Analyze each term by writing the prefix, root, combining vowel, and suffix separated by vertical slashes. Based on the meaning of the word parts, write a definition for each term. Check the definition in a medical dictionary. Note that some terms might have more than one root.

1. audiologist

prefix	root	combining vowel	suffix

DEFINITION: _____

2. audiology

prefix	root	combining vowel	suffix

DEFINITION: _____

3. otologist

prefix	root	combining vowel	suffix

DEFINITION: _____

4. otology

prefix	root	combining vowel	suffix

DEFINITION: _____

5. otorhinolaryngologist

prefix	root	combining vowel	suffix

DEFINITION: _____

6. otorhinolaryngology

prefix	root	combining vowel	suffix

DEFINITION: _____

7. otoscope

prefix	root	combining vowel	suffix

DEFINITION: _____

8. acoustic

prefix	root	combining vowel	suffix

DEFINITION: _____

9. cochlear

prefix	root	combining vowel	suffix

DEFINITION: _____

10. auditory

prefix	root	combining vowel	suffix

DEFINITION: _____

11. otoscopy

prefix	root	combining vowel	suffix

DEFINITION: _____

Disease and Disorder Terms Related to the Ear

Ear diseases and disorders include familiar problems such as an earache as well as more complex, less familiar diagnoses such as acoustic neuroma. Review the pronunciation and definition of the terms in Table 15-11 and complete the exercises.

TABLE 15-11   DISEASE AND DISORDER TERMS RELATED TO THE EAR

Term with Pronunciation	Definition
acoustic neuroma (ah-**KOO**-stik noo-**ROO**-mah) acoust/o = hearing -ic = pertaining to neur/o = nerve -oma = tumor; mass	benign tumor of the acoustic nerve
cholesteatoma (**koh**-lee-**stee**-ah-**TOH**-mah)	slow-growth cystic mass or tumor made up of epithelial cell debris and cholesterol; commonly occurs in the middle ear

(continues)

TABLE 15-11 DISEASE AND DISORDER TERMS RELATED TO THE EAR
(continued)

Term with Pronunciation	Definition
conductive deafness	hearing loss caused by impaired transmission of sound waves through the middle or external ear
impacted cerumen (seh-**ROO**-men)	excessive accumulation of cerumen (earwax)
labyrinthitis (**lab**-ih-rin-**THIGH**-tis) labyrinth/o = labyrinth -itis = inflammation	inflammation or infection of the labyrinth or inner ear
Meniere's disease (man-ee-**AYRZ**)	chronic inner ear disorder characterized by episodes of vertigo, a sensation of a spinning moition, intermittent hearing loss, tinnitus (ringing in the ears), and a feeling of fullness or pressure in the ear
myringitis (mir-in-**JIGH**-tis) myring/o = tympanic membrane; eardrum -itis = inflammation	inflammation of the tympanic membrane (eardrum)
otalgia (oh-**TAL**-jee-ah) ot/o = ear -algia = pain	pain in the ear; earache
otitis externa (oh-**TIGH**-tis eks-**TER**-nah) ot/o = ear -itis = inflammation	inflammation of the external ear canal; commonly called *swimmer's ear*
otitis media (oh-**TIGH**-tis **MEE**-dee-ah) ot/o = ear -itis = inflammation	infection and inflammation of the middle ear; commonly called a *middle ear infection*
otomycosis (**oh**-toh-my-**KOH**-sis) ot/o = ear myc/o = fungus -osis = condition	fungal infection of the external auditory meatus (opening)
otorrhea (oh-toh-**REE**-ah) ot/o = ear -(r)rhea = flow; discharge	discharge or drainage from the ear

(continues)

TABLE 15-11   DISEASE AND DISORDER TERMS RELATED TO THE EAR
(continued)

Term with Pronunciation	Definition
otosclerosis (**oh**-toh-sklair-**OH**-sis) ot/o = ear -sclerosis = hardening	hereditary condition characterized by irregular ossification of the bones of the middle ear, especially the stapes, causing tinnitus and deafness
perforation of the tympanic membrane	rupture or development of holes in the eardrum
presbycusis (prez-bee-**KOO**-sis) presby- = old -cusis = hearing	impaired hearing related to the aging process
sensorineural deafness (**sen**-soh-ree-**NOO**-ral)	loss of hearing resulting from impaired or damaged auditory nerve cells or tissue
serous otitis media (**SEER**-us oh-**TIGH**-tis) ot/o = ear -itis = inflammation	middle ear infection characterized by an accumulation of serous fluid and air bubbles behind the tympanic membrane (Figure 15-16)

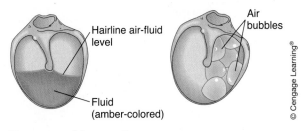

Figure 15-16   Serous otitis media.

suppurative otitis media (**SOO**-per-ah-tiv oh-**TIGH**-tis) ot/o = ear -itis = inflammation	middle ear infection characterized by an accumulation of purulent (pus-filled) fluid behind the tympanic membrane; symptoms might include dizziness and tinnitus (Figure 15-17)

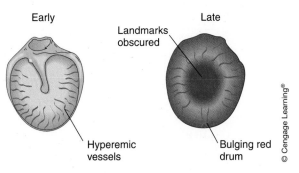

Figure 15-17   Suppurative otitis media.

TABLE 15-11 DISEASE AND DISORDER TERMS RELATED TO THE EAR
(continued)

Term with Pronunciation	Definition
tinnitus (tin-**NIGH**-tus)	ringing or tinkling sensation in the ears
tympanitis (**tim**-pah-**NIGH**-tis) tympan/o = eardrum -itis = inflammation	inflammation of the tympanic membrane (eardrum); often associated with otitis media
vertigo (**VER**-tih-goh)	sensation of spinning or dizziness, usually a result of a disturbance of equilibrium

© 2016 Cengage Learning®

EXERCISE 22

Analyze each term by writing the prefix, root, combining vowel, and suffix separated by vertical slashes. Based on the meaning of the word parts, write a definition for each term. Check the definition in a medical dictionary. Note that some terms might have more than one root.

1. labyrinthitis

prefix	root	combining vowel	suffix

DEFINITION: _____

2. myringitis

prefix	root	combining vowel	suffix

DEFINITION: _____

3. otalgia

prefix	root	combining vowel	suffix

DEFINITION: _____

4. otomycosis

prefix	root	combining vowel	suffix

DEFINITION: _____

5. otorrhea

prefix	root	combining vowel	suffix

DEFINITION: _____

6. otosclerosis

prefix	root	combining vowel	suffix

DEFINITION: _____

7. presbycusis

prefix	root	combining vowel	suffix

DEFINITION: _____

8. tympanitis

prefix	*root*	*combining vowel*	*suffix*

DEFINITION: _____

EXERCISE 23

Replace the italicized phrase with the correct medical term.

1. Felipe's hearing loss was caused by a *benign tumor of the acoustic nerve.*

    _____

2. *Excessive earwax* should be removed by a health care professional.

    _____

3. Many hours in the pool caused Tawnia's *swimmer's ear.*

    _____

4. *Middle ear infection* is a common childhood problem.

    _____

5. *Excessive fluid in the inner ear* leads to profound dizziness.

    _____

6. A hearing aid often improves *hearing loss due to impaired transmission of sound waves through the middle ear.*

    _____

7. Chronic otitis media might lead to a *cystic mass of cell debris and cholesterol.*

    _____

8. Many individuals experience *dizziness* in high places.

    _____

9. Recurrent *pus-filled middle ear infections* might require surgical intervention.

    _____

10. *Ringing in the ears* might be a symptom of inner ear problems.

    _____

11. Li's *benign acoustic nerve tumor* was successfully treated with radiation.

    _____

12. Marta's *inner ear infection* did not respond to antibiotic therapy.

    _____

13. *Chronic inner ear disease* is characterized by nausea, vomiting, and loss of balance.

    _____

14. Bart had *an excessive accumulation of earwax* removed by his family physician.

    _____

Diagnostic and Treatment Terms Related to the Ear

Review the pronunciation and definition of the diagnostic and treatment terms in Table 15-12 and complete the exercises.

TABLE 15-12 DIAGNOSTIC AND TREATMENT TERMS RELATED TO THE EAR

Term with Pronunciation	Definition
audiogram (**AW**-dee-oh-gram) audi/o = hearing -gram = record	graphic record of hearing
audiometry (aw-dee-**OM**-eh-tree) audi/o = hearing -metry = to measure	measuring the sense of hearing
myringoplasty (mir-**IN**-goh-**plass**-tee) myring/o = tympanic membrane; eardrum -plasty = surgical repair	surgical repair of the tympanic membrane
myringotomy (mir-in-**GOT**-oh-mee) myring/o = tympanic membrane; eardrum -(o)tomy = incision into	incision into the tympanic membrane
myringotomy and tubes (mir-in**GOT**-oh-mee) myring/o = tympanic membrane; eardrum -(o)tomy = incision into	incision into the tympanic membrane and insertion of tubes to allow drainage of fluid that might accumulate behind the eardrum (Figure 15-18)

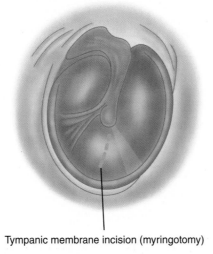

Tympanic membrane incision (myringotomy)

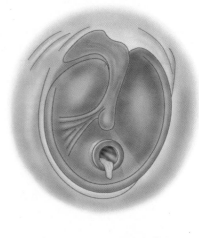

Tube placement to drain fluid

© Cengage Learning®

Figure 15-18 Myringotomy with tube placement.

TABLE 15-12   DIAGNOSTIC AND TREATMENT TERMS RELATED TO THE EAR (continued)

Term with Pronunciation	Definition
otoplasty (**OH**-toh-**plass**-tee) ot/o = ear -plasty = surgical repair	surgical repair of one or both of the ears, usually refers to repair of the outer ear
otoscopy (oh-**TOSS**-koh-pee) ot/o = ear -scopy = examination with a scope	visualization and examination of the tympanic membrane using an otoscope
Rinne test (**RIN**-nee)	hearing examination that compares bone and air conduction of sound waves using a vibrating tuning fork
stapedectomy (**stay**-pee-**DEK**-toh-mee) staped/o = stapes -ectomy = surgical removal	excision of the stapes
tympanoplasty (**tim**-pan-oh-**PLASS**-tee) tympan/o = tympanic membrane; eardrum -plasty = surgical repair	surgical repair of the tympanic membrane
tympanotomy (**tim**-pan-**OT**-oh-mee) tympan/o = tympanic membrane; eardrum -(o)tomy = incision into	incision into the tympanic membrane
Weber test	examination of auditory acuity to determine whether a hearing deficit is conductive or sensorineural

© 2016 Cengage Learning®

EXERCISE 24

Analyze each term by writing the prefix, root, combining vowel, and suffix separated by vertical slashes. Based on the meaning of the word parts, write a definition for each term. Check the definition in a medical dictionary.

1. audiogram

prefix	root	combining vowel	suffix

DEFINITION: _____

2. audiometry

prefix	root	combining vowel	suffix

DEFINITION: _____

3. myringoplasty

prefix	root	combining vowel	suffix

DEFINITION: _____

4. myringotomy

prefix	root	combining vowel	suffix

DEFINITION: _____

5. otoplasty

prefix	root	combining vowel	suffix

DEFINITION: _____

6. otoscopy

prefix	root	combining vowel	suffix

DEFINITION: _____

7. stapedectomy

prefix	root	combining vowel	suffix

DEFINITION: _____

8. tympanoplasty

prefix	root	combining vowel	suffix

DEFINITION: _____

9. tympanotomy

prefix	root	combining vowel	suffix

DEFINITION: _____

EXERCISE 25

Circle the term that best fits the definition.

DEFINITION	**CIRCLE ONE TERM**
1. surgical repair of the tympanic membrane	*myringotomy* OR *myringoplasty*
2. incision into the tympanic membrane	*myringotomy* OR *myringoplasty*
3. surgical repair of the ear(s)	*otoplasty* OR *otomy*
4. measurement of hearing	*otometery* OR *audiometry*
5. graphic record of hearing	*audiogram* OR *audiometry*
6. conductive, sensorial hearing loss test	*Weber test* OR *Rinne test*
7. visualization of the inner ear	*otography* OR *otoscopy*
8. bone and air conduction sound test	*Weber test* OR *Rinne test*

Abbreviations

Review the abbreviations in Table 15-13. Practice writing the meaning of each abbreviation.

TABLE 15-13   ABBREVIATIONS

Abbreviation	Meaning
AC	air conduction
AD	right ear (auris dextra)
AS	left ear (auris sinistra)
AU	each ear (auris unitas)
BC	bone conduction
BOM	bilateral otitis media
EENT	eyes, ears, nose, throat
ENT	ears, nose, throat
TM	tympanic membrane

© 2016 Cengage Learning®

CHAPTER REVIEW

The Chapter Review can be used as a self-test. Go through each exercise and answer as many questions as you can without referring to previous exercises or earlier discussions within this chapter. Check your answers and fill in any blanks. Practice writing any terms you might have misspelled.

EXERCISE 26

Write the medical term for each definition.

1. within the eye _____

2. physician who specializes in diseases and treatment of the eye _____

3. inflammation of the eyelids _____

4. inflammation of the conjunctiva _____

5. abnormal protrusion of the eyeballs _____

6. farsightedness _____

7. nearsightedness _____

8. impaired vision related to aging _____

9. surgical repair of the eyelid _____

10. abnormal sensitivity to light _____

11. pertaining to hearing _____

12. specialist who evaluates hearing loss _____

13. ear, nose, and throat physician specialist _____

14. excessive accumulation of earwax _____

15. inflammation of the eardrum _____

16. fungal infection of the ear   _____

17. AS   _____

18. ringing sensation in the ears   _____

19. dizziness   _____

20. incision into the eardrum   _____

EXERCISE 27

Write a brief definition for each medical term.

1. nasolacrimal   _____

2. ophthalmology   _____

3. blepharoptosis   _____

4. diplopia   _____

5. glaucoma   _____

6. keratitis   _____

7. nyctalopia   _____

8. retinopathy   _____

9. ophthalmoscope   _____

10. cochlear   _____

11. labyrinthitis   _____

12. otalgia   _____

13. otorrhea   _____

14. presbycusis   _____

15. audiometry   _____

16. tympanoplasty   _____

EXERCISE 28

Circle the medical term that best fits the definition.

DEFINITION	CIRCLE ONE TERM
1. agent that constricts the pupil	*mydriatic* OR *miotic*
2. cyst caused by an obstructed meibomian gland	*hordeolum* OR *chalazion*
3. divergent strabismus	*ectropion* OR *exotropia*
4. turning inward of the eyelash margin	*esotropia* OR *entropion*
5. increased intraocular pressure	*glaucoma* OR *cataract*
6. agent that dilates the pupil	*miotic* OR *mydriatic*
7. convergent strabismus	*esotropia* OR *entropion*
8. bacterial infection of an eyelash follicle	*pterygium* OR *hordeolum*

9. progressive cloudiness of the lens *glaucoma* OR *cataract*
10. turning outward of the eyelash margins *pterygium* OR *ectropion*
11. chronic, contagious conjunctivitis *trachoma* OR *hordeolum*
12. inability of the eyes to gaze in the same direction *nystagmus* OR *strabismus*
13. irregular thickening of the conjunctiva *chalazion* OR *pterygium*
14. involuntary movement of the eyes *nystagmus* OR *strabismus*

EXERCISE 29

Match the term or abbreviation in Column 1 with the description in Column 2

COLUMN 1

_____ 1. astigmatism
_____ 2. audiogram
_____ 3. audiology
_____ 4. BOM
_____ 5. chalazion
_____ 6. cholesteatoma
_____ 7. hordeolum
_____ 8. Meniere's disease
_____ 9. otitis externa
_____ 10. otitis media
_____ 11. otology
_____ 12. otoplasty
_____ 13. otorhinolaryngologist
_____ 14. retinoblastoma
_____ 15. uveitis

COLUMN 2

a. bilateral otitis media
b. chronic inner ear disorder with fluid accumulation
c. swimmer's ear
d. surgical repair of the ear
e. graphic record of hearing
f. infection of the middle ear
g. mass of cellular debris and cholesterol
h. specialist of the ear, nose, and throat
i. study of diseases and treatments of the ear
j. study of hearing
k. inflammation of the iris, ciliary body, and choroid
l. irregularly focused light rays, abnormally shaped cornea
m. sty
n. cyst due to obstructed meibomian gland
o. malignant tumor of the retina

EXERCISE 30

Read the following operative report. Write out the abbreviations and provide a brief definition of the italicized medical terms. Use a medical dictionary to look up the meaning of the terms.

PREOPERATIVE DIAGNOSIS: Nuclear (1) *cataract* with cortical spoking, (2) *OD*.
POSTOPERATIVE DIAGNOSIS: Nuclear cataract with cortical spoking, OD.
OPERATION PERFORMED: (3) *ECCE* with a posterior chamber (4) *intraocular* lens implant, OD.

DESCRIPTION OF PROCEDURE: The patient was placed in the supine position, and (5) *periorbital* anesthesia was achieved. The patient's periorbital areas were prepped and the right eye draped in the usual fashion for an (6) *ophthalmic* surgical procedure. The lids of the right eye were retracted, an 8-0 black silk bridle suture was passed under the superior rectus tendon, and the globe was retracted downward. A (7) *conjunctival* peritomy was then performed for 180 degrees. A (8) *corneoscleral* groove was then formed. Two preplaced 8-0 black silk sutures were then passed through the groove. The (9) *anterior chamber* was then entered with a razor blade incision through the groove and filled with Healon. The anterior (10) *capsulotomy* was then performed. The nucleus was then expressed without difficulty. The patient tolerated the procedure well and was transferred to the recovery room in excellent condition.

1. _____
2. _____
3. _____
4. _____
5. _____
6. _____
7. _____
8. _____
9. _____
10. _____

EXERCISE 31

Read the progress note and write a brief definition for each italicized medical term, abbreviation, or phrase.

PROGRESS NOTE
The patient is a 9-month-old infant who presents with tenderness, (1) *AU*. His mother states that he has been "fussy during feeding and does not have a fever." (2) *Otoscopic* examination reveals (3) *suppurative otitis media*, more pronounced in the left ear. The (4) *tympanic membrane* is edematous and bulging. I explained to mom due to recurring episodes of (5) *serous otitis media* and today's problem, she should consider bilateral (6) *myringotomy* and (7) *tympanostomy* with placement of tubes. We briefly discussed the pros and cons of this procedure and mom understands my concern related to (8) *labyrinthitis*. I prescribed (9) *otic* drops to be administered three times per day. A two-week follow-up visit will be scheduled.

1. _____
2. _____
3. _____

4. _____

5. _____

6. _____

7. _____

8. _____

9. _____

EXERCISE 32

Select the best answer for each question or statement.

1. Select the term for involuntary movements of the eyes.
   a. astigmatism
   b. nystagmus
   c. hordeolum
   d. pterygium

2. Which term means impaired vision related to aging?
   a. myopia
   b. hyperopia
   c. presbyopia
   d. esotropia

3. Select the term for abnormal cloudiness of the lens.
   a. cataract
   b. hordeolum
   c. glaucoma
   d. pterygium

4. Select the medical term for the condition commonly known as *cross-eyed*.
   a. ectropion
   b. entropion
   c. exotropia
   d. esotropia

5. Which medical term describes an irregular thickening of the conjunctiva?
   a. conjunctivitis
   b. pterygium
   c. hordeolum
   d. nystagmus

6. Choose the medical term for nearsightedness.
   a. myopia
   b. hyperopia
   c. nyctalopia
   d. exotropia

7. Select the medical term for the condition commonly known as a *sty*.
   a. pterygium
   b. hordeolum
   c. entropion
   d. dacryocystitis

8. Which medical term describes an abnormal protrusion of the eyeballs?
   a. exotropia
   b. hyperopia
   c. esotropia
   d. exophthalmia

9. Select the medical term for a drooping eyelid.
   a. blepharoptosis
   b. ectropion
   c. entropion
   d. hordeolum

10. Which term best describes the condition commonly known as *walleyed*?
    a. exophthalmia
    b. exotropia
    c. hyperopia
    d. esotropia

11. The structures of the inner ear are collectively known as which term?
    a. ossicles
    b. semicircular canals
    c. vestibule
    d. labyrinth

12. Which term describes the structure(s) of the ear that play a role in balance and equilibrium?
    a. labyrinth
    b. ossicles
    c. semicircular canals
    d. eustachian tube

13. Select the term for the structure(s) of the ear that house the organ of Corti.
    a. cochlea
    b. ossicles
    c. labyrinth
    d. eustachian tube

14. Collectively, what term describes the bones of the middle ear?
    a. ossicles
    b. labyrinth
    c. cochlea
    d. semicircular canals

15. Which term describes the ear structure(s) that help equalize the pressure between the ear and the atmosphere?
    a. cochlea
    b. labyrinth
    c. semicircular canals
    d. eustachian tube

16. Which abbreviation means left ear?
    a. AS
    b. AD
    c. LE
    d. AU

17. Which term names the structure that separates the middle ear from the inner ear?
    a. cochlea
    b. labyrinth
    c. oval window
    d. tympanic membrane

18. Select the term for a ringing sensation in the ears.
    a. tympanitis
    b. vertigo
    c. otosclerosis
    d. tinnitus

19. Select the correct abbreviation for right ear.
    a. AS
    b. AD
    c. RE
    d. AU

20. Which term is the test that uses a tuning fork to measure the conduction of sound waves?
    a. otoscopy
    b. Weber test
    c. sensorineural test
    d. Rinne test

CHALLENGE EXERCISES

1. *Laser surgery to correct various vision problems has been widely publicized. Visit a local ophthalmologist and gather information about the types of surgery being performed, the vision problems that can be corrected with each type of surgery, and the risks and benefits of the surgery. If you do not have access to a local*

ophthalmologist, search the Internet for the information, using the keywords "laser surgery" and "eye."

2. *Interview a local audiologist or search the Internet using the keywords audiology or audiologist for specific information about the profession. What are the educational requirements? Is there a national or state certification or licensing examination? What type of equipment does an audiologist use? Are there many employment opportunities in the field?*

Pronunciation Review

Review the terms in the chapter. Pronounce each term using the following phonetic pronunciations. Check off the term when you are comfortable saying it.

TERM	PRONUNCIATION
□ acoustic neuroma	ah-**KOO**-stik noo-**ROH**-mah
□ aqueous humor	**AY**-kwee-us humor
□ astigmatism	ah-**STIG**-mah-tizm
□ audiogram	**AW**-dee-oh-gram
□ audiologist	aw-dee-**ALL**-oh-jist
□ audiology	aw-dee-**ALL**-oh-jee
□ audiometry	aw-dee-**OM**-eh-tree
□ auditory	**AW**-dih-tor-ee
□ auricle	**OR**-ih-kal
□ blepharitis	bleh-fah-**RIGH**-tis
□ blepharoplasty	**BLEFF**-ah-roh-**plass**-tee
□ blepharoptosis	bleh-fah-roh-**TOH**-sis
□ cataract	**KAT**-ah-rakt
□ cerumen	seh-**ROO**-men
□ ceruminous gland	seh-**ROOM**-ih-nus gland
□ chalazion	kah-**LAY**-zee-on
□ cholesteatoma	koh-lee-**stee**-ah-**TOH**-mah
□ choroid	**KOH**-royd
□ cilia	**SILL**-ee-ah
□ ciliary body	**SILL**-ee-air-ee body
□ cochlea	**KOK**-lee-ah
□ cochlear	**KOK**-lee-ar
□ conductive deafness	kon-**DUK**-tiv deafness
□ conjunctiva	kon-junk-**TIGH**-vah
□ conjunctivitis	kon-**junk**-tih-**VIGH**-tis
□ cornea	**KOR**-nee-ah
□ corneal transplant	**KOR**-nee-al transplant
□ cryoextraction of the lens	**krigh**-oh-eks-**TRAK**-shun of the lens
□ crystalline lens	**KRIS**-tah-lin lens

☐ dacryocystitis — **dak**-ree-oh-sis-**TIGH**-tis

☐ diabetic retinopathy — **digh**-ah-**BET**-ik **reh**-tin-**OP**-ah-thee

☐ diplopia — dih-**PLOH**-pee-ah

☐ ectropion — ek-**TROH**-pee-on

☐ entropion — en-**TROH**-pee-on

☐ enucleation of the eye — ee-**noo**-klee-**AY**-shun of the eye

☐ esotropia — es-oh-**TROH**-pee-ah

☐ eustachian tube — yoo-**STAY**-shun tube

☐ exophthalmia — **eks**-off-**THAL**-mee-ah

☐ exotropia — **eks**-oh-**TROH**-pee-ah

☐ extracapsular cataract extraction — **eks**-trah-**KAPS**-yoo-lar **KAT**-ah-rakt extraction

☐ funduscopy — fun-**DUSS**-koh-pee

☐ glaucoma — glaw-**KOH**-mah

☐ hordeolum — hor-**DEE**-oh-lum

☐ hyperopia — **high**-per-**OH**-pee-ah

☐ impacted cerumen — impacted seh-**ROO**-men

☐ incus — **INK**-us

☐ intraocular — **in**-trah-**OK**-yoo-lar

☐ intraocular lens implant — **in**-trah-**OK**-yoo-lar lens implant

☐ iridectomy — ir-id-**EK**-toh-mee

☐ iris — **EYE**-ris

☐ iritis — ir-**EYE**-tis

☐ keratitis — **kair**-ah-**TIGH**-tis

☐ keratoplasty — **KAIR**-ah-toh-**plass**-tee

☐ labyrinth — **LAB**-ih-rinth

☐ labyrinthitis — **lab**-ih-rin-**THIGH**-tis

☐ lacrimal — **LAK**-rih-mal

☐ lacrimal duct — **LAK**-rih-mal duct

☐ lacrimal fluid — **LAK**-rih-mal fluid

☐ lacrimal gland — **LAK**-rih-mal gland

☐ lacrimal sac — **LAK**-rih-mal sac

☐ malleus — **MAL**-lee-us

☐ meibomian glands — migh-**BOH**-mee-an glands

☐ Meniere's disease — man-ee-**AYRZ** disease

☐ miotic — migh-**OT**-ik

☐ mydriatic — mid-ree-**AT**-ik

☐ myopia — migh-**OH**-pee-ah

☐ myringitis — mir-in-**JIGH**-tis

☐ myringoplasty   mir-**IN**-goh-**plass**-tee

☐ myringotomy   mir-in-**GOT**-oh-mee

☐ nasolacrimal   **nay**-zoh-**LAK**-ree-mal

☐ nyctalopia   **nik**-toh-**LOH**-pee-ah

☐ nystagmus   nih-**STAG**-mus

☐ ophthalmologist   **off**-thall-**MALL**-oh-jist

☐ ophthalmology   **off**-thall-**MALL**-oh-jee

☐ ophthalmoscope   off-**THAL**-moh-skohp

☐ ophthalmoscopy   **off**-thal-**MOSS**-koh-pee

☐ optician   op-**TIH**-shun

☐ optometrist   op-**TOM**-eh-trist

☐ optometry   op-**TOM**-eh-tree

☐ organ of Corti   organ of **KOR**-tee

☐ ossicles   **OSS**-ih-kulz

☐ otalgia   oh-**TAL**-jee-ah

☐ otitis externa   oh-**TIGH**-tis eks-**TER**-nah

☐ otitis media   oh-**TIGH**-tis **MEE**-dee-ah

☐ otologist   oh-**TALL**-oh-jist

☐ otology   oh-**TALL**-oh-jee

☐ otomycosis   **oh**-toh-migh-**KOH**-sis

☐ otoplasty   **OH**-toh-**plass**-tee

☐ otorhinolaryngologist   **oh**-toh-**righ**-noh-**lair**-in-**GALL**-oh-jist

☐ otorhinolaryngology   **oh**-toh-**righ**-noh-**lair**-in-**GALL**-oh-jee

☐ otorrhea   oh-toh-**REE**-ah

☐ otosclerosis   **oh**-toh-sklair-**OH**-sis

☐ otoscope   **OH**-toh-skohp

☐ otoscopy   oh-**TOSS**-koh-pee

☐ phacoemulsification   **fak**-oh-ee-**MULL**-sih-fih-**kay**-shun

☐ photo-refractive keratectomy   **FOH**-toh ree-**FRAK**-tiv **kair**-ah-**TEK**-toh-mee

☐ photophobia   foh-toh-**FOH**-bee-ah

☐ photoretinitis   **foh**-toh-reh-tih-**NIGH-tis**

☐ presbycusis   prez-bee-**KOO**-sis

☐ presbyopia   prez-bee-**OH**-pee-ah

☐ pterygium   ter-**IJ**-ee-um

☐ radial keratotomy   **RAY**-dee-al **kair**-ah-**TOT**-oh-mee

☐ retina   **RET**-ih-nah

☐ retinal photocoagulation   **REH**-tin-al **foh**-toh-koh-**ag**-yoo-**LAY**-shun

☐ retinitis pigmentosa **reh**-tih-**NIGH**-tis **pig**-men-**TOH**-sah

☐ retinoblastoma **reh**-tin-oh-blass-**TOH**-mah

☐ retinopathy **reh**-tin-**OP**-ah-thee

☐ Rinne test **RIN**-nee test

☐ sensorineural deafness **sen**-soh-ree-**NOO**-ral deafness

☐ serous otitis media **SEER**-us oh-**TIGH**-tis media

☐ sclera **SKLAIR**-ah

☐ scleral buckling **SKLAIR**-al buckling

☐ stapedectomy **stay**-pee-**DEK**-doh-mee

☐ stapes **STAY**-peez

☐ strabismus strah-**BIZ**-mus

☐ suppurative otitis media **SOO**-per-ah-tiv oh-**TIGH**-tis media

☐ suspensatory ligaments suh-**SPEN**-sah-tor-ee ligaments

☐ tinnitus tin-**NIGH**-tus

☐ trabeculectomy trah-**bek**-yoo-**LEK**-toh-mee

☐ trachoma tray-**KOH**-mah

☐ tympanic membrane tim-**PAN**-ik membrane

☐ tympanitis **tim**-pah-**NIGH**-tis

☐ tympanoplasty **tim**-pan-oh-**PLASS**-tee

☐ tympanotomy **tim**-pan-**OT**-toh-mee

☐ uveitis yoo-vee-**EYE**-tis

☐ vertigo **VER**-tih-goh

☐ vestibule **VESS**-tih-byool

☐ vitrectomy vih-**TREK**-toh-mee

☐ vitreous humor **VIH**-tree-us humor

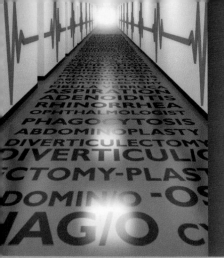

16 Specialty Terminology

OBJECTIVES

At the completion of this chapter, the student should be able to:

1. Define and spell medical terms related to oncology, pharmacology, and surgery.
2. Describe the difference between benign and malignant tumors.
3. Discuss four cancer treatment methods.
4. Compare five diagnostic methods related to cancer.
5. Interpret commonly used prescription medication abbreviations.
6. Differentiate between medication actions and medication effects.
7. Compare four types of anesthesia.
8. Describe six surgical positions.

OVERVIEW

This chapter introduces you to frequently used medical terminology related to the following: (1) **oncology** (on-**KALL**-oh-jee), the medical specialty for the study, diagnosis, and treatment of cancer; (2) **pharmacology** (**farm**-ah-**KALL**-oh-jee), the study of the nature, uses, and effects of drugs used for medicinal purposes; and (3) surgery. Some of the body system terms related to these topics have been presented in previous chapters. The terms presented in this chapter are more general and add to your knowledge of the language of the health care industry.

Oncology

As stated in the overview, oncology is the medical specialty dedicated for the study, diagnosis, and treatment of cancer. Physicians who specialize in this field are called **oncologists** (on-**KALL**-oh-jists). A **radiation oncologist** is a physician who specializes in using radiation to treat cancer. A **radiation therapist** is an individual who administers highly focused forms of radiation to treat cancer and other diseases.

Some texts define oncology as the sum of knowledge regarding tumors. Tumors, described as abnormal masses of tissue due to excessive cell growth, are generally classified as **benign** (bee-**NIGHN**) or **malignant** (mah-**LIG**-nant). Benign tumors are seldom life-threatening and do not spread to other parts of the body. Malignant tumors are referred to as cancer because they can be life-threatening, and are characterized by uncontrollable growth and **metastasis** (meh-**TASS**-tah-sis). According to the American Cancer Society (ACS), metastasis is the spread of cancer cells to other parts of the body.

Cancer

Cancer develops when cells in the body begin growing in an uncontrolled manner and continue to grow and form new abnormal cells. Cancer cells develop when the **DNA** (deoxyribonucleic acid) of our normal cells becomes damaged. DNA is in every cell and is responsible for directing all cellular activities, including cellular reproduction. Under normal conditions, the body is able to repair damaged DNA. In cancer cells, the DNA is not repairable, resulting in abnormal, uncontrolled cell growth and reproduction.

Damaged DNA can be inherited from genetic mutations in maternal or paternal chromosomes. About 5% of cancers in the United States are the result of inherited genetic mutations. According to the ACS, an individual's DNA becomes damaged by exposure to **carcinogens** (**kar**-**SIN**-oh-jenz), which are any substances that cause cancer or help cancer grow, such as the substances in tobacco products. Other environmental carcinogens include prolonged exposure to sunlight, exhaust fumes from vehicles, insecticides, and other chemicals. Regardless of the origin, cancer is the second leading cause of death in the United States.

Types of Cancer

There are two main categories of cancer that are classified according to the type of tissue where the tumor arises, or begins. The categories are **carcinomas** (**kar**-sin-**OH**-mahz) and **sarcomas** (sar-**KOH**-mahz).

Carcinomas are made up of epithelial cells and often infiltrate surrounding tissue. This is the largest group of malignant tumors and 80–90% of all cancers are carcinomas. In the early stages, this type of cancer might present as **carcinoma in situ** (**kar**-sin-**OH**-mah in **SIGH**-too), which means the tumor is confined to the organ where it first developed. The cancer has not metastasized and often is highly curable. Two types of carcinoma are **squamous** (**SKWAY**-mus) **cell carcinoma** and **adenocarcinoma** (**add**-in-noh-**kar**-sin-**OH**-mah). Squamous cell carcinoma begins in nonglandular cells such as the skin, as illustrated in Figure 16-1.

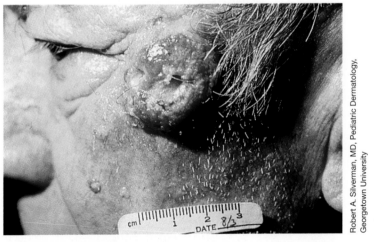

Robert A. Silverman, MD, Pediatric Dermatology, Georgetown University

Figure 16-1 Squamous cell carcinoma (Robert A. Silverman, MD, Pediatric Dermatology, Georgetown University).

Adenocarcinoma begins in glandular tissue such as the ducts or lobules of the breast. Adenocarcinomas can also arise from the tissue of organs such as the stomach, colon, pancreas, and kidneys. Figure 16-2 illustrates adenocarcinoma of the colon.

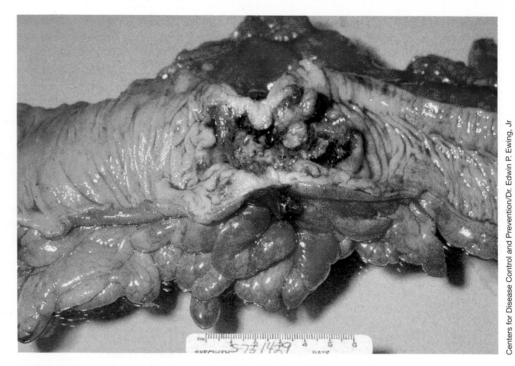

Centers for Disease Control and Prevention/Dr. Edwin P. Ewing, Jr

Figure 16-2   Adenocarcinoma of the colon (Centers for Disease Control and Prevention/Dr. Edwin P. Ewing Jr.).

Sarcomas begin in connective tissue such as bone, cartilage, and muscles. Recall that smooth muscle cancer is called leiomyosarcoma, and skeletal muscle cancer is called rhabdomyosarcoma.

Diagnostic Methods

Several **biopsy** methods are available to confirm a cancer diagnosis. All methods involve removing or withdrawing a sample of the suspicious tissue or tumor. The sample is then examined under a microscope to asses the type of cellular growth associated with the tumor. Diagnostic methods include:

- **Fine needle aspiration biopsy** (FNAB)—A very thin needle attached to a syringe is used to withdraw a small amount of tissue from the suspected tumor.
- **Needle core biopsy**—A slightly larger needle is used in this type of biopsy. The larger needle allows the physician to withdraw a larger sample of tissue.
- **Excisional** or **incisional biopsy**—A surgeon cuts through the skin and removes the entire tumor, which is known as an excisional biopsy; or the surgeon removes a small part of a large tumor, which is known as an incisional biopsy. These biopsies are often done with local or regional anesthesia.
- **Endoscopic biopsy**—During an endoscopic biopsy, a flexible tube is inserted into a natural body opening. The tube contains a viewing lens or camera, a fiber-optic light, and small instruments for removing samples of the tumor or suspicious tissue.
- **Laparoscopy**, **thoracoscopy**, or **mediastinoscopy**—These methods are similar to an endoscopic biopsy, but each requires a small incision to introduce the endoscope into the body. When the sample is taken from tumors

or tissue in the abdominal or pelvic cavities, the procedure is called *laparoscopy*. If the procedure involves the chest, it is called a *thoracoscopy* or *mediastinoscopy*.

- **Open surgical exploration**—When a needle or endoscopic biopsy method does not or will not provide enough information about a suspected malignancy, a *laparotomy* might be necessary. Laparotomy requires general anesthesia and often involves an incision from the lower end of the sternum to the lower part of the abdomen. With this method, the physician can visually examine the size of the tumor as well as take biopsies. If this procedure involves the chest, it is called *thoracotomy* or *mediastinotomy*.

Grading and Staging Malignant Tumors

To determine the best course of treatment, oncologists must know the characteristics of malignant tumors or cancers. This information is obtained through gross and microscopic examinations of the tumor and its cells. After these examinations are completed, the tumor is assigned a **grade** on a scale from 1 to 4, which measures the extent to which malignant cells and tissue resemble the "normal," or parent cells. Grade 1 tumors have cells that are very much like normal cells; grade 4 tumors have cells that are the least like normal cells. The term **differentiation** (**diff**-er-en-shee-**AY**-shun), which means the cells have developed into what they are supposed to be, is also used when tumors are graded. Therefore, a tumor that is categorized as *grade 1* is composed of cells that are very close to normal. Table 16-1 lists tumor grades and their definitions.

TABLE 16-1   TUMOR GRADES

Grade	Description
GX	grade cannot be assessed
G1	well-differentiated cells; tumor cells look very much like parent cells
G2	moderately differentiated; tumor cells resemble parent cells
G3	poorly differentiated; tumor cells barely resemble parent cells
G4	undifferentiated; tumor cells are unlike parent cells

© 2016 Cengage Learning®

Staging is used in conjunction with grading to further identify the characteristics of malignant tumors. Staging tells the oncologist the relative size of the tumor and the extent to which the tumor has metastasized. The **TNM staging system** is an internationally recognized method for staging malignant tumors. In this system, *T* refers to the size of the primary tumor, *N* refers to the involvement of regional lymph nodes, and *M* refers to how far the tumor has metastasized. Numerical values for staging range from 0 to 4, with 0 indicating the least involvement or size, and 4 indicating the highest degree of size and metastasis. Table 16-2 lists tumor stages and their definitions.

TABLE 16-2 TNM STAGING SYSTEM

Tumor	Description
T_0	no evidence of a primary tumor
T_{IS}	carcinoma in situ
T_1, T_2, T_3, T_4	progressive size of the tumor: T_1 is the smallest; T_4 is the largest
T_x	tumor cannot be assessed
Node	**Description**
N_0	regional lymph nodes not abnormal or not involved
N_1, N_2, N_3, N_4	increasing lymph node involvement: regional or distant; N_1 is the least number of involved lymph nodes; N_4 is the highest lymph node involvement
N_x	regional lymph nodes cannot be clinically assessed
Metastasis	**Description**
M_0	no evidence of metastasis
M_1, M_2, M_3	ascending degrees of metastasis: M_1 indicates less metastasis than M_2, which indicates less metastasis than M_3

© 2016 Cengage Learning®

EXERCISE 1

Write a brief definition for each term.

1. benign _____

2. biopsy _____

3. carcinogen _____

4. carcinoma in situ _____

5. differentiation _____

6. fine needle aspiration biopsy _____

7. malignant _____

8. metastasis _____

9. oncology _____

10. radiation oncologist _____

11. sarcoma _____

12. undifferentiated _____

EXERCISE 2

Read the following statements and write the meaning of the grade and stage for each malignant tumor.

1. adenocarcinoma of the stomach; G3, T_2, N_0, M_0

_____

2. osteosarcoma; G4, T_3, N_2, M_1

_____

3. adenocarcinoma of the lung; G4, T_4, N_4, M_4

_____

Treating Cancer

Surgery is the most common way to treat cancer and offers the greatest chance for curing cancers that have not metastasized. **Curative** surgery is described as a primary cancer treatment when the tumor is *in situ* and can be removed in total. **Debulking** surgery means the surgeon removes as much of the tumor as possible, but total removal would cause significant damage to organs or tissue near the tumor. The remainder of the tumor or cancer is then treated with chemotherapy or radiation therapy, and sometimes with both.

Radiation therapy is defined as treating cancer with high-energy rays (such as x-rays) to kill or shrink cancer cells. There are two general categories of radiation therapy: external and internal. **External beam radiation** is the most widely used type of radiation therapy. As the name implies, the radiation is delivered from a source outside the body and the beams are focused on the area affected by cancer. The equipment that delivers the beams is called a **linear accelerator**. External beam radiation provides treatment for large areas of the body such as the area of the main tumor and nearby lymph nodes.

Internal radiation therapy is also called **brachytherapy** (**brack**-ee-**THEH**-rah-pee), which means short-distance therapy. With this treatment method, the radiation source is placed directly into the tumor or into a cavity close to the tumor. There are two main types of internal radiation: (1) **interstitial** (in-ter-**STISH**-al) **radiation**, during which small pellets, wires, tubes, or containers of radioactive material are placed directly into, or close to, the tumor; and (2) **intracavity radiation**, during which a container of radioactive material is placed in a body cavity, such as the vagina. Radioactive material is intended to destroy cancer cells, but also affects normal body tissue and cells, such as bone marrow, the gastrointestinal tract, and reproductive organs.

Chemotherapy involves using anticancer drugs either alone or in combinations to treat cancer. This type of treatment has been available since the early 1950s. As with all cancer treatments, the objective of chemotherapy is to destroy cancer cells and tissue. The medications used in chemotherapy also have an effect on bone marrow, the gastrointestinal tract, reproductive organs, and hair follicles. Chemotherapy medications are given in the following ways:

- **Intravenous** (**IV**)—Medication is injected directly into a vein via a small catheter.

- **Vascular access device** (**VAD**)—A catheter is surgically placed under the skin into a blood vessel usually in the chest area; medications are injected into the VAD.
- **Orally**— Medications in the form of a pill, capsule, or liquid are taken by mouth.

Chemotherapy is usually given over the course of several weeks. The time between treatments allows the body's normal tissue, specifically the bone marrow, a recovery period. The chemotherapy medications travel throughout the bloodstream and can destroy cancer cells that have metastasized. Side effects of chemotherapy include nausea, vomiting, hair loss, and **neutropenia** (noo-troh-**PEE**-nee-ah), which is a decrease in the number of neutrophils (white blood cells). The action of chemotherapeutic agents on bone marrow is responsible for neutropenia.

EXERCISE 3

Write the medical term for each definition or abbreviation.

1. treatment method to totally remove an *in situ* tumor

    _____

2. surgical removal of as much of the tumor as possible

    _____

3. most commonly used type of radiation therapy

    _____

4. another term for internal radiation therapy

    _____

5. radioactive material is placed directly into or near the tumor

    _____

6. using medications to treat cancer

    _____

7. VAD

    _____

Pharmacology

Pharmacology is the study of the nature, uses, and effects of drugs for medicinal purposes. A **pharmacist** is a specialist who is licensed to formulate and dispense medications. A basic understanding of the special terms related to pharmacology will add to your knowledge of the language of the health care industry. This section covers the following topics:

- The difference between prescription and over-the-counter medications
- Routes of medication administration
- Medical terms related to medication action and effects
- Abbreviations related to medications

Some health care professionals refer to medications as drugs. To differentiate between legal and illegal drugs, this text refers to all substances taken to treat or relieve the signs or symptoms of illness as **medications**.

Medications are dispensed under one of two names: the **generic name** or the **brand name**. The federal government assigns the generic name, which can be used by any manufacturer. Levothyroxine is the generic name for a medication prescribed to replace certain thyroid hormones. The brand name, also called the trade or private name, indicates ownership by a specific manufacturer. Synthroid is a brand name for levothyroxine; both medications are used to replace the same thyroid hormone.

Prescription and Over-the-Counter Medications

A **prescription** (**Rx**) is an order for medication, therapy, or other intervention that must be authorized by a licensed health care professional. Prescriptions are usually given in writing by a physician. In some states, health care professionals such as nurse practitioners or physician assistants can write prescriptions. Some prescriptions can be refilled by telephone.

A **prescription medication** is a medication that may be dispensed only with a prescription from an appropriately licensed health care professional. A pharmacist or **pharmacy technician**, an individual who works under the direct supervision of a pharmacist, must dispense the medication. Erythromycin is an example of a familiar prescription medication.

An **over-the-counter** (**OTC**) **medication** is a medication that may be dispensed without a written prescription. Aspirin is an example of a familiar OTC medication. Many prescription medications are available in a less potent form as an OTC. Motrin is an example of a medication that is available as both an OTC and a prescription medication.

All medications must be taken as directed by the prescription or according to the product directions. Abbreviations are often used to note the time and frequency for administering or taking prescription medications. However, health care professionals and various health care organizations have identified abbreviations and other symbols that contribute to medication errors. Therefore, the Joint Commission, an agency that accredits health care organizations, has issued an official "do not use" list of abbreviations and symbols. The Institute for Safe Medication Practices (ISMP) has published the ISMP List of Error-Prone Abbreviations, Symbols, and Dosage Designations. Table 16-3, which lists some of the commonly used abbreviations related to the time and frequency of administration for prescription medications, includes the "do not use" and error-prone abbreviations. Abbreviations from the Joint Commission's "do not use" list are flagged with an asterisk. Abbreviations from the ISMP's list are flagged with two asterisks. Even though these abbreviations should not be in current use, they are present in medical reports that were generated before the lists were published. Note that the abbreviations are taken from the Latin phrases that describe time and frequency.

TABLE 16-3 TIME AND FREQUENCY OF ADMINISTRATION

Abbreviation	Meaning	Latin Phrase
ac	before meals	*ante cibum*
ad lib	as desired	*ad libitum*
bid	twice a day	*bis in die*
h, hr	hour	(none)
pc	after meals	*post cibum*
**hs	at bedtime	*hor somni*
po	by mouth	*per os*
prn	as needed	*pro re nata*

(continues)

TABLE 16-3   TIME AND FREQUENCY OF ADMINISTRATION (continued)

Abbreviation	Meaning	Latin Phrase
q	every	*quaque*
qam	every morning	(none)
*qd	every day	*quaque die*
qh	every hour	*quaque hora*
q2h, q3h, etc.	every 2 hours, etc.	(none)
qid	four times a day	*quarter in die*
*qod	every other day	(none)
sos	if necessary	(none)
stat	immediately	(none)
tid	three times a day	*ter in die*

* Joint Commission - Do Not Use
** ISMP - Error-Prone Abbreviations
© 2016 Cengage Learning®

The **dosage**, which is the amount taken, of the medication is also written as an abbreviation. Some of these abbreviations are familiar, such as **cc** to indicate cubic centimeter; others are less familiar, such as **dr** to indicate dram. Table 16-4 lists some of the commonly used abbreviations related to dosage. As in Table 16-3, abbreviations from the Joint Commission's "do not use" list are flagged with an asterisk. Abbreviations from the ISMP's list are flagged with two asterisks.

TABLE 16-4   ABBREVIATIONS FOR MEDICATION DOSAGE

Abbreviation	Meaning
**cc	cubic centimeter
cm	centimeter
dr	dram
Gm, g, gm	gram
gr	grain
gtt	drops
kg	kilogram
mg	milligram
mEq	millequivalent
mL	milliliter
oz	ounce
**$\overline{ss}$	one-half
T, Tbsp	tablespoon
t, tsp	teaspoon

* Joint Commission - Do Not Use
** ISMP - Error-Prone Abbreviations
© 2016 Cengage Learning®

EXERCISE 4

Write the abbreviation for each definition.

1. after meals   _____

2. as desired   _____

3. as needed   _____

4. at bedtime   _____

5. before meals   _____

6. by mouth   _____

7. every   _____

8. four times a day   _____

9. three times a day   _____

10. twice a day   _____

EXERCISE 5

Write the meaning for each abbreviation.

1. cc   _____

2. cm   _____

3. dr   _____

4. Gm, g, gm   _____

5. gr   _____

6. gtt   _____

7. kg   _____

8. L   _____

9. mg   _____

10. mEq   _____

11. mL   _____

12. oz   _____

13. T, Tbsp   _____

14. t, tsp   _____

Routes of Administration

For a medication to be effective, it must be introduced into the body. Medications can be delivered through the digestive tract or bypassing the digestive tract. Table 16-5 lists the most common digestive tract routes of administration.

TABLE 16-5 DIGESTIVE TRACT ROUTES OF ADMINISTRATION

Route	Description	Advantages/Disadvantages
oral	given by mouth, swallowed	+ easy, safe, economical – slow absorption; might be destroyed by digestive juices
rectal	inserted into the rectum	+ patient does not have to swallow – slow irregular absorption
nasogastric	delivered through a tube placed through the nose and into the stomach	+ patient does not have to swallow – slow absorption; might be destroyed by digestive juices

© 2016 Cengage Learning®

Parenteral (pah-**REN**-ter-al) **routes** of administration bypass the digestive tract. These routes deliver medication through mucous membranes, the skin, muscle tissue, and veins. **Intravenous** (**IV**) administration delivers the medication directly into the bloodstream. Table 16-6 lists commonly used parenteral routes of medication administration. Three types of injections are illustrated in Figure 16-3.

TABLE 16-6 PARENTERAL ROUTES OF ADMINISTRATION

Route	Description	Examples
inhalation	taken through the nose or mouth; absorbed into the bloodstream through the lungs	asthma and anesthesia medications
intradermal (ID) intra- = within derm/o = skin, dermis -al = pertaining to	injection into the dermis of the skin	vaccinations, tuberculosis, and allergy tests
intramuscular (IM) intra- = within muscul/o = muscle -ar = pertaining to	injection into muscle tissue	antibiotics
intravenous (IV) intra- = within ven/o = vein -ous = pertaining to	injection directly into a vein	antibiotics
sublingual sub- = under, beneath, below ling/o = tongue -ual = pertaining to	under the tongue; absorbed through the mucous membranes of the mouth	nitroglycerin

(continues)

TABLE 16-6 PARENTERAL ROUTES OF ADMINISTRATION (continued)

Route	Description	Examples
**subcutaneous (SC, SQ, SubQ) sub- = under, beneath, below cutane/o = skin -ous = pertaining to	injection into the fatty layer of the skin, just below the dermis	insulin, hormones, local anesthetics
topical	on the skin or mucous membrane	ointments, sprays, powders
transdermal trans- = through, across derm/o = skin -al = pertaining to	through the skin; continuous administration via a patch or disk	hormones, nitroglycerin

* Joint Commission - Do Not Use
** ISMP - Error-Prone Abbreviations
© 2016 Cengage Learning®

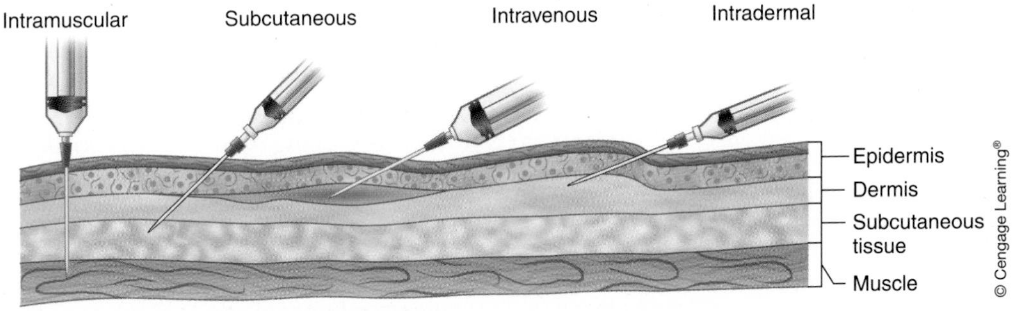

Figure 16-3 Types of Injections.

EXERCISE 6

With the exception of pharmac/o, *which means drug, the roots, prefixes, and suffixes associated with pharmacology were covered in previous chapters. Using your knowledge of these word parts, analyze the listed terms by separating the prefix, root, combining vowel, and suffix with vertical slashes. Write a brief definition for each term. Some terms have more than one root.*

1. intradermal

prefix	*root*	*combining vowel*	*suffix*

2. intramuscular

prefix	*root*	*combining vowel*	*suffix*

3. intravenous

prefix	*root*	*combining vowel*	*suffix*

4. nasogastric

prefix	*root*	*combining vowel*	*suffix*

5. oral

prefix	root	combining vowel	suffix

6. rectal

prefix	root	combining vowel	suffix

7. sublingual

prefix	root	combining vowel	suffix

8. subcutaneous

prefix	root	combining vowel	suffix

9. transdermal

prefix	root	combining vowel	suffix

Medication Actions and Effects

Once taken, all medications have an effect on the body. Of course, we want the medication to have the **desired effect**, to act as it was intended to act. For example, antibiotics should reduce or eliminate disease-causing bacteria; sedatives should induce a state of relaxation; anticoagulants should prevent abnormal blood clotting.

There are times, however, when medications produce an undesired or unanticipated effect. Table 16-7 lists both desirable and undesirable effects of medications.

TABLE 16-7   MEDICATION EFFECTS

Effect	Description
addiction	compulsive, uncontrollable dependence on a medication, or other substances
adverse reaction	an unexpected effect of taking a medication
anaphylactic (**an**-ah-fih-**LAK**-tik) shock	serious and profound state of shock caused by an adverse reaction to a medication
cumulation (**KYOOM**-yoo-**lay**-shun)	medication levels accumulate in body tissues because the medication is not completely excreted before the next dose is given
local effect	response to a medication is confined to a specific body area, organ, or part
potentiation (poh-**ten**-she-**AY**-shun)	effect of one medication is increased when taken in combination with another medication

(continues)

TABLE 16-7   MEDICATION EFFECTS (continued)

Effect	Description
side effect	additional, expected effect of a medication that is not part of the intended effect; nausea is a common side effect
systemic effect	medication has a widespread effect on more than one body system

© 2016 Cengage Learning®

Medications are prescribed with a specific action in mind. Medication actions range from curing a disease by eliminating bacteria from the body to providing relief from the symptoms of diseases that cannot be cured. Table 16-8 lists and describes four types of medication actions.

TABLE 16-8   MEDICATION ACTIONS

Action	Description	Example
palliative (**PAL**-ee-ah-tiv)	relieves the symptoms of a disease, but does not cure	aspirin relieves pain and reduces fever
placebo (plah-**SEE**- boh)	no action on the disease or its symptoms; commonly called a *sugar pill*	inactive substance given to some participants involved in testing new medications
prophylactic (proh-fih-**LAK**-tik)	prevents disease	immunizations
therapeutic (**thair**-ah-**PYOO**-tik)	cures or treats the disease or cause of the disease	antibiotics, hormone replacements

© 2016 Cengage Learning®

EXERCISE 7

Replace each italicized phrase with the correct medical term.

1. Demerol has a high potential for developing an *uncontrollable dependence on a medication.*

   _____

2. Vaccinations are intended to act as a *medication that prevents disease.*

   _____

3. After taking penicillin for the third time, Ellen experienced *a serious and profound state of shock.*

   _____

4. A topical medication's response to disease is defined as a *response that is confined to a specific body area.*

   _____

5. Philip had an *unexpected response* while taking Prozac for depression.

   _____

6. Because the bacteria causing Marietta's fever could not be isolated, her physician prescribed a medication that had a *widespread effect throughout her body.*

   _____

7. During clinical testing of a new hypertension medication, some participants received a *sugar pill*.

   _____

Abbreviations

Many pharmacology abbreviations are listed in Tables 16-3 and 16-4. Additional abbreviations are listed in Table 16-9. Abbreviations from the Joint Commission's "do not use" list are flagged with an asterisk. Abbreviations from the ISMP's list are flagged with two asterisks. Review these abbreviations and practice writing them and their meanings.

TABLE 16-9 ABBREVIATIONS

Abbreviation	Meaning	Abbreviation	Meaning
c	with	s̄	without
caps	capsules	sig	written on label
ID	intradermal	sol	solution
IM	intramuscular	supp	suppository
inj	injection	tab	tablet
*IU	international unit	tinct	tincture
IV	intravenous	TO	telephone order
oint, ung	ointment	*U	unit
Rx	treatment; prescription	VO	verbal order

* Joint Commission - Do Not Use
** ISMP - Error-Prone Abbreviations
© 2016 Cengage Learning®

Surgery

Surgical terminology related to each body system has been presented in the specific system chapters. There are additional medical terms that are unique to surgery or operative procedures. This chapter includes commonly used medical terms related to:

- Anesthesia
- Surgical positions
- Surgical instruments
- Suture materials
- Suture techniques

In addition to these topics, a brief review of surgical suffixes is also presented.

Surgical Suffixes

Surgical suffixes identify exactly what the surgeon is doing for the patient. Review the suffixes in Table 16-10 and complete the exercises.

TABLE 16-10   SURGICAL SUFFIXES

Suffix	Meaning
-desis	binding; fixation
-ectomy	surgical removal; excision
-pexy	surgical fixation
-plasty	surgical correction or repair
-(r)rhaphy	suture of
-(o)stomy	creation of a new or artificial opening
-(o)tomy	incision into
-tripsy	crushing

© 2016 Cengage Learning®

EXERCISE 8

Use the word roots and suffixes to create 20 surgical terms. Write a definition based on the meanings of the roots and suffixes. Using a medical dictionary, look up the full meaning of each term.

WORD ROOTS: arthr/o; card/i, cardi/o; crani/o; cyst/o; derm/o, dermat/o; gastr/o; hepat/o; lith/o; and nephr/o.
SUFFIXES: -desis; -ectomy; -(o)stomy; -(o)tomy; -plasty; -(r)rhaphy; -tripsy.

TERM	DEFINITION
1. _____	_____
2. _____	_____
3. _____	_____
4. _____	_____
5. _____	_____
6. _____	_____
7. _____	_____
8. _____	_____
9. _____	_____
10. _____	_____
11. _____	_____
12. _____	_____
13. _____	_____
14. _____	_____

15. _____ _____
16. _____ _____
17. _____ _____
18. _____ _____
19. _____ _____
20. _____ _____

Anesthesia Terms

Anesthesiology (**an**-es-thee-zee-**ALL**-oh-jee) is the study of medications and procedures intended to produce a lack of feeling or sensation. An **anesthesiologist** (**an**-ess-thee-zee-**ALL**-oh-jist) is a physician specialist who administers anesthetic agents and studies the effects. An **anesthetist** (ah-**NESS**-theh-tist) is a nurse who has special training related to the administration of anesthetic agents.

There are four categories of **anesthesia** (an-ess-**THEE**-zee-ah) that include: (1) general anesthesia; (2) regional anesthesia; (3) local anesthesia; and (4) topical anesthesia. Table 16-11 provides a description and example of each type of anesthesia.

TABLE 16-11 TYPES OF ANESTHESIA

Anesthesia	Description	Example
general anesthesia	complete loss of consciousness and sensation; respiratory support is necessary	inhalation: gaseous agents intravenous; liquid agents; mastectomy
regional anesthesia	interrupts nerve conduction to a body area; patient is conscious	injection; liquid agents surgery; cesarean section
local anesthesia	confined to one part of the body; may or may not involve the nerves	subcutaneous; liquid or gaseous agents; removal of skin lesions
topical anesthesia	type of local anesthesia applied directly to the surface of the involved body part	surface area; creams, gas, ointments; removal of warts or moles

Modes of Induction

The methods used to introduce anesthetic agents into the body are called **modes of induction**, and are dependent on the type of anesthesia. Table 16-12 lists the general modes of induction for each type of anesthesia. Review these terms and complete the exercises.

TABLE 16-12   MODES OF INDUCTION

Mode of Induction	Description
endobronchial (**en**-doh-**BRONG**-kee-al) endo- = within bronch/o = bronchus -al = pertaining to	administration of anesthetic gas through a tube placed in the bronchus; general anesthesia
endotracheal (**en**-doh-**TRAY**-kee-al) endo- = within trache/o = trachea -al = pertaining to	administration of anesthetic gas through a tube in the trachea; general anesthesia
epidural block (ep-ih-**DOO**-ral) epi- = above dur/a = dura mater -al = pertaining to	anesthetic agent is injected into the epidural space of the spinal column; anesthetizes the pelvic, abdominal, or genital area; regional anesthesia
infiltration	injection of an anesthetic agent into tissues; local anesthesia
inhalation	the patient breathes or inhales an anesthetic gas into the lungs; general anesthesia
insufflation (in-soo-**FLAY**-shun)	anesthetic gas is administered by way of a tube placed someplace in the respiratory tract; general anesthesia
intercostal inter- = between cost/o = rib -al = pertaining to	anesthetic agent is injected into an intercostal nerve (located near the ribs); regional anesthesia
intravenous intra- = within ven/o = vein -ous = pertaining to	anesthetic agent is injected directly into a vein; general anesthesia
saddle block	anesthetic agent is injected into the area of the spinal cord that affects the buttocks, perineum, and inner aspects of the thighs; regional anesthesia
spinal block	anesthetic agent is injected along any area of the spinal cord, and the structures beneath the point of injection are affected; regional anesthesia
topical	application of an anesthetic agent directly to the surface of the area involved in the surgery; the integrity of the skin or membranes is not compromised; local anesthesia

Place a "G" next to the mode of induction associated with general anesthesia, an "R" for regional anesthesia, and an "X" for local or topical anesthesia.

1. endobronchial _____
2. endotracheal _____
3. epidural block _____
4. infiltration _____
5. inhalation _____
6. insufflation _____
7. intercostal _____
8. intravenous _____
9. saddle block _____
10. spinal block _____

Sedation

Sedation is defined as the act of calming by administration of a **sedative**, a medication that is used to calm the nervous system. Sedation is used to relieve an individual's anxiety and discomfort that might be associated with unpleasant diagnostic or surgical procedures. Dental procedures provide a good example of using sedation. The need for a root canal provokes anxiety in many individuals. In this situation, the dentist injects a medication to anesthetize the root canal area (local anesthesia) and might also give the patient an inhaled medication, usually nitrous oxide, that allows the patient to remain calm during the procedure. Sedation is also used for diagnostic tests that require prolonged immobilization such as magnetic resonance imaging (MRI) and computed axial tomography (CAT) scanning.

Conscious Sedation

Conscious sedation is described as the use of sedatives and **analgesic** (an-al-**GEE**-sik) medication to induce a semiconscious state that allows an individual to better tolerate various surgical and diagnostic procedures. Analgesic medications provide pain relief during the procedure. Conscious sedation is also called *sedation analgesia*. Under conscious sedation, the patient is able to breathe independently and respond appropriately to verbal directions or gentle stimulation. The medications used during conscious sedation are usually administered intravenously.

Colonoscopy, an endoscopic examination of the large intestine, provides an excellent example of conscious sedation. Before the physician advances the colonoscope, an intravenous (IV) sedative is administered to relax the patient. The sedative might also act to lessen the patient's memory about any discomfort related to the procedure. Once the patient is relaxed, an analgesic is added to the IV for pain relief. During the colonoscopy, the patient remains semialert, is able to breathe independently, and can communicate with the physician. Under conscious sedation, the patient will feel drowsy and might even sleep through some of the procedure, but can be aroused when spoken to or touched.

Surgical Positions

Surgical positions describe how the patient is placed on the operating table. Surgical positions take their names from the medical terms for body positions. For example: Dorsal and supine pertain to the back, or lying on one's back. A *dorsal surgical position* indicates that the patient is lying on his or her back. Depending on the type of surgery and the organ or body part involved, the patient might be placed on his or her back, stomach, side, and at times even in a sitting position. Review the surgical position terms and their descriptions in Table 16-13.

TABLE 16-13 SURGICAL POSITIONS

Position	Description	Type of Surgery
dorsal, supine	flat on the back with legs extended (Figure 16-4)	abdominal surgery

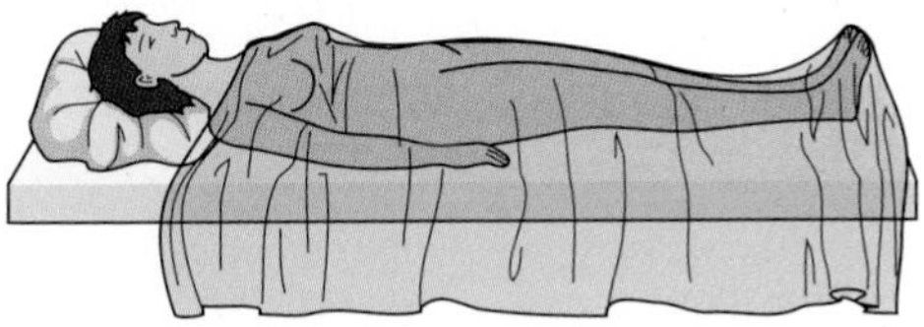

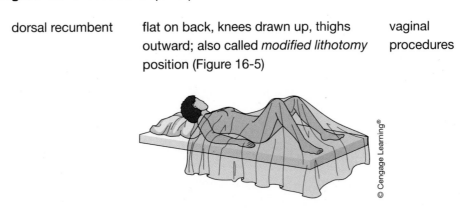

Figure 16-4 Dorsal supine position.

Position	Description	Type of Surgery
dorsal recumbent	flat on back, knees drawn up, thighs outward; also called *modified lithotomy* position (Figure 16-5)	vaginal procedures

Figure 16-5 Dorsal recumbent position.

Position	Description	Type of Surgery
knee-chest	face down with hips flexed so that the knees and chest rest on the examination table (Figure 16-6)	rectal procedures

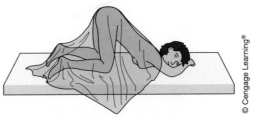

Figure 16-6 Knee-chest position.

(continues)

TABLE 16-13   SURGICAL POSITIONS (continued)

Position	Description	Type of Surgery
lithotomy	on back, legs in stirrups, buttocks near edge of table (Figure 16-7)	obstetric and gynecologic procedures

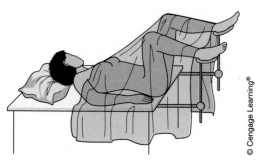

Figure 16-7   Lithotomy position.

| prone | flat on abdomen, head turned to one side (Figure 16-8) | back surgery |

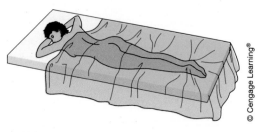

Figure 16-8   Prone position.

| Sims' | on left side, with left arm back, right knee drawn up (Figure 16-9) | rectal surgery |

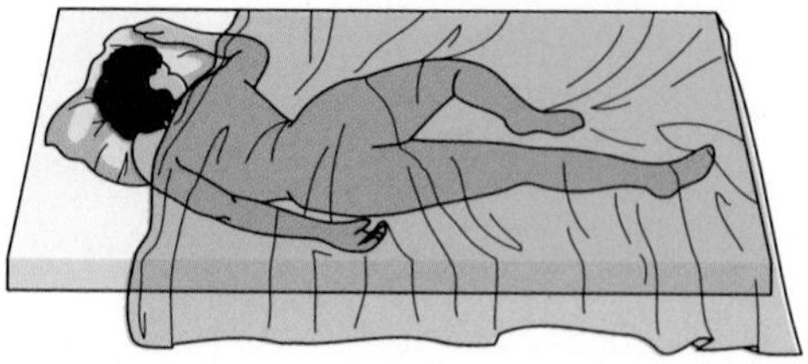

Figure 16-9   Sims' position.

| Trendelenburg (tren-**DELL**-en-burg) | on back, table tilted with the head lower than the feet | pelvic surgery |

Surgical Instruments

Naming all the surgical instruments in this text is, of course, impossible. Entire catalogs are devoted to types of cutting instruments alone. Surgical instruments are named for their action, for example, saws, drills, needles, and clamps. Other surgical instruments are named for the individual who invented or perfected the instrument. A limited number of the more commonly known surgical instruments, descriptions, and intended uses are presented in Table 16-14.

TABLE 16-14 COMMON SURGICAL INSTRUMENT TERMS

Instrument	Description/Use
aspirator (**ASS**-per-ay-tor)	any instrument that suctions fluids or gas
catheter (**KATH**-eh-ter)	tubular instrument inserted into a vessel or body cavity
clamp	instrument for gripping, joining, supporting, or compressing an organ or vessel (Figure 16-10)

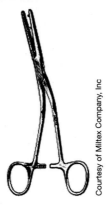

Courtesy of Miltex Company, Inc

Figure 16-10 Muscle clamp (Miltex Company Inc.).

curette, curet (**KOO**-ret)	spoon-shaped instrument for scraping and removing tissue (Figure 16-11)

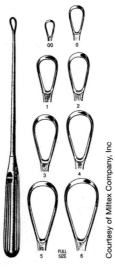

Courtesy of Miltex Company, Inc

Figure 16-11 Curette (Miltex Company Inc.).

(continues)

TABLE 16-14 COMMON SURGICAL INSTRUMENT TERMS (continued)

Instrument	Description/Use
dilator (digh-**LAY**-tor)	instrument for increasing the diameter of a body part by stretching (Figure 16-12)

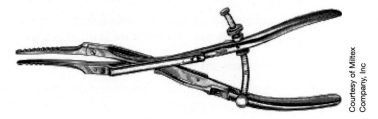

Courtesy of Miltex Company, Inc

Figure 16-12 Dilator (Miltex Company Inc.).

forceps (**FOR**-seps)　　　instrument with two blades and a handle for pulling, grasping, and compressing (Figure 16-13)

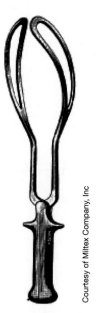

Courtesy of Miltex Company, Inc

Figure 16-13 Forceps (Miltex Company Inc.).

(continues)

TABLE 16-14   COMMON SURGICAL INSTRUMENT TERMS (continued)

Instrument	Description/Use
hemostat (**HEE**-moh-stat)	instrument used to stop the flow of blood
retractor (ree-**TRAK**-tor)	instrument for pulling back the edges of a wound, incision, or body parts (Figure 16-14)

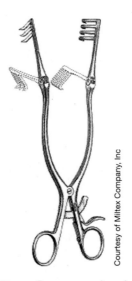

Figure 16-14   Retractor (Miltex Company Inc.).

scalpel (**SKAL**-pal)	surgical knife with both a blunt and sharp edge (Figure 16-15)

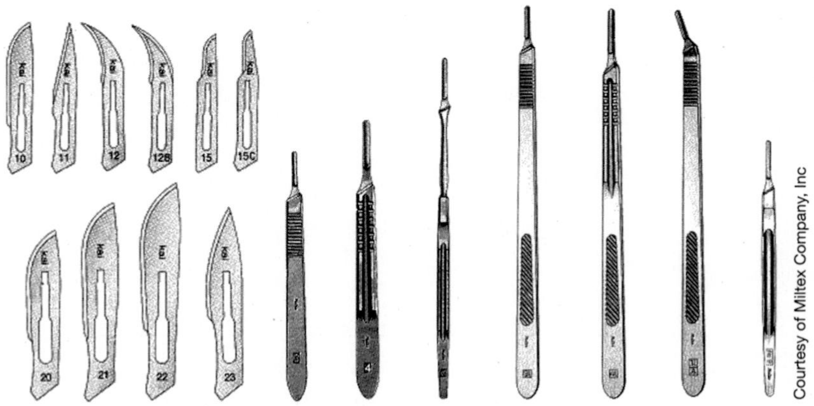

Figure 16-15   Scalpels (Miltex Company Inc.).

tenaculum (teh-**NAK**-yoo-lum)	hooklike instrument for seizing, holding, grasping, and pulling

Suture Materials

Suture material is any substance used to hold any part of the body together. Some suture materials are **absorbable**. These sutures dissolve during the healing process and do not need to be removed. **Nonabsorbable suture materials** remain intact until removed. Size and composition describe suture materials.

Suture material size refers to the diameter of the material. Size has been standardized by governmental regulations. Numbers 3, 2, 1, and 0 are used to express suture size. Material sized as #3 is the thickest and strongest. Size #2 is thicker than #1, and size #1 is thicker than size #0.

As suture material *decreases* in diameter, the number of 0s that describe the suture size *increases*. Therefore, the more 0s, the finer the suture. The number of 0s is written as a hyphenated number. For example, suture material sized 000000 is written as 6-0. Following this pattern, 12-0 suture material is finer (has a smaller diameter) than 6-0 suture material.

Natural and synthetic products are used for sutures. Natural materials might include catgut, silk, and linen. Synthetic materials include nylon, polyester, Teflon, plastic, and surgical steel. Each type of tissue requires suture material appropriate to the tissue. For example, a surgeon will not staple a new cornea to your eye. By the same token, 12-0 suture material is not appropriate for repairing or closing muscle wounds and layers. Tevdek, Vicryl, silk, cotton, Prolene, and Dermalon are examples of suture materials.

Suture Techniques

Suture technique refers to the method used to unite body parts, repair body parts, or close an incision. The two basic types of techniques are **continuous** and **interrupted**. As the names imply, a continuous suture technique means the suture starts in one place and ends in another, without being cut or tied between those places. An interrupted technique means that each suture is independent of the other sutures. Suture techniques are often named for the general appearance of the final product or for the person who developed or perfected a specific technique. Imagine what the suture techniques listed in Table 16-15 look like.

TABLE 16-15   SUTURE TECHNIQUES

baseball	chain	fishhook	purse string
blanket	circular	mattress	sliding
button	crown	noose	zipper

© 2016 Cengage Learning®

CHAPTER REVIEW

The Chapter Review can be used as a self-test. Go through each exercise and answer as many questions as you can without referring to previous exercises or information in the chapter. Check your answers and fill in any blanks. Practice writing any terms you might have misspelled.

EXERCISE 10

Write the medical term for each description.

1. flat on the back with legs extended   _____

2. flat on back, knees drawn up, thighs outward   _____

3. on one side, toward the abdomen, body elevated   _____

4. on back, legs in stirrups, buttocks near the edge
   of the table   _____

5. flat on abdomen, head turned to one side   _____

6. on back, table tilted at a 45-degree angle toward
   the head, bent at the knee   _____

7. instrument for gripping or compressing an organ
   or vessel   _____

8. any instrument that suctions fluids or gas   _____

9. spoon-shaped instrument for scraping and
   removing tissue   _____

10. instrument that increases the diameter of a body
    part by stretching   _____

11. instrument for pulling back the edges of a wound,
    incision, or body part   _____

12. any substance used to hold any part of the body
    together   _____

13. sutures that dissolve during the healing process   _____

14. suture starts at one point and ends at another
    without being cut or tied between points   _____

15. each suture is independent of other sutures   _____

EXERCISE 11

Write a brief description for each term or abbreviation.

1. adenocarcinoma   _____

2. adverse reaction   _____

3. anaphylactic shock   _____

4. anesthesiology   _____

5. anesthetist   _____

6. radiation therapy   _____

7. brachytherapy   _____

8. brand, trade name   _____

9. carcinogen _____

10. cumulation _____

11. generic name _____

12. grading _____

13. in situ _____

14. metastasis _____

15. palliative effect _____

16. parenteral administration _____

17. pharmacist _____

18. placebo _____

19. potentiation _____

20. staging _____

EXERCISE 13

Write the correct term or phrase for the abbreviations.

1. ACS _____

2. FNB _____

3. IM _____

4. IU _____

5. OTC _____

6. R$_x$ _____

7. TNM _____

8. TO _____

9. VAD _____

10. VO _____

EXERCISE 14

Write out the following prescriptions.

EXAMPLE: Zyloprim, po 200 mg every day
Zyloprim, by mouth, 200 milligrams every day

1. Xanax, po 0.5 mg tid

_____

2. Elavil, IM 200 mg qid

_____

3. Elavil, IM 120 mg hs

_____

4. Micronase, 2.5 mg tab bid

_____

5. Propulsid, po 10 mg qid at least 15 min ac

_____

6. Zocor, po 30 mg bid in pm

_____

7. Nitro-Bid sublingual tabs 0.3 mg, may repeat q5min, no more than 3 tabs/15 min

_____

8. Tyzine, 2 gtt q4h prn. in each nostril

_____

9. Monistat, 200 mg supp at bedtime × 3 days or 100 mg supp at bedtime × 1 week

_____

10. Insulin, SC 0.5 Units qid given 30 min ac

_____

EXERCISE 15

Write a brief description that compares the difference(s) between the listed pairs of terms.

1. chemotherapy and brachytherapy

_____

2. fine needle biopsy and needle core biopsy

_____

3. excisional biopsy and incisional biopsy

_____

4. endoscopic biopsy and laparoscopy

_____

5. open surgical exploration and endoscopic biopsy

_____

6. general anesthesia and conscious sedation

_____

EXERCISE 16

Read the following excerpt from an operative report. Use a medical dictionary and this chapter to write a brief description or definition of the italicized medical terms and phrases.

OPERATIONS PERFORMED: 1. Full-thickness wedge resection of the (1) *squamous cell carcinoma* of the left upper lip. 2. (2) *Incisional biopsy* of an actinic keratosis of the left nasal fold.

DESCRIPTION OF PROCEDURE: The patient was taken to the operating room and placed in the (3) *supine* position and given 2 (4) *mg* of Versed (5) *intravenously* for (6) *conscious sedation*. The lesion was marked off in a full-thickness wedge in an inverted W-shape, with margins appearing to have adequate normal skin around the lesion. The lesion was excised through a full-thickness wedge of the lip, with the upper part of the wedge being just at the columella and at the base of the left nasal border. The specimen was sent to pathologist; she reported this to be a squamous cell carcinoma with margins clear and adequately excised. We also did an (7) *excisional biopsy* of a crusty lesion near the nasal fold. The wound was closed with 4-0 Vicryl with final closure of the skin done with multiple (8) *interrupted sutures* of 6-0 black silk. Blood loss was minimal.

1. _____
2. _____
3. _____
4. _____
5. _____
6. _____
7. _____
8. _____

EXERCISE 17

Write the abbreviations. Complete as many as you can without referencing information in the chapter.

1. ac   _____
2. ACS   _____
3. ad lib   _____
4. FNAB   _____
5. gtt   _____
6. ID   _____
7. IM   _____
8. IV   _____

9. mEq   _____

10. OTC   _____

11. pc   _____

12. prn   _____

13. qam   _____

14. R$_x$ _____

15. sol   _____

16. stat   _____

17. tab   _____

18. TNM   _____

19. tinct   _____

20. VO   _____

CHALLENGE EXERCISE

Cancer is the second leading cause of death in the United States. Researchers are discovering important information about the genetic and hereditary links to cancer. Access the American Cancer Society website at www.cancer.org and search the site for genetic or hereditary cancer links. Use the keywords genetic cancer _or_ hereditary cancer. _What types of cancer appear to have a hereditary or genetic connection?_

Pronunciation Review

Review the terms in the chapter. Pronounce each term using the following phonetic pronunciations. Check off the term when you are comfortable saying it.

TERM	PRONUNCIATION
☐ addiction	ah-**DIK**-shun
☐ adenocarcinoma	**add**-ih-no-**kar**-sin-**OH**-mah
☐ anaphylactic shock	**an**-ah-fih-**LAK**-tik shock
☐ anesthesia	**an**-ess-**THEE**-zee-ah
☐ anesthesiologist	**an**-ess-thee-zee-**ALL**-oh-jist
☐ anesthesiology	**an**-ess-thee-zee-**ALL**-oh-jee
☐ anesthetist	ah-**NESS**-theh-tist
☐ aspirator	**ASS**-per-ay-tor
☐ benign	bee-**NIGHN**
☐ brachytherapy	**brack**-ee-**THEH**-rah-pee
☐ carcinogen	**kar**-sin-**OH**-jen
☐ carcinoma	**kar**-sin-**OH**-mah

☐ carcinoma in situ	**kar**-sin-**OH**-mah in **SIGH**-too
☐ catheter	**KATH**-eh-ter
☐ cumulation	**KYOOM**-yoo-**lay**-shun
☐ curette, curet	**KOO**-ret
☐ differentiation	**diff**-er-en-shee-**AY**-shun
☐ dilator	**DIGH**-lay-tor
☐ dorsal	**DOOR**-sall
☐ dorsal recumbent	**DOOR**-sall ree-**KUM**-bent
☐ endobronchial	**en**-doh-**BRONG**-kee-al
☐ endotracheal	**en**-doh-**TRAY**-kee-al
☐ epidural	ep-ih-**DOO**-ral
☐ forceps	**FOR**-seps
☐ hemostat	**HEE**-moh-stat
☐ inhalation	**in**-hah-**LAY**-shun
☐ insufflation	in-soo-**FLAY**-shun
☐ interstitial	in-ter-**STISH**-al
☐ intradermal	**in**-trah-**DERM**-al
☐ intramuscular	**in**-trah-**MUSS**-kyoo-lar
☐ intravenous	**in**-trah-**VEE**-nus
☐ malignant	mah-**LIG**-nant
☐ metastasis	meh-**TASS**-tah-sis
☐ neutropenia	noo-troh-**PEE**-nee-ah
☐ oncologist	on-**KALL**-oh-jist
☐ oncology	on-**KALL**-oh-jee
☐ palliative	**PAL**-ee-ah-tiv
☐ parenteral	pah-**REN**-ter-al
☐ pharmacist	**FARM**-ah-sist
☐ pharmacologist	**far**-mah-**KALL**-oh-jist
☐ pharmacology	**far**-mah-**KALL**-oh-jee
☐ placebo	plah-**SEE**-boh
☐ potentiation	poh-**ten**-she-**AY**-shun
☐ prophylactic	proh-fih-**LAK**-tik
☐ retractor	ree-**TRAK**-tor
☐ scalpel	**SKAL**-pal
☐ squamous	**SKWAY**-mus
☐ subcutaneous	**sub**-kyoo-**TAY**-nee-us
☐ sublingual	sub-**LING**-wall
☐ tenaculum	teh-**NAK**-yoo-lum
☐ therapeutic	**thair**-ah-**PYOO**-tik
☐ Trendelenburg	tren-**DELL**-en-burg

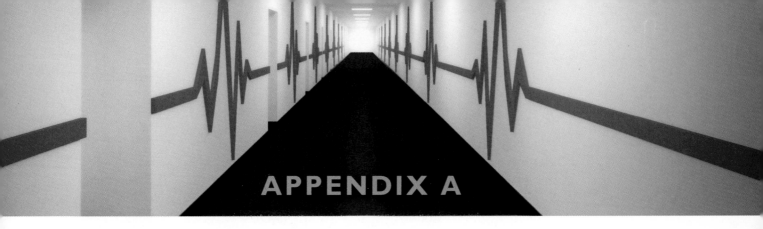

Part I Word Element to Meaning

WORD ROOTS

Root	Meaning	Root	Meaning
abdomin/o	abdomen	bas/o	base
acid/o	sour; bitter	bil/i	bile; gall
acoust/o	hearing	blast/o	immature
acr/o	extremities	blephar/o	eyelid
aden/o	gland	bronch/o;	bronchus
adenoid/o	adenoid	bronch/i	
adip/o	fat	bronchiol/o	bronchiole
adren/o	adrenal glands	bucc/o	cheek
adrenal/o	adrenal glands	burs/o	bursa; sac
agglutin/o	to clump	calc/i	calcium
alveol/o	alveolus	cardi/o	heart
amni/o	amnion	carp/o	wrist bones
amnion/o	amnion	cec/o	cecum
an/o	anus	celi/o	abdomen
andr/o	male; man	cephal/o	head
aneurysm/o	aneurysm	cerebell/o	cerebellum
angi/o	vessel	cerebr/o	cerebrum
ankyl/o	stiff	cervic/o	cervix
anthrac/o	coal	cheil/o	lips
append/o	appendix	chol/e	bile; gall
appendic/o	appendix	cholangi/o	bile duct
aque/o	watery	cholecyst/o	gallbladder
arachn/o	spider	choledoch/o	common bile duct
arter/o	artery	chondr/o	cartilage
arteri/o	artery	chori/o	chorion
arteriol/o	arteriole	clavicul/o	clavicle;
arthr/o	joint		collarbone
articul/o	joint	coagul/o	clotting
atel/o	incomplete	coccyg/o	coccyx; tailbone
ather/o	fat; fatty plaque;	cochle/o	cochlea
	fatty, yellowish	col/o	colon
	plaque	colon/o	colon
audi/o	hearing; sound	colp/o	vagina
balan/o	glans penis	coni/o	dust

Root	Meaning	Root	Meaning
conjunctiv/o	conjunctiva	glomerul/o	glomerulus
cor/o	heart	gloss/o	tongue
corne/o	cornea	gluc/o	glucose; sugar; sweet
coron/o	heart		
cortic/o	cortex	glyc/o	glucose; sugar; sweet
cost/o	rib		
crani/o	cranium; skull	gonad/o	sex glands
cry/o	cold	granul/o	granules
crypt/o	hidden	gravid/o	pregnancy
cut/o	skin	gyn/o	woman
cutane/o	skin	gynec/o	woman
cyan/o	blue; bluish	hem/o	blood
cyst/o	bladder; sac; urinary bladder	hemat/o	blood
		hepat/o	liver
dacry/o	tears	hidr/o	sweat
dacryocyst/o	tear sac	humer/o	humerus; upper arm bone
dendr/o	branching		
derm/o	skin	hydr/o	water; fluid
dermat/o	skin	hyster/o	uterus
dipl/o	two; double	ile/o	ileum
dips/o	thirst	ili/o	ilium; pelvic bone
duoden/o	duodenum	immun/o	protection
electr/o	electricity	ir/o	iris
embry/o	embryo	irid/o	iris
encephal/o	brain	is/o	equal
endocrin/o	endocrine	ischi/o	ischium; pelvic bone
enter/o	intestines		
eosin/o	rosy red; rosy	jejun/o	jejunum
epididym/o	epididymis	kal/i	potassium
epiglott/o	epiglottis	kary/o	nucleus
episi/o	vulva	kerat/o	cornea; horny tissue; hard
esophag/o	esophagus		
fasci/o	fascia; fibrous tissue	ket/o	ketone bodies
		kyph/o	humpback
femor/o	femur; thigh bone	labyrinth/o	inner ear; labyrinth
fet/o; fet/i	fetus		
fibr/o	fiber; fibrous tissue	lacrim/o	tears
		lact/o	milk
fibul/o	fibula; outer lower leg bone	lamin/o	lamina; thin flat plate or layer
fund/o	fundus	lapar/o	abdominal wall
gastr/o	stomach	laryng/o	larynx
gingiv/o	gums	leiomy/o	smooth muscle
glauc/o	silver; gray	leuk/o	white
gli/o	neuroglia; nerve cell	ligament/o	ligament
		lingu/o	tongue

Root	Meaning	Root	Meaning
lip/o	fat	orth/o	straight
lith/o	stone	oste/o	bone
lord/o	swayback	ot/o	ear
lumb/o	lower back	ovari/o	ovary
lymph/o	lymph	ox/i	oxygen
lymphaden/o	lymph gland	pachy/o	thick
lymphangi/o	lymph vessel	palpebr/o	eyelid
mamm/o	breast	pancreat/o	pancreas
mandibul/o	mandible; lower jawbone	par/o	bear; give birth to; labor; childbirth
mast/o	breast	part/o	bear; give birth to; labor; childbirth
maxill/o	maxilla; upper jaw bone	patell/o	patella; kneecap
meat/o	meatus; opening	pector/o	chest
melan/o	black	pelv/i	pelvis
men/o	menses; menstruation	perine/o	perineum
		peritone/o	peritoneum
mening/o	meninges	phac/o	lens
metacarp/o	hand bones	phag/o	to eat
metatars/o	foot bones	phak/o	lens
metr/i; metr/o	uterus	phalang/o	finger and toe bones
morph/o	form; shape		
muc/o	mucus	pharyng/o	pharynx
my/o	muscle	phleb/o	vein
myc/o	fungus	phot/o	light
myel/o	bone marrow; spinal cord	phren/o	diaphragm
		pil/o	hair
myring/o	eardrum	pleur/o	pleura
nas/o	nose	pneum/o	lung; air
nat/o	birth	poikil/o	varied; irregular
natr/o	sodium	polyp/o	polyp
nephr/o	kidney	proct/o	rectum
neur/o	nerve	prostat/o	prostate gland
noct/o	night	pub/o	pubis; pelvic bone
nucle/o	nucleus	pubi/o	pubis; pelvic bone
nyctal/o	night	puerper/o	childbirth
ocul/o	eye	pulmon/o	lungs
olig/o	few; diminished	pupill/o	pupil
onych/o	nail	py/o	pus
oophor/o	ovary	pyel/o	renal pelvis
ophthalm/o	eye	quadr/i	four
opt/o	vision; eye	radi/o	radius; outer lower arm bone
or/o	mouth		
orch/o	testis; testicle	rect/o	rectum
orchi/o	testis; testicle	ren/o	kidney
orchid/o	testis; testicle	retin/o	retina

Root	Meaning	Root	Meaning
rhabdomy/o	skeletal muscle; striated muscle	tars/o	ankle bones
		ten/o	tendon
rhin/o	nose	tend/o	tendon
rhytid/o	wrinkles	tendin/o	tendon
salping/o	fallopian tubes; oviducts	tenosynov/o	tendon sheath
		test/o	testis; testicle
sarc/o	flesh	testicul/o	testis; testicle
scapula/o	scapula; shoulder blade	thec/o	sheath
		thorac/o	chest
scler/o	sclera; hard	thromb/o	clot; thrombus
scoli/o	crooked; bent	thym/o	thymus gland
seb/o	sebum	thyr/o	thyroid gland
semin/i	semen	thyroid/o	thyroid gland
sial/o	salivary gland; saliva	tonsill/o	tonsils
		toxic/o	poison
sigmoid/o	sigmoid colon	trache/o	trachea
sinus/o	sinus	trich/o	hair
somat/o	body	tympan/o	eardrum
sperm/o	sperm; spermatic cord	ungu/o	nail
		ur/o	urine; urinary system
spermat/o	sperm; spermatic cord	ureter/o	ureter
		urethr/o	urethra
spher/o	sphere; round	uter/o	uterus
sphygm/o	pulse	uve/o	uvea
spir/o	breathe; breath	vagin/o	vagina
splen/o	spleen	vas/o	vessel; vas deferens
spondyl/o	vertebra; vertebral column		
squam/o	scale	ven/o	vein
staped/o	stapes; middle ear bone	ventricul/o	ventricle
		vertebr/o	vertebra; vertebral column
stern/o	sternum; breastbone		
		vesic/o	urinary bladder
steth/o	chest	vitre/o	glassy; jelly-like
stomat/o	mouth	vulv/o	vulva
sud/o	sweat	xanth/o	yellow
sudor/o	sweat	xer/o	dry

PREFIXES

Prefix	Meaning	Prefix	Meaning
a-	no; not; without	anti-	against
ab-	away from	astr-	star
an-	no; not; without	auto-	self
ana-	no; not; without	bi-	two; double; both
ante-	before; forward	brady-	slow

Prefix	Meaning	Prefix	Meaning
carcin-	cancer; malignant	neo-	new
contra-	against; opposite	non-	not
dura-	hard	nulli-	none
dys-	abnormal; painful; difficult	oxy-	sharp; quick
echo-	sound	pan-	all
ect-	outside; out	para-	beside; around
en-	within; in; inward	per-	through
endo-	within; inner	peri-	around; surrounding
epi-	above; upon	poly-	many; excessive
eso-	within; in; inward	post-	after
eu-	same; normal	pre-	before; in front of
ex-	out; outward	presby-	old
hemi-	half	primi-	first; one
hyper-	above; excessive	retro-	backward; behind; upward
hypo-	deficient; below		
infra-	below; inferior	semi-	half
inter-	between	sub-	under; below; beneath
intra-	within		
iso-	same; equal	super-	above; over; excess
macro-	large		
mal-	bad; poor; abnormal	supra-	above; on top of
		sym-	with; association
meta-	change; after; beyond	syn-	together; with; union
micro-	small	tachy-	fast
mono-	one	tri-	three
multi-	many	uni-	one

SUFFIXES

Suffix	Meaning	Suffix	Meaning
-ac	pertaining to	-crine	to secrete
-al	pertaining to	-crit	to separate
-algia	pain	-cusia	hearing
-ary	pertaining to	-cusis	hearing
-asthenia	without feeling or sensation	-cytosis	condition of cells
		-desis	binding; fixation
-blast	immature; embryonic	-dynia	pain
-capnia	carbon dioxide	-ectasis	stretching; dilatation
-cele	hernia; protrusion		
-centesis	surgical puncture to remove fluid	-ectomy	surgical removal; excision
		-emesis	vomiting
-clasia	surgical breaking	-emia	blood condition
-clasis	surgical breaking	-gen	producing; forming

Suffix	Meaning	Suffix	Meaning
-genesis	producing; forming	-philia	attraction to
-genic	producing; forming	-phonia	sound; voice
-globin	protein	-phoresis	carrying; transmission
-globulin	protein		
-gram	record; picture; x-ray film	-phoria	feeling; mental state
		-plasty	surgical repair
-graph	instrument for recording	-plegia	paralysis
		-pnea	breathing
-graphy	process of recording	-poiesis	formation; production of
-ia	condition; abnormal condition	-ptosis	drooping; sagging
		-ptysis	spitting up
-iac	pertaining to	-(r)rhagia	hemorrhage
-iasis	condition; abnormal condition	-(r)rhaphy	suture of
		-(r)rhea	discharge; flow
-ic	pertaining to	-(r)rhexis	rupture
-itis	inflammation	-sclerosis	hardening
-kinesia	movement	-scope	instrument for viewing
-(o)logist	specialist		
-(o)logy	study of	-scopy	visualization with a scope
-lysis	destruction; break down	-somnia	sleep
-lytic	destruction; break down	-stasis	control; stop; stopping or controlling
-malacia	softening		
-megaly	enlarged; enlargement	-stenosis	narrowing
		-(o)stomy	creating a new or artificial opening
-meter	instrument to measure		
		-therapy	treatment
-metry	measuring; to measure	-thorax	chest; pleural cavity
-oid	like; resembling	-tocia	labor; birth
-oma	tumor	-(o)tomy	incision into
-opia	vision	-tonia	muscle tone
-osis	condition; abnormal condition	-tresia	opening
		-tripsy	crushing
-ous	pertaining to	-trophy	growth; development
-paresis	partial paralysis		
-pathy	disease; illness	-tropia	to turn; turning
-penia	deficiency; decreased number	-tropin	stimulating effect of a hormone
-pepsia	digestion	-tropion	to turn; turning
-pexy	surgical fixation	-uria	urine; urination
-phagia	eating; swallowing	-version	to turn

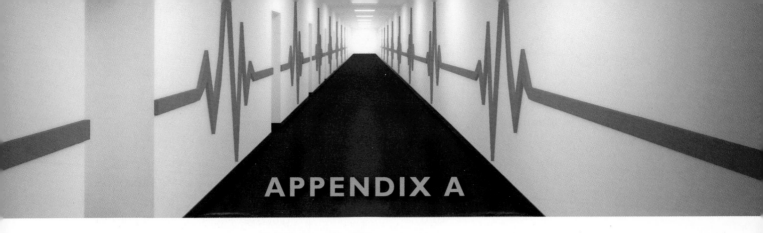

Part 2 Meaning to Word Element

WORD ROOTS

Meaning	Root	Meaning	Root
abdomen	abdomin/o; celi/o	breathe	spir/o
abdominal wall	lapar/o	bronchiole	bronchiol/o
adenoid	adenoid/o	bronchus	bronch/o; bronch/i
adrenal glands	adren/o; adrenal/o	bursa	burs/o
air	pneum/o	calcium	calc/i
alveolus	alveol/o	cartilage	chondr/o
amnion	amni/o; amnion/o	cecum	cec/o
aneurysm	aneurysm/o	cerebellum	cerebell/o
ankle bones	tars/o	cerebrum	cerebr/o
anus	an/o	cervix	cervic/o
appendix	append/o; appendic/o	cheek	bucc/o
arteriole	arteriol/o	chest	pector/o; steth/o; thorac/o
artery	arter/o; arteri/o	childbirth	par/o; part/o; puerper/o
base	bas/o		
bear	par/o; part/o	chorion	chori/o
bent	scoli/o	clavicle	clavicul/o
bile	bil/i; chol/e	clot	thromb/o
bile duct	cholangi/o	clotting	coagul/o
birth	nat/o	to clump	agglutin/o
bitter	acid/o	coal	anthrac/o
black	melan/o	coccyx	coccyg/o
bladder	cyst/o	cochlea	cochle/o
blood	hem/o; hemat/o	cold	cry/o
blue	cyan/o	collarbone	clavicul/o
bluish	cyan/o	colon	col/o; colon/o
body	somat/o	common bile duct	choledoch/o
bone	oste/o	conjunctiva	conjunctiv/o
bone marrow	myel/o	cornea	corne/o; kerat/o
brain	encephal/o	cortex	cortic/o
branching	dendr/o	cranium	crani/o
breast	mamm/o; mast/o	crooked	scoli/o
breastbone	stern/o	diaphragm	phren/o
breath	spir/o	diminished	olig/o

Meaning	Root
double	dipl/o
dry	xer/o
duodenum	duoden/o
dust	coni/o
ear	ot/o
eardrum	myring/o; tympan/o
to eat	phag/o
electricity	electr/o
embryo	embry/o
endocrine	endocrin/o
epididymis	epididym/o
epiglottis	epiglott/o
equal	is/o
esophagus	esophag/o
extremities	acr/o
eye	ocul/o; ophthalm/o; opt/o
eyelid	blephar/o; palpebr/o
fallopian tubes	salping/o
fascia	fasci/o
fat	adip/o; lip/o
fatty, yellowish plaque	ather/o
femur	femor/o
fetus	fet/o; fet/i
few	olig/o
fiber	fibr/o
fibrous tissue	fasci/o; fibr/o
fibula	fibul/o
finger and toe bones	phalang/o
flesh	sarc/o
fluid	hydr/o
foot bones	metatars/o
form	morph/o
four	quadr/i
fundus	fund/o
fungus	myc/o
gall	bil/i; chol/e
gallbladder	cholecyst/o
give birth to	par/o; part/o

Meaning	Root
gland	aden/o
glans penis	balan/o
glassy	vitre/o
glomerulus	glomerul/o
glucose	gluc/o; glyc/o
granules	granul/o
gray	glauc/o
gums	gingiv/o
hair	pil/o; trich/o
hand bones	metacarp/o
hard	kerat/o; scler/o
head	cephal/o
hearing	acoust/o; audi/o
heart	cardi/o; cor/o; coron/o
hidden	crypt/o
horny tissue	kerat/o
humerus	humer/o
humpback	kyph/o
ileum	ile/o
ilium	ili/o
immature	blast/o
incomplete	atel/o
inner ear	labyrinth/o
intestines	enter/o
iris	ir/o; irid/o
irregular	poikil/o
ischium	ischi/o
jejunum	jejun/o
jelly-like	vitre/o
joint	arthr/o; articul/o
ketone bodies	ket/o
kidney	ren/o; nephr/o
kneecap	patell/o
labor	par/o; part/o
labyrinth	labyrinth/o
lamina	lamin/o
larynx	laryng/o
lens	phac/o; phak/o
ligament	ligament/o
light	phot/o
lips	cheil/o
liver	hepat/o

Meaning	Root	Meaning	Root
lower back	lumb/o	pleura	pleur/o
lower jawbone	mandibul/o	poison	toxic/o
lung	pneum/o	polyp	polyp/o
lungs	pulmon/o	potassium	kal/i
lymph	lymph/o	pregnancy	gravid/o
lymph gland	lymphaden/o	prostate gland	prostat/o
lymph vessel	lymphangi/o	protection	immun/o
male	andr/o	pubis	pubi/o; pub/o
man	andr/o	pulse	sphygm/o
mandible	mandibul/o	pupil	pupill/o
maxilla	maxill/o	pus	py/o
meatus	meat/o	radius	radi/o
meninges	mening/o	rectum	proct/o; rect/o
menses	men/o	renal pelvis	pyel/o
menstruation	men/o	retina	retin/o
milk	lact/o	rib	cost/o
mouth	or/o; stomat/o	rosy	eosin/o
mucus	muc/o	rosy red	eosin/o
muscle	my/o	round	spher/o
nail	onych/o; ungu/o	sac	cyst/o; burs/o
nerve	neur/o	saliva	sial/o
nerve cell	gli/o	salivary gland	sial/o
neuroglia	gli/o	scale	squam/o
night	noct/o; nyctal/o	scapula	scapula/o
nose	nas/o; rhin/o	sclera	scler/o
nucleus	kary/o; nucle/o	sebum	seb/o
opening	meat/o	semen	semin/i
outer lower arm bone	radi/o	sex glands	gonad/o
outer lower leg bone	fibul/o	shape	morph/o
		sheath	thec/o
ovary	oophor/o; ovari/o	shoulder blade	scapula/o
oviducts	salping/o	sigmoid colon	sigmoid/o
oxygen	ox/i	silver	glauc/o
pancreas	pancreat/o	sinus	sinus/o
patella	patell/o	skeletal muscle	rhabdomy/o
pelvic bone	ili/o; ischi/o; pubi/o; pub/o	skin	cut/o; cutane/o; derm/o; dermat/o
pelvis	pelv/i	skull	crani/o
perineum	perine/o	smooth muscle	leiomy/o
peritoneum	peritone/o	sodium	natr/o
pharynx	pharyng/o	sound	acoust/o; audi/o; ech/o
		sour	acid/o

Meaning	Root
sperm	sperm/o; spermat/o
spermatic cord	sperm/o; spermat/o
sphere	spher/o
spider	arachn/o
spinal cord	myel/o
spleen	splen/o
stapes	staped/o
sternum	stern/o
stiff	ankyl/o
stomach	gastr/o
stone	lith/o
straight	orth/o
striated muscle	rhabdomy/o
sugar	gluc/o; glyc/o
swayback	lord/o
sweat	hidr/o; sud/o; sudor/o
sweet	gluc/o; glyc/o
tailbone	coccyg/o
tear sac	dacryocyst/o
tears	dacry/o; lacrim/o
tendon	ten/o; tend/o; tendin/o
tendon sheath	tenosynov/o
testicle	orch/o; orchi/o; orchid/o; test/o; testicul/o
testis	orch/o; orchi/o; orchid/o; test/o; testicul/o
thick	pachy/o
thigh bone	femor/o
thin flat plate or layer	lamin/o
thirst	dips/o

Meaning	Root
thrombus	thromb/o
thymus gland	thym/o
thyroid gland	thyr/o; thyroid/o
tongue	gloss/o; lingu/o
tonsils	tonsill/o
trachea	trache/o
two	dipl/o
upper arm bone	humer/o
upper jawbone	maxill/o
ureter	ureter/o
urethra	urethr/o
urinary bladder	vesic/o; cyst/o
urinary system	ur/o
urine	ur/o
uterus	hyster/o; metr/i; metr/o; uter/o
uvea	uve/o
vagina	colp/o; vagin/o
varied	poikil/o
vas deferens	vas/o
vein	phleb/o; ven/o
ventricle	ventricul/o
vertebra	spondyl/o; vertebr/o
vertebral column	spondyl/o; vertebr/o
vessel	angi/o; vas/o
vision	opt/o
vulva	epis/o; vulv/o
water	hydr/o
watery	aque/o
white	leuk/o
woman	gyn/o; gynec/o
wrinkles	rhytid/o
wrist bones	carp/o
yellow	xanth/o

PREFIXES

Meaning	Prefix
abnormal	dys-; mal-
above; on top of; upon	supra-; epi-
above; over; excess; excessive	super-; hyper-
after	post-; meta-

Meaning	Prefix
against	anti-; contra-
all	pan-
around	para-; peri-
association	sym-
away from	ab-
backward	retro-

Meaning	Prefix
bad	mal-
before	ante-; pre-
behind	retro-
below	infra-; hypo-; sub-
beneath	sub-
beside	para-
between	inter-
beyond	meta-
both	bi-
cancer	carcin-
change	meta-
deficient	hypo-
difficult	dys-
double	bi-
equal	iso-
excessive	poly-; hyper-; super-
fast	tachy-
first	primi-
forward	ante-
half	hemi-; semi-
hard	dura-
in	en-; eso-
in front of	pre-
inferior	infra-
inner	endo-
inward	en-; eso-
large	macro-
malignant	carcin-
many	multi-; poly-
new	neo-
no	a-; an-; ana-

Meaning	Prefix
none	nulli-
normal	eu-
not	a-; an-; ana-; non-
old	presby-
one	mono-; primi-; uni-
opposite	contra-
out	ect-; ex-
outside	ect-
outward	ex-
painful	dys-
poor	mal-
quick	oxy-
same	eu-; iso-
self	auto-
sharp	oxy-
slow	brady-
small	micro-
sound	echo-
star	astr-
surrounding	peri-
three	tri-
through	per-
together	syn-
two	bi-
under	sub-
union	syn-
upward	retro-
with	syn-; sym-
within	en-; eso-; endo-; intra-
without	a-; an-; ana-

SUFFIXES

Meaning	Suffix
abnormal condition	-ia; -iasis; -osis
attraction to	-philia
binding	-desis
birth	-tocia
blood condition	-emia
break down	-lysis; -lytic
breathing	-pnea
carbon dioxide	-capnia

Meaning	Suffix
carrying	-phoresis
chest	-thorax
condition	-ia; -iasis; -osis
condition of cells	-cytosis;
control controlling	-stasis
creating a new or artificial opening	-(o)stomy
crushing	-tripsy
decreased number	-penia

Meaning	Suffix	Meaning	Suffix
deficiency	-penia	picture	-gram
destruction	-lysis; -lytic	pleural cavity	-thorax
development	-trophy	process of recording	-graphy
digestion	-pepsia		
dilatation	-ectasis	producing	-genesis; -genic; -gen
discharge	-(r)rhea		
disease	-pathy	production of	-poiesis
drooping	-ptosis	protein	-globin; -globulin
eating	-phagia	protrusion	-cele
embryonic	-blast	record	-gram
enlarged	-megaly	resembling	-oid
excision	-ectomy	rupture	-(r)rhexis
feeling	-phoria	sagging	-ptosis
fixation	-desis	to secrete	-crine
flow	-(r)rhea	to separate	-crit
formation	-poiesis	sleep	-somnia
forming	-genesis; -genic; -gen	softening	-malacia
		sound	-phonia
growth	-trophy	specialist	-(o)logist
hardening	-sclerosis	spitting up	-ptysis
hearing	-cusis; cusia	stimulating effect of a hormone	-tropin
hemorrhage	-(r)rhagia		
hernia	-cele	stop; stopping	-stasis
illness	-pathy	stretching	-ectasis
immature	-blast	study of	-(o)logy
incision into	-(o)tomy	surgical breaking	-clasis; -clasia
inflammation	-itis	surgical fixation	-pexy
instrument for recording	-graph	surgical puncture to remove fluid	-centesis
instrument for viewing	-scope	surgical removal	-ectomy
		surgical repair	-plasty
instrument to measure	-meter	suture of	-(r)rhaphy
		swallowing	-phagia
labor	-tocia	transmission	-phoresis
like	-oid	treatment	-therapy
to measure; measuring	-metry	tumor	-oma
		to turn; turning	-tropia; -tropion; -version
mental state	-phoria		
movement	-kinesia	urine; urination	-uria
muscle tone	-tonia	vision	-opia
narrowing	-stenosis	visualization with a scope	-scopy
opening	-tresia		
pain	-algia; -dynia	voice	-phonia
paralysis	-plegia	vomiting	-emesis
partial paralysis	-paresis	without feeling or sensation	-asthenia
pertaining to	-ac; -al; -ary; -iac; -ic; -ous	x-ray film	-gram

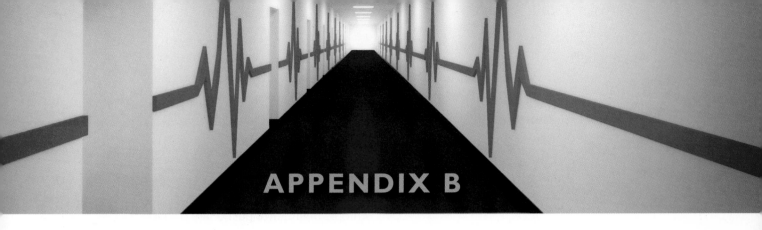

APPENDIX B

Abbreviation List

Abbreviation	Meaning
ac	before meals
ABG	arterial blood gases
AC	air conduction
ACTH	adrenocorticotropic hormone
ad lib	as desired
AD	right ear (auris dextra)
ADH	antidiuretic hormone
AIDS	acquired immune deficiency syndrome
ALS	amyotrophic lateral sclerosis
ANS	autonomic nervous system
ARD	acute respiratory distress
ARDS	adult respiratory distress syndrome
ARF	acute respiratory failure
AS	left ear (auris sinistra)
ASHD	arteriosclerotic heart disease
AU	each ear (auris unitas)
AV node	atrioventricular node
BBB	bundle branch block
bid	twice a day
BC	bone conduction
BE	barium enema
BOM	bilateral otitis media
BP	blood pressure
BPH	benign prostatic hypertrophy
BUN	blood urea nitrogen
bx; Bx	biopsy
$\bar{c}$	with
CABG	coronary artery bypass graft
CAD	coronary artery disease
CAPD	continuous ambulatory peritoneal dialysis
CAT	computed axial tomography
CBC	complete blood count
cc	cubic centimeter
CCPD	continuous cycler-assisted peritoneal dialysis
CF	cystic fibrosis

Abbreviation	Meaning
CHF	congestive heart failure
cm	centimeter
CNS	central nervous system
CO_2	carbon dioxide
COPD	chronic obstructive pulmonary disease
CP	cerebral palsy
CPR	cardiopulmonary resuscitation
C-section	cesarean section
CSF	cerebrospinal fluid
CST	contraction stimulation test
CVA	cerebrovascular accident
CVS	chorionic villus sampling
D&C	dilatation and curettage
DEXA	duel-energy x-ray absorptiometry
DIP	distal interphalangeal
dr	dram
DTR	deep tendon reflexes
DVT	deep vein thrombosis
ECCE	extracapsular cataract extraction
EDB	expected date of birth
EDC	expected or estimated date of confinement
EDD	expected date of delivery
EEG	electroencephalography
EENT	eyes, ears, nose, throat
EGD	esophagogastroduodenoscopy
EKG, ECG	electrocardiogram
EMG	electromyography
ENT	ears, nose, throat
EOM	extraocular movement
ERCP	endoscopic retrograde cholangiopancreatography
ESR	erythrocyte sedimentation rate
FBS	fasting blood sugar
FHR	fetal heart rate
FM	fibromyalgia
FSH	follicle-stimulating hormone
fx	fracture
GERD	gastroesophageal reflux disease
GH	growth hormone
GI	gastrointestinal
GI series	gastrointestinal series
Gm, g, gm	gram
gr	grain
gtt	drops

Abbreviation	Meaning
GTT	glucose tolerance test
GYN	gynecology
h, hr	hour
hs	at bedtime
HD	Huntington's disease
Hct	hematocrit
Hgb	hemoglobin
HHD	hypertensive heart disease
HIV	human immunodeficiency virus
HPV	human papillomavirus
HSV	herpes simplex virus
ICCE	intracapsular cataract extraction
ICP	intracranial pressure
ID	intradermal
IDDM	insulin-dependent diabetes mellitus
IM	intramuscular
inj	injection
IOL	intraocular lens
IOP	intraocular pressure
IU	international unit
IV	intravenous
IVP	intravenous pyelography
kg	kilogram
KUB	kidneys, ureters, and bladder
L	liter
LAGBP	laparoscopic adjustable gastric bypass
LASIK	laser in situ keratomileusis
L&D	labor and delivery
LH	luteinizing hormone
LLQ	left lower quadrant
LMP	last menstrual period
LP	lumbar puncture
LUQ	left upper quadrant
MCH	mean corpuscular hemoglobin
MCHC	mean corpuscular hemoglobin concentration
MCP	metacarpophalangeal
MCV	mean corpuscular volume
MD	muscular dystrophy
mEq	milliequivalent
mg	milligram
MI	myocardial infarction
mL	milliliter
MRI	magnetic resonance imaging

Abbreviation	Meaning
MS	multiple sclerosis
MSH	melanocyte-stimulating hormone
MTP	metatarsophalangeal
NG	nasogastric
NHL	non-Hodgkin's lymphoma
NIDDM	non-insulin-dependent diabetes mellitus
NIPD	nocturnal intermittent peritomeal dialysis
NPO, npo	nothing by mouth
NSD	normal spontaneous delivery
OB	obstetrics
OD	right eye (oculus dexter)
oint., ung	ointment
ORIF	open reduction internal fixation
OS	left eye (oculus sinister)
OTC	over-the-counter
OU	each eye (oculus uterque)
oz	ounce
pc	after meals
po	by mouth
prn	as needed
PAC	premature atrial contraction
PAP	prostatic acid phosphatase
Pap smear	Papanicolaou smear
PAT	paroxysmal atrial tachycardia
PCP	*Pneumocystis carinii* pneumonia
PEG	pneumoencephalogram
PERRLA	pupils equal, round, reactive to light and accommodation
PFTs	pulmonary function tests
PID	pelvic inflammatory disease
PIH	pregnancy-induced hypertension
PIP	proximal interphalangeal
PMS	premenstrual syndrome
PNS	peripheral nervous system
PPS	postpolio syndrome
PRK	photo-refractive keratectomy
PSA	prostate-specific antigen
PT	prothrombin time
PTCA	percutaneous transluminal coronary angioplasty
PTH	parathyroid hormone
PVC	premature ventricular contraction
q	every
q2h	every 2 hours
qam	every morning

Abbreviation	Meaning
qd	every day
qh	every hour
qid	four times a day
qod	every other day
RA	rheumatoid arthritis
RAIU	radioactive iodine uptake test
RBC	red blood cell
RDS	respiratory distress syndrome
REM	rapid eye movement
RF	rheumatoid factor
RHD	rheumatic heart disease
RK	radial keratotomy
RLQ	right lower quadrant
RUQ	right upper quadrant
Rx	treatment; prescription
RYGBP	Roux-en-y gastric bypass
$\bar{s}$	without
SA node	sinoatrial node
SBF	small bowel follow-through
SC	subcutaneous
sig	write on label
SNS	somatic nervous system
SOB	shortness of breath
sol	solution
sos	if necessary
$\bar{\bar{ss}}$	one-half
stat	immediately
STD	sexually transmitted disease
STH	somatotropin hormone
STI	sexually transmitted infection
subQ	subcutaneous
supp	suppository
SVD	spontaneous vaginal delivery
T, Tbsp	tablespoon
t, tsp	teaspoon
tid	three times a day
T_3	triiodothyronine
T_4	thyroxine
tab	tablet
TAH	total abdominal hysterectomy
TB	tuberculosis
TEE	transesophageal echocardiogram
TENS	transcutaneous electrical nerve stimulation
THR	total hip replacement

Abbreviation	Meaning
TIA	transient ischemic attack
tinct	tincture
TM	tympanic membrane
TO	telephone order
TPN	total parenteral nutrition
TSH	thyroid-stimulating hormone
TSS	toxic shock syndrome
TURP	transurethral resection of the prostate
TVH	total vaginal hysterectomy
U	unit
UA	urinalysis
UGI	upper gastrointestinal series
UPPP	uvulopalatopharyngoplasty
URI	upper respiratory tract infection
UTI	urinary tract infection
VA	visual acuity
VAD	vascular access device
VF	visual field
VO	verbal order
V/Q scan	ventilation/perfusion scan
WBC	white blood cell

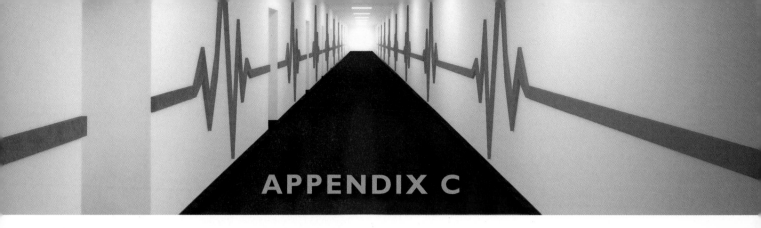

Health-Related Websites

Name	Web Address	Brief Description
American Cancer Society	www.cancer.org	primary resource for information about cancer prevention, detection, and treatment
Centers for Disease Control and Prevention	www.cdc.gov	primary resource for information about current activities related to prevention and control of communicable diseases
Discovery Health	http://health.discovery.com	Discovery Channel's health website; user-friendly information about a wide variety of health issues
Mayo Clinic	www.mayohealth.org/home	Mayo Clinic home page; user-friendly access to information from a highly respected leading institution in health care
Medical Dictionary	www.medicaldictionary.com	A comprehensive medical dictionary
Medline	www.medlineplus.gov	A subservice of the National Library of Medicine; information available by subject
Merck Manual Home Edition	www.merck.com/mmhe/index.html	consumer-friendly, online version of the widely used medical reference *The Merck Manual*
WebMD	http://health.msn.com	MSN health website; user-friendly alphabetic index of diseases, conditions, and more

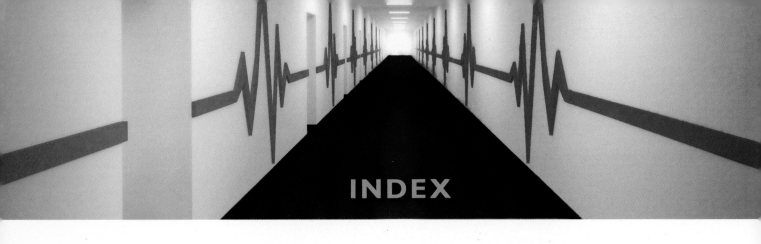

INDEX